ADVANCES
IN
ENVIRONMENTAL
PSYCHOLOGY
Volume 4
Environment and Health

ADVANCES IN ENVIRONMENTAL PSYCHOLOGY

Volume 4
Environment and Health

Edited by **ANDREW BAUM**
JEROME E. SINGER
Uniformed Services University
of the Health Sciences

LEA LAWRENCE ERLBAUM ASSOCIATES, PUBLISHERS
1982   Hillsdale, New Jersey

Lawrence Erlbaum Associates, Inc., Publishers
365 Broadway
Hillsdale, New Jersey 07642

Library of Congress Cataloging in Publication Data

Environment and health.

   (Advances in environmental psychology; v. 4)
   Bibliography: p.
   Includes indexes.
   1. Environmental psychology.   I. Baum, Andrew.
II. Singer, Jerome E.   III. Series.   [DNLM: 1. Environ-
mental health.   2. Public health.   WA 30 E6051]
BF353.E484   1982   155.9   82-8792
ISBN 0-89859-174-0   AACR2

Printed in the United States of America

Contents

Preface

The term "applied psychology" has always covered a variety of areas and fields of study and use. Although often thought of primarily as industrial psychology or organizational development, it has become increasingly clear, if it ever was in doubt, that applied psychology covers an enormous number of ways in which psychologists take their basic research findings and utilize them in the world outside the laboratory. In recent years two of the most rapidly developing areas of applied psychology have been those united in this volume: health behavior and environmental studies.

The field of environmental studies in psychology has been a product, by and large, of the last decade. The history of its development has been chronicled (Altman, 1976).[1] And though the roots of the topic extend well back into time, serious concerted study of the environment is a recent phenomenon. Environment is such a pervasive thing, that with only a minimum of rhetorical dexterity, almost all psychology could be called environmental. Some clinicians have made the case that clinical psychology is environmental psychology, for example. After all, if most behavior disturbances are not genetic, where else could they arise but from human interactions with the environment? In actual practice, however, environmental psychology has meant the study of noise, crowding, architecture, and a minor amount of attention to those conditions of concern to the Environmental Protection Agency and the Council on Environmental Quality.

The field of health psychology has an equally long history of concern, and a much longer span of practice. Psychologists have been integral parts of the health care system for years, with an especial boost in participation following the post World War II expansion and systematization of graduate training. But again, many psychologists working in hospitals and other health care settings as researchers and practitioners were, if not isolated from mainstream psychology, not organized as an interest group or recognized subfield either. The last decade

---

[1]Altman, I. *The environment and social behavior.* Monterey, CA: Brooks/Cole, 1976.

has seen a major change in this area also. Health psychology has been organized into a separate subfield, and new books and journals abound with health and medical studies by psychologists.

These two newly emerging areas share one important feature. Both have kept a foot in the basic research camp. Such concepts as perceived control, selective attention, and learned helplessness have shuttled back and forth from the experimental and social psychological literature to that on health and environment to the benefit of both the basic and applied camps—quite often the same researchers worked both sides of the street. This mixture of basic and applied is reflected in the present volume. Several of the chapters could equally well have been retitled, slightly rewritten to change emphases and been published as equally cogent contributions to the study of a variety of basic processes.

More importantly, health and environment have broadened each other's horizons. Not too long ago, people did not talk about health psychology, they referred to medical psychology. The shift from medical issues to the broader set of health concerns reflects, in part, the influence of the consideration of environmental factors on human welfare. The effects of noise, crowding, or air pollution are ones that pull the investigator out of the physician's milieu and into a larger arena of concern. But in reciprocal fashion, attention to health issues and outcomes has involved the scope of the environmental investigators. Without such interests, it is highly probable that environmental studies would be almost entirely devoted to the mainstream of density, crowding, and architecture. Those interests are, of course, represented in this volume. But so too are daily experiences, extreme environments, air pollution, and noise. In fact, the reality of environmental settings and the importance of health outcomes combine to produce a particularly interesting psychological collection of studies combining these fields and the present volume is one which we hope will be the precursor of a stream of valuable reports.

As with every volume, the final product is the work of more people than just the editors and authors. For her otherwise anonymous, but nevertheless vital contributions, we would like to extend our sincere thanks to Martha Gisriel, a paragon of organization, indexing, and the general keeping of things straight.

Andrew Baum
Jerome E. Singer

ADVANCES
IN
ENVIRONMENTAL
PSYCHOLOGY
Volume 4
Environment and Health

1 Quality of the Residential Environment and Mental Health

Stanislav V. Kasl
Yale University School of Medicine

Julie Will
Yale University School of Medicine

Marni White
Columbia University

Peter Marcuse
Columbia University School of Urban Planning

> *"What a wretched lodging you have, Rodya! It's like a tomb,"* said Pulcheria Alexandrovna, suddenly breaking the oppressive silence. *"I am sure it's quite half through your lodging you have become so melancholy."*
>
> *"My lodging,"* he answered, listlessly. *"Yes, the lodging had a great deal to do with it ... I thought that, too ... If only you knew, though, what a strange thing you said just now, mother,"* he said, laughing strangely.
>
> —Dostoyevsky, *Crime and Punishment*
> (Constance Garnett translation)

INTRODUCTION TO THE PROBLEM AND PREVIOUS WORK

It has been a common observation of workers in various social and welfare agencies for over 40 years that there exist "problem families" that consume a highly disproportionate amount of resources of the various agencies. These "problem families" are defined by coexistence or co-occurrence of a large number of interrelated problems: physical illness, mental illness, low income, unemployment, social disorganization, racial discrimination, broken families, poor housing, slum location, crime and delinquency, alcoholism and drug abuse, and so on. This packaging of the many sides of poverty and social inequality, and their many correlates, is an indisputable empirical observation. Many disciplines and areas of investigation have gotten a lot of mileage out of this basic phenomenon: They study only a limited fragment of it, and they impute strong causal inferences to their observations. Thus, we have a rise of the "stress and disease" set of studies in social science and medicine, the rise of psychiatric epidemiology with its emphasis on social disorganization and mental illness, and the whole set of housing and health studies with inferences about the pathogenecity of inadequate housing. These fields have flourished and gained visibility by simplifying the problem and by studying only part of it.

However, the dilemma here is a real one, both for the reformer and the scientist. The planner or social activist wishes to avoid having to reform all aspects of society simultaneously; but he must also avoid changing such a small part of the overall rich causal network that other causal influences easily "take over," and status quo is quickly restored. Similarly, it is a basic strategy of the scientist to try to isolate the various causes and effects and to study them separately; but he must avoid distorting the phenomenon by his attempts to subdivide and isolate.

If the whole package of poverty, illness, and social problems could be unravelled into a single long causal chain with housing as one of the early links, then it would be reasonable to expect large impact of housing variables and many benefits of housing interventions. But it is more likely that the package is a mess of interconnected causal relationships and feedback loops, so that a single intervention or a single causal influence evaporates into ineffectiveness.

Over the years, the public health, social science, and urban planning literature on the residential environment has included many writers who were unravelling a single causal chain with housing as an early link. Frequently, their faith in the self-evident link between poor housing and pathology obliterated any felt need for documentation. Such ecological determinism is perhaps not totally naive because, in a few instances, the power of logical reasoning alone can produce defensible statements of relationships, such as the presence of rats is a necessary (but not sufficient!) condition for rat bites. Conversely, the absence of rats leads to a confident prediction about the absence of rat bites. However, deductive reasoning alone is rarely sufficient to detect and describe empirical associations, and such logical statements have to be precise and carefully hedged. Moreover, what once was (or appeared to have been) a "self-evident" or "obvious" association, such as between crowding and tuberculosis, may no longer hold because of a changing picture regarding the pathology in question, as well as, possibly, the changing range of the independent variable within which the respondents are to be found.

The accumulating empirical literature on the health and mental health effects of the residential environment was not readily supportive of wide claims about such effects. For example, in *Slums and Social Insecurity* (1963), Schorr painted a broad picture of the presumed adverse effects of poor housing and "slum" neighborhood settings on physical and mental health of the residents, including assertions about effects on self-perceptions, pessimism, and passivity. At about the same time, Wilner published the results of his classical study of improved housing (Wilner, Walkley, Pinkerton, & Tayback, 1962). The findings revealed minimal benefits of improved housing on mental health (mood, nervousness, general morale, self-esteem, general anxiety), on aspirations, and on various self-promotive activities. Such minimal effects or negative findings were altogether too common (Kasl, 1976, 1977; Kasl & Rosenfield, 1980) and provided scant support for the position of the various reviewers (Gilbertson & Mood, 1964; Rosow, 1961; Schorr, 1963), whose a priori belief appeared to be that the physical–residential environment does—indeed, perhaps, must—influence mental health and behavior in significant and meaningful ways.

One response to the minimal or negative findings reported in the literature was to condemn the scope of the independent variable being studied. For example, Wilner has been criticized (Pynoos, Schafer, & Hartman, 1973) for using a much too-limited notion of housing (heat and plumbing, more dwelling space, structural safety, modernity) and for not attempting: "to improve other dimensions of the housing services bundle, such as the social environment, status, and location [p. 132]." Many other expressions of the need to take an adequately broad view of housing can be found. For example, the Report of the President's Committee on Urban Housing (1969) takes the position that: "The most successful programs for bettering housing conditions and economic opportunities cannot, in themselves, produce better environments. Good neighbors are vital for preserving good neighborhoods [p. 12]." The intertwining of the social and the physical parameters is also seen in the following quote from Downs (1973), who talks of the "critical mass effect" of concentrating poor people in the inner city slums: "compelling thousands of such households to become concentrated in the worst urban housing causes a reverberation of their problems, greatly magnifying the total negative effects [p. 10]."

The preceding quotes are getting at the same theme: the embeddedness of housing variables in a larger social context or matrix; the intertwining of housing effects with other effects; the need for a broad approach to housing both at the conceptual as well as the empirical level; the need to understand the "meaning" of housing in the experiential sense rather than as a set of physical parameters; the inability to assess the impact of housing by studying housing alone. The emerging dictum for the social planner is: Poor housing is an obstacle to well-being and self-fulfillment, but remedying only poor housing is not enough.

One problem with this broadening of the concept of housing and residential environment is that it is not clear whether it represents a desirable redefinition of the independent variable and an appropriate redirection of our research efforts, or whether it is just a way of sweeping the minimal and negative findings under the rug.

From the viewpoint of research strategy, there are a number of possible disadvantages to broadening the concept of the residential environment to include, beyond the physical parameters, the psychosocial dimensions as well. When the two become inextricably mixed, we can no longer tell how the two sets of dimensions interact with each other, or, even, whether the observed impact in fact may not be due solely to the social dimensions, and the physical parameters have no impact, either independent or interactive. Furthermore, interventions in the psychosocial environment may be much more difficult to implement than those in the physical–residential environment, but with data on impact coming from studies using a very broad operational definition of residential environment, the design-oriented planner or architect may not be able to infer what the called-for modifications of the physical parameters are, if any.

In short, just because it is agreed that the impact of the physical parameters of the residential setting must be studied in a rich network of psychosocial-environmental variables, this does not mean that the operational definition of the residential environment should inextricably confound the physical and psychosocial components. In fact, the primary effort of such research must be to attempt to disentangle the many interrelated influences and the many interrelated outcomes.

Although it is not our intent to review the empirical literature on the residential environment and mental health, we do wish to take advantage of some recent reviews (Hinkle & Loring, 1977; Kasl, 1976; Kasl & Rosenfield, 1980) to suggest a number of conclusions that appear to us both justifiable and worth the reader's attention. Overall, it would seem that the impact of the residential environment is greatest on indices of well-being or satisfaction that deal specifically with residential parameters, and weakest on the more traditional indicators of mental health, such as symptom checklists or diagnostic classifications; effects of intermediate magnitude tend to be seen for indices of social and leisure activity and general evaluations of one's current life circumstances. In other words, the strongest link is with various indices of residential satisfaction, impact criteria that have numerous conceptual and methodological problems, and a tenuous link to mental health as conventionally conceived. It also appears likely, though close documentation has in fact not yet been carried out, that the residential environment has a greater impact on those members of the society with the fewest social and personal resources, such as children, the elderly, female heads of household, and so on.

However, the most appropriate statement regarding the empirical evidence on the impact of the residential environment on mental health is that we have a large set of more or less trustworthy findings that do not yet permit any kind of closure. The recent debate on crowding/density, the most busily researched of the residential parameters, is a good illustration supporting this conclusion (Baldassare, 1979; Booth & Edwards, 1976; Booth, Johnson, & Edwards, 1980a,b; Gove & Hughes, 1980a,b; Gove, Hughes, & Galle, 1979). Fundamental issues regarding conceptualization, assessment, and study design are still being debated, in spite of a great advance in research sophistication of the crowding/density studies of the last 30 years.

There is nowadays a near-universal agreement among investigators that simple, direct effects of a large magnitude from the residential environment to mental health should not be expected; instead, one should expect the residential variables to be richly embedded in a large matrix of individual and social variables that condition and attenuate the impact of the residential environment. Given this view—which is certainly a most sensible one at this point—then it is difficult to see just how much closure one should expect when reviewing the diversity of empirical data. Stated somewhat differently, how does one distinguish a high order of specificity of impacts of weak magnitude from inconsistency, nonreplication, and spuriousness of findings? One kind of help here would be a comprehensive and compelling theoretical framework that is sufficiently detailed to spell out the many interactive relationships between the individual-social variables and the housing parameters that are to be expected or suspected. However, no such theory exists or can be reasonably expected to exist, because it would have to include large chunks of behavioral science (development over the life cycle, parent–child relations, aspiration–goal setting–achievement, needs fulfillment, attribution processes, adaptation processes, and so on) and would have to solve the problem of bridging the physicalistic description of the environment and the psychological description of the cognitions and behavior of the people. The great diversity of ideas about how crowding/density ought to be conceptualized and measured again illustrates how difficult the problem of a comprehensive theory is even on a scale smaller than the whole residential environment.

Another source of help with distinguishing inconsistency from specificity of findings could come from having criteria for a "definitive" research design for examining the impact of the residential environment on mental health. Then one could review only studies that reasonably satisfy such criteria and thus generate trustworthy findings. However, here too, like our comprehensive theory, such a "definitive" design can only be a distant aspiration. It is simply impossible to put together a design that: uses a widely representative subject population with all vulnerable subgroups identified and oversampled, examines a sufficient range of values on diverse residential parameters combined to form a spectrum of residential settings, is adequately free of self-selection biases, is sufficiently longitudinal to detect effects at different points in time, overcomes long-standing measurement problems, and collects such richness of data that important adaptation processes are thereby described and major conditioning/intervening/buffering variables are thereby revealed.

In the absence of a comprehensive theoretical framework linking the residential environment to mental health outcomes and the absence of a "definitive" research design that is feasible under ordinary field research conditions, we have precious few guidelines with which to organize existing evidence, settle controversies, and decide on the most useful next set of studies. We have to resign ourselves to piecemeal and tentative conceptualizations and piecemeal studies; they will add to our knowledge provided that they do not repeat all the limitations of previous studies. And it is too early to engage in controversies that attempt to settle once and for all the definitive conceptualization or the evidence (viz. Booth versus Gove, earlier, regarding crowding/density).

It seems particularly important to retain a strategy of studying the effects of the residential parameters, physicalistically defined, in interaction with a rich set of psychosocial variables, subjective perceptions, and behavioral reactions. We may not be able to disentangle the various components of the "independent" variable that we are studying at any one time (e.g., improved housing versus social uprooting from the neighborhood's social networks; housing deficiencies versus lack of influence over indifferent management; residential stability versus subjective inability to find improved housing; housing satisfaction versus curtailed aspirations; and so on), but we shall be able to state more precisely the specific conditions under which the effects of such compound "independent" variables are manifest. And when different studies do not include the potential for the same confounding variables, then we may begin to disentangle some of the component effects.

On the other hand, it would seem undesirable and premature to take a particular residential parameter, such as crowding/density, and translate it into a specific psychological process or construct, such as deficit of privacy or perceived lack of control (Altman, 1975; Stokols, 1972). This tends to commit us to a single intervening process between some physical aspect of the residential environment and behavioral outcomes, when we have not yet fully explored the many possible ways of operationalizing crowding/density, and the many ways in which various psychosocial variables can condition or attenuate the effects in various subgroups. If one juxtaposes the many theoretical formulations that have been proposed in connection with crowding/density (Baldassare, 1979; Stokols, 1978) and the *field* studies on the impact of the residential environment on mental health, one is quickly impressed by the fact that the empirical studies carried out thus far haven't begun to deal with the richness and variety of intervening processes that have been proposed. Much of the empirical work is carried out at the level of opaque indices, such as persons/room, and it is difficult to determine what theoretical construct(s) is (are) operationalized by this index, and what are the possible confounding or correlated variables: marital status, social isolation, stage of life cycle, number of dependent children, use of available space, interference with home-based activities, and so on. Ultimately, we are asking: How are significant human experiences, such as loneliness, or failure, or family conflict dependent on spatial characteristics of the dwelling unit captured by persons/room.

In concluding this section, we enlarge the discussion of the residential environment and mental health by considering briefly certain interesting parallels in the literature on work environment and mental health (Kasl, 1974, 1978). These are the two classes of (physical) environment determinants of mental health that have been most richly explored (that is, other than those environments that are primarily psychosocial, such as parent–child relations or husband–wife interactions). The parallels are several:

1. The strongest effect of work environment is on various components of job satisfaction, and only sporadic or weak effects have been demonstrated for traditional indicators of mental health, such as symptom check-lists or diagnostic classifications; job satisfaction is at best weakly related to such indicators of mental health.

2. A satisfactory bridging of the physicalistic description of the demands of the work environment with the psychological description of the cognitions of this environment and reactions to it has not been accomplished, and the short-circuiting of this problem by dealing only with subjective perceptions and evaluations has been a popular "solution."

3. National survey data on human concerns and quality of life (Cambell, Converse, & Rogers, 1976; Cantril & Roll, 1971) indicate that neither the residential setting nor the work environment can compare in judged importance to health, marriage, and family life as influences on well-being.

These parallels are noted in order to suggest that in trying to trace the effects of the residential environment on mental health, we encounter problems of theory and evidence that may not be unique to this one area of investigation.

METHODS

The findings to be reported in the following come from the initial interview wave data from a longitudinal, 3-year panel study of 337 Black and Hispanic women living in Waterbury, Connecticut, a city of some 130,000. Respondents were selected on the basis of four specific housing situations. The primary target population for this study were the families living in a recently built, federally funded low-income housing project in downtown Waterbury. This housing project, The "Inner City Housing," was built to conform to the maximum HUD standards for federally subsidized housing and was selected for study because it incorporates design alternatives to previously build low-income housing projects: The structures are two-story condominium style and the complex is small-scale (69 units); it is built in a downtown location, close to the previous housing of its residents; it is managed by a Black nonprofit corporation.

In addition to the primary target population, four comparison groups were selected. The first were *applicants* from the waiting list for the "Inner City Housing" project who had not received housing in the project, and who could be located in the Waterbury area. They were located on the basis of addresses and information from the official applications on file for the test housing. However, a review of these applications showed that some were up to 3 years out of date. A search for all applicants on the waiting list ($N = 213$) revealed that only one third of these applicants could be located at the time of Wave I interviewing. Because of this high rate of loss, there is question as to the extent to which the applicants who could be located are representative of the total applicant pool. Analysis of the limited information available from the official application form showed that applicants who could not be located for interviewing were more likely to be younger, single, poorer, and unemployed or on welfare, than those who were located for interviews. There was also some evidence that Black applicants were more likely to obtain project housing than Hispanic applicants. Previous research has shown that housing authority officials may act as "gatekeepers" in the selection of tenants from the applicant pool, selecting intact families with higher incomes over husbandless, lower-income residents (Kriesberg, 1970).

The second comparison group were socioeconomically and racially similar families living in the neighborhoods where project residents had lived prior to moving to the test project who had *not* applied for project housing. This group of *"Neighborhood residents"* was obtained by a block-quota sampling procedure. Respondents were neighborhood residents who had not applied to the Inner City housing project but were living at the same residence or on the same blocks as either the applicants to the Inner City project, or at the former addresses of the current residents of this project. This group was based on the addresses of both the target and applicant groups and is therefore the largest of the control groups.

The third comparison group were socioeconomically and radically similar residents occupying project housing that is structurally similar to "Inner City Housing" but is located in outlying suburban areas of Waterbury; they are referred to as *"Other Projects."* Locating the respondents for this group also proved to be rather difficult. Only a small number of minority-group members presently live in these surburban projects. Out of four housing project sites in suburban Waterbury, with 1053 units, only 76 Black or Hispanic families could be located. Because of this small number of respondents, a decision was made to include in the survey an additional suburban housing project that was somewhat different from the original suburban sites, and from the target housing project. This became the fourth comparison group referred to as "Scott Gardens." It is an older project with two-story buildings and shared entranceways. A higher proportion of minority-group residents live at this project than at the other suburban projects. Also, because of a delay in the interviewing at this housing site, interviews took place at a different time of year. Because of these physical, social, and possible seasonal differences, the data on respondents living in this older suburban housing project were not merged with the data from respondents living in the other suburban projects.

This rather cumbersome design with several comparison groups was set up in order to permit a variety of contrasts: (1) residence in project housing (Inner City, Other Projects, Scott Gardens) versus nonproject housing (Applicants and Neighborhood), which is essentially a contrast on quality of housing; (2) Inner city versus suburban location (Inner City versus Other Projects and Scott Gardens), which is within better housing groups but also involves a contrast on type of management; (3) applying versus not applying for project housing (Applicants versus Neighborhood), which presumably reflects level of housing satisfaction, aspirations, and (for some) blocked residential mobility—among those in poorer housing. The final contrast (which is orthogonal to the previous three and completes the partitioning of four degrees of freedom from a five-group one-way ANOVA) compares Scott Gardens (somewhat older, more balanced racially) and Other Projects (somewhat newer, predominantly white).

Only women were interviewed and any household with no woman present was excluded. There were two reasons for this decision. One was to eliminate the sex of respondent as a variable that would further reduce the numbers in statistical analysis. A second reason concerned the nature of the information to be obtained on the outcome measures for children's health and mental health. Women would be more likely to be living with their children and therefore more likely to know of health problems in the family, childhood disease and illness, and better able to answer questions about their children on these scales.

Structured personal interviews lasting approximately 1 1/2 hours were given. An effort was made to match interviewers for race–ethnic status with the respondents and all interviewers were Black- or Hispanic-background persons. All initial interviewing was done during the summer of 1977, except for Scott Gardens, where the interview took place in February–March, 1978. At the time of data collection, the respondents in the primary target-study group (Inner City) had lived in their new housing approximately 20 months.

Table 1.1 summarizes the basic descriptive information about the study respondents. The overall participation rate of 90% varies little across the study groups but has different meanings for these groups. For those in the better housing (Inner City, Other Projects, Scott Gardens), participation rate is based on those eligible for study: all Inner City residents or Black/Hispanic women in the other two groups. For Applicants, it is based on those who were located at the time of attempted contact. For Neighborhood, it is based on those who were found at home at the time the contact was attempted at a given address.

The other information in Table 1.1 merits the following comments: (1) On mean age, only Scott Gardens respondent are notably different (younger); (2) on family income, Other Projects and Scott Gardens are higher; this is presumably associated with the somewhat greater percent of currently employed and married (i.e., two incomes in the family); (3) the lower percent currently employed among the Neighborhood respondents is a reflection of the quota-sampling procedure that would favor those not working being located; (4) the greater percent

TABLE 1.1

Social and Demographic Characteristics of Female
Respondents in Waterbury Study of Residential Environment

Study Group*	Initial Interview		Mean Age +	Mean Family Income	Mean years of Education	Percent Married	Percent Currently Employed	Percent Black
	N	Particip. Rate**						
"Inner City"	62	90%	2.55	$ 6,500	10	37%	54%	90%
Applicants	65	86%	2.45	$ 6,200	9	38%	51%	71%
Neighborhood	104	91%	2.21	$ 6,000	10	40%	33%	76%
Other Projects	70	90%	2.52	$ 9,900	12	64%	64%	91%
"Scott Gardens"	36	86%	1.77	$10,700	12	50%	60%	81%

*Study Groups
1) *"Inner City*: test population which moved into a new federally assisted housing project in downtown Waterbury
2) *Applicants*: applicants to test site who had *not* become residents
3) *Neighborhood*: residents living in housing similar to prior housing of "inner city" residents, did not apply for project housing
4) *Other projects*: socioeconomically similar families living in housing structurally similar to "inner city" but located in suburban areas of Waterbury; respondents a racial minority
5) *"Scott Gardens"*: like one of the "other projects", but somewhat older and racially balanced
**See text for different meanings of participation rate
+ Age groupings: 1 = <25; 2 = 25–39; 3 = 40–59; 4 = >59

of Hispanics among the Applicants is, in part, a reflection of selection processes (discussed previously) of who got into Inner City housing.

Overall, the study groups are not fully comparable on sociodemographic characteristics; in particular, the two groups in suburban projects are somewhat higher on socioeconomic status. However, this is not a volunteering or sampling frame effect; these subjects reflect the universe of Black and Hispanic Waterbury residents in these projects. The lack of homogeneity on Table 1.1 variables are handled in data analysis with statistical controls for these effects.

Let us now turn to a brief characterization of the *data collected*. Two major indices were used to measure the quality of the residential environment. The quality of the housing unit was measured by a 29-item *Housing Index*. This index is composed of items selected from the more extensive American Public Health Association's "Appraisal Method for Measuring the Quality of Housing" (A.P.H.A., 1950) and is similar to the "shortened version" of the "Appraisal Method" used by Wilner et al. (1962). There is also considerable overlap of items with the current Annual Housing Survey: Indicators of Housing and Neighborhood Quality (U.S. Department of Commerce, 1975) so that comparison with data from a national sample can be obtained.

The Housing Index includes items that assess housing conditions in five areas. The quality of housing in four areas was rated on the basis of information supplied by the respondent. These four areas include: "unit facilities" (8 items: complete kitchen and bath, kitchen and bath plumbing, running water in unit, central heat, laundry facilities, rooms in unit that lack heat); "unit maintenance" (8 items: peeling paint, leaky pipes, heat, plumbing, or toilet breakdowns, adequate garbage collection, presence of cockroaches, mice or rats in unit); "unit structure" (1 item: location of unit); and "crowding" (2 items: persons per room, use of living room as bedroom). A fifth area in which housing quality was rated, "deficiencies in the exterior and interior structure" of the unit, was evaluated by the interviewer for the presence of 10 specific conditions: large holes, open cracks, rotted, loose or missing materials of floors, walls of interior and exterior of unit, sagging of interior or exterior walls, small exterior holes, open cracks in walls, shaky porch or railings, broken or missing window panes, rotted window frames, deep wear of doors or steps.

Each item on the Housing Index was scored on a 5-point scale graded as to the severity of the condition, with 1 indicating good qualtiy housing and 5 indicating the maximum score for poor quality housing. Unlike the original A.P.H.A. "Appraisal Method," and the shortened version of this measure used by Wilner, no attempt was made to weight individual items, or to assign scores based on perceptions of the relative health hazard of specific conditions.

The second major index used to assess the quality of the residential environment was a 9-item index of *Neighborhood Conditions*. Items on this index were selected from the current Annual Housing Survey (U.S. Department of Commerce, 1975), and from the American Public Health Association's "Appraisal

Method (A.P.H.A., 1950)." The Neighborhood Conditions Index was based on respondent's reports on traffic and street noise, upkeep of the neighborhood (trash or litter on streets, boarded up or abandoned buildings), and quality of neighborhood services (inadequate street lighting, streets in need of repair). For each condition the respondent was asked if the condition exists on their immediate block or street, and, if present, the extent to which they were "bothered" by this condition. Scoring for the index was from 1 (no condition present) to 5 (the condition is present and bothers the respondent).

A comparison of selected items from the Housing Index and the Neighborhood Conditions Index for the Waterbury respondents and national sample data from the 1976 Annual Housing Survey for housing units headed by Black or Hispanic persons revealed that the Waterbury respondents have housing facilities that are similar to those reported by the national sample. However, the Waterbury group reports more maintenance problems and more breakdowns in the plumbing and heating equipment in the home, and more problems with insufficient heat in the winter. Because insufficient heat may be a regional problem, the Waterbury data were further compared to Northeast regional data. Even then the proportion of the Waterbury group reporting insufficient heat is high. Location may also be a factor in the poorer quality of neighborhood conditions reported by the Waterbury group. Particularly in the areas of neighborhood upkeep and services, this group is worse off than comparable households in the national sample, and this high incidence may reflect conditions of older urban areas.

The major *dependent variables* in this study are based on mother's reports on the health and behavior of one preselected child in the family (closest to age 10), on her and her partner's parenting behavior, and on her own mental health. The information on the child and on parenting behavior are based on instruments developed by T.S. Langner and his collaborators (Gersten, 1976; Langner, Gersten, & Eisenberg, 1973; Langner, Gersten, McCarthy, Eisenberg, Greene, Herson, & Jameson, 1976). The relevant scales are as follows:

1. *Child's Mild Chronic Illnesses:* 8 items dealing with frequency of stomach aches, sore throat, headaches, colds, etc.
2. *Child's Anger-Conflict with Parents:* 6 items dealing with child's expression of anger or temper, disobedience, etc., directed at a parent.
3. *Child's Depressed-Resentful Mood:* 6 items dealing with moodiness, saddness, crying spells, withdrawal, etc.
4. *Child's Poor School Adjustment:* 6 items concerned with child's happiness at school, conflict with teachers, teacher's complaints, etc.
5. *Peer Conflict-Excitability:* 7 items dealing with the child's restlessness, fighting, excitability, and so on, when he/she is with age mates.
6. *Parental Coldness:* 7 items essentially dealing with how much affection each parent shows to the child.

7. *Parental Punitiveness:* 5 items concerned with use of physical punishment and strict discipline.

8. *Mother Excitable-Rejecting:* 5 items dealing with lack of emotional control when disciplining the child.

9. *Parental Inadequacy:* summary of previous 3 scales.

The woman respondent's reports on her own mental health and well-being included four factors from the SCL-90, a self-report symptom inventory (Derogatis, Lipman, & Covi, 1973; Derogatis, Lipman, Rickels, Uhlenhuth, & Covi, 1974):

1. *Agitated Depression:* 9 symptoms, such as trembling, poor appetite, crying easily.

2. *Phobic Anxiety:* 9 symptoms, such as being afraid of open spaces, uneasy in crowds, sudden fears.

3. *Somatization:* 14 items that include the typical psychophysiological symptoms: headache, dizziness, upset stomach, heart pounding, etc.

4. *Anger-Hostility:* 12 items denoting irritation, temper outbursts, urgency to smash things, etc.

In addition to these, the 20-item Zung Depression Scale (Zung, 1965) and the Srole Anomia Scale (Srole, 1956) were included.

These 15 scales are the focus of this report. Their internal consistency (coefficient alpha) appears adequate for most (i.e., $\geq .70$). The three exceptions are Parental Coldness (.51), Parental Punitiveness (.42), and Mother Excitable-Rejecting (.49); because two of the three combine the behavior of both parents, this could be one reason for their low internal consistency.

The intercorrelations among the scales reveal, not unexpectedly, that these are not fully independent constructs: (1) the four SCL-90 factors and the Zung scale show an average intercorrelation of .50; the five scales, however, are not substantially associated with Anomia Scale (average $r = .24$); (2) the three parenting scales show an average intercorrelation of .33, whereas for the five scales describing the child, the average value is .27; (3) of the 30 correlations, created by the matrix of six scales of mother's self-report of mental health with five scales reporting on the child, only six are over .20 and the highest is only .32 (between Peer Conflict-Excitability and Anger-Hostility); this does not suggest a substantial influence of mother's self-perceived mental health on the reporting of the behavior of her child.

There are additional variables and measures that are utilized in this report. The necessary information about such measures is provided as they are introduced in the section on results.

The primary approach to the *data analysis* relied heavily on the General Linear Models (GLM) procedure of the Statistical Analysis System (SAS); specifically, we used the Type-IV Sum of Squares procedure (SAS User's Guide, 1979). In this approach, we first introduced the following (potential) predictors: age, income, race, years of residence in Waterbury, number of children, whether married or single, education, monthly rent, and age and sex of child on whom data were collected. Then the two major residential variables were introduced, Housing index and Neighborhood conditions. The final predictor was "Sample," that is, the study group to which the respondent belonged; the four degrees of freedom attributable to this variable were partitioned into four orthogonal contrasts, discussed earlier.

This basic approach to the data analysis was then elaborated and made more complex, when additional predictors of interest were introduced, or when we were examining specific interactions among predictors.

The strategy and logic of this type of analysis merits a comment. From the technical point, the analysis permits two types of statements: (1) What is the contribution of a particular predictor (i.e., variance accounted for in the dependent variable), given that a certain set of preceding predictors has been introduced first; (2) what is the unique contribution of a predictor, given the effects of a whole set of other predictors, irrespective of the order in which they were introduced. From the conceptual viewpoint, this approach reflects the notion that the dependent variables in these analyses have certain known correlates (e.g., social status or marital status in relation to mental health) and that we are seeking to establish the contribution of residential parameters *above and beyond* the effects of these known influences. The variable "Sample" is also used as a predictor, because we do not believe that the Housing Index and Neighborhood Conditions can exhaustively characterize the residential setting of the five study groups. However, variance accounted for by "Sample" may not be easy to interpret to the extent that unmeasured and subtle influences may be encompassed by belonging to one or another study group.

The preceding approach to data analysis does not provide definitive clues to appropriate causal interpretations. Furthermore, the strategy is a "conservative" one with respect to estimating the effects of residential parameters; that is, housing and sociodemographic variables are associated with each other, and we don't really know how much of an effect, more properly attributable to housing, we are removing by introducing a variety of sociodemographic predictors into the analysis first and then looking only at the residual (or incremental) contribution of housing.

RESULTS

Before proceeding with the presentation of results, we wish to characterize briefly the five study samples on the two major residential parameters. On Housing Index, the five study groups account for 28.7% of the total variance; moreover, nearly all (98%) of this between-group variance is represented by the single contrast, residence in project versus nonproject housing. On Neighborhood Conditions, the five groups account for 12.0% of the total variance; moreover, nearly all (96%) of this between-group variance is represented by a single contrast, which compares suburban housing (other Projects, Scott Gardens) versus downtown housing (Inner City, Applicants, Neighborhood). In other words, the target-study sample, "Inner City," shares good quality housing with the other two projects and poor neighborhood conditions with the applicants and neighborhood residents.

The next three tables present the major findings from the primary data-analysis approach, described previously. In Table 1.2 we have the data on the five scales that represent the mother's reports on the health and behavior of one preselected child. Of the 10 sociodemographic variables introduced first in the analysis, only the six listed in Table 1.2 explained some significant variance in the five dependent variables. The findings may be summarized as follows:

1. For Child's Mild Chronic Illnesses, only one variable shows a significant association: Older children are described as having more symptoms.

TABLE 1.2

Amount of Variance in Children's Mental Health
Explained by Socio-Demographic and Major
Residential Variables

		Child's Mild Chronic Illnesses	Anger-Conflict With Parents	Depressed-Resentful Mood	Poor School Adjustment	Peer Conflict-Excitability
Age of Child		6.7	–	–	–	1.7
Age of Respondent		–	5.7	6.2	5.9	–
Marital Status						
(1 = married, 2 = other)		–	6.1	–	–	7.6
Race (1 = Black, 2 =						
Puerto Rican)		–	–	–	5.8	–
Respondent's Education		–	–	–	1.9	–
Sex of Child (1 = Female,						
2 = Male)		–	–	–	2.6	–
Housing Index		–	3.1	–	–	–
Neighborhood Conditions		–	–	–	–	–
Study Group		–	5.7	4.6	–	–
Inner City	Adjusted Group	-.16	-.57	-.51	-.08	-.32
Applicants	Means, in Standard	-.30	.05	-.51	.04	-.40
Neighborhood	Scores, With Scott	-.51	-.59	-.82	-.19	-.46
Other Projects	Gardens Set	-.47	-.20	-.47	-.24	-.27
Scott Gardens	at .00	.00	.00	.00	.00	.00
Housing by Neighborhood Interaction?		No	No	No	No	No

2. For Anger–Conflict with Parents, age and marital status of the mother make a difference. In the case of age, the association is curvilinear with lowest anger reported in the intermediate age groups; also, married women report more anger. In addition to sociodemographic correlates, less-adequate housing is related to more reports of anger. The significant variance due to Study Groups reflects primarily the low mean values for Inner City and Neighborhood residents.

3. For Depressed–Resentful Mood, age of respondent shows a significant association, with lowest values shown in the intermediate age group. The significant variance due to Study Groups reflects primarily the high mean value for the Scott Gardens respondents.

4. For Poor School Adjustment, several sociodemographic variables are significantly associated. More school problems are reported by older respondents, Blacks, those with more education, and for female children.

5. For Peer Conflict–Excitability, reporting on a younger child and being married is associated with reporting more problems.

Because the focus of this analysis is on the residential variables, we do not comment further on the pattern of sociodemographic correlates. The data in Table 1.2 show no impact of Neighborhood Conditions and only one significant association with the Housing Index, involving Anger–Conflict with Parents. Two variables show an association with Study Group; the one group that stands apart in both instances are the residents in Scott Gardens. Because neither housing quality nor conditions of the neighborhood are producing this effect, one must turn to the unique aspects of the Scott Gardens group: (1) a mid-winter interview; (2) a more even black–white residential split; (3) a less-friendly and less-open management (which resisted any cooperation with the study). It is, of course, impossible to pin down how reasonable an explanation one or another of these aspects may be. The winter interviewing would presumably not be a simple "seasonal effect" but might operate via increased time children spend at home with the mother during cold weather. The more even racial integration could lead to greater conflict with neighbors (especially given the structural characteristics of shared entranceways), but this effect should either show up with another scale (Peer Conflict), or it should have a greater impact on the adult's reports on her own mental health (see Table 1.4). The possible effects of an unfriendly management are also more likely to impact on the mother than the child.

The last line in Table 1.2 refers to results of additional multivariate analyses in which an interaction term, involving Housing Index and Neighborhood Conditions, was introduced as another predictor. None of the five dependent variables revealed a significant effect, ruling out the possibility that the effects of one residential parameter were conditioned by the level of the other residential parameter.

Table 1.3 summarizes the results for the scales that describe parenting behavior. The main findings are:

TABLE 1.3
Amount of Variance in Parenting Behavior Explained by
Socio-Demographic and Major Residential Variables

		Parental Coldness	Parental Punitive-ness	Mother Excitable-Rejecting	Parental Inadequacy
Age of Respondent		5.6	7.0	3.4	6.5
Number of Children		2.0	—.	2.5	–
Sex of Child (1 = Female, 2 = Male)		–	1.7	–	–
Age of Child		–	–	–	2.1
Housing Index		2.2	2.1	–	2.8
Neighborhood Conditions		2.0	–	–	–
Study Group		7.8	–	–	–
Inner City	Adjusted Group	.18	.17	.22	.21
Applicants	Means, in Standard	.86	-.44	.14	-.01
Neighborhood	Scores, With Scott	-.11	-.16	.10	-.03
Other Projects	Gardens Set	.39	-.22	.35	-.04
Scott Gardens	at .00	.00	.00	.00	.00
Housing by Neighborhood Interaction?		Yes	No	No	No

1. On Parental Coldness, higher scores are found among older respondents, and those who have more children. Both residential variables show an association: Greater parental coldness is related to lower quality of housing but *better* neighborhood conditions. The significant variance attributable to Study Groups is primarily due to the contrast between Applicants and Neighborhood Residents. The significant interaction effect between Housing Index and Neighborhood Conditions suggested that, within good neighborhood conditions, housing quality makes little difference and the values on Parental Coldness are intermediate; however, under poor neighborhood conditions, the negative effects of poor housing on Parental Coldness are enhanced.

2. Parental Punitiveness shows a significant association with age, but this is not interpretable, because with only four age groupings, a quadratic effect is evident. Reporting on a female child is associated with higher punitiveness. The association with Housing Index reveals more punitiveness under poor housing conditions.

3. Mother Excitable–Rejecting shows significant associations only with the sociodemographic variables: Being older and having more children is associated with more excitable-rejecting behavior.

4. The overall Parental Inadequacy scale reveals poorer parenting among older respondents reporting on younger children. Poor housing is also related to poor parenting.

Overall, the results in Table 1.3 concerning the residential parameters suggest a modest adverse effect of housing conditions on parenting behavior. The possi-

TABLE 1.4
Amount of Variance in Respondent's Mental Health Explained by Socio-Demographic and Major Residential Variables

		Agitated Depression	Phobic Anxiety	Soma-tization	Anger-Hostility	Zung Depression	Anomia
Family Income		3.0	–	3.1	–	–	7.8
Respondent's Education		2.0	2.2	2.8	–	–	–
Working for Pay		–	1.2	–	–	2.1	–
Age of Respondent		–	–	2.2	–	2.2	–
Number of Children		–	–	–	–	3.7	–
Marital Status		–	–	–	–	2.3	–
Race		–	–	–	–	–	4.0
Housing Index		–	–	1.6	–	2.1	–
Neighborhood Conditions		2.4	2.3	–	1.2	1.7	2.0
Study Group		4.2	–	–	8.1	12.4	–
Inner City	Adjusted Group	-.45	-.29	-.26	-.69	-1.24	-.10
Applicants	Means, in Standard	-.20	-.03	-.18	-.34	-.99	.00
Neighborhood	Scores, With Scott	-.70	-.44	-.54	-.94	-1.47	-.27
Other Projects	Gardens Set	-.32	-.26	-.25	-.41	-1.09	-.16
Scott Gardens	at .00	.00	.00	.00	.00	.00	.00
Housing by Neighborhood Interaction?		Yes	No	No	Yes	No	No

bly paradoxical association between good neighborhood conditions and greater parental coldness are better seen in terms of the interaction effects of the two residential parameters: Poor neighborhood conditions enhance the adverse effects of poor housing, and good neighborhood conditions buffer such housing effects.

Among the Study Groups, the Applicants stand out for two reasons: (1) The contrast between Applicants and Neighborhood residents accounts for most of the between group variance on Parental Coldness; (2) the Applicants are the highest on Parental Coldness and the Lowest on Parental Punitiveness, even though the two scales are moderately positively correlated (r = .29) when the five Study Groups are combined. This finding appears somewhat puzzling, but perhaps the Parental Punitiveness scale is somewhat ambiguous: A low score could indicate either a benevolent (lenient) style of disciplining, or parental indifference that leads to absence of discipline of any kind.

In Table 1.4 we present the data on respondent's own mental health. Because of the substantial intercorrelation among the first five scales (excluding Anomia), we do not summarize the results for each scale separately. The highlights of the findings are:

1. Indicators of socioeconomic status (income, education) show the expected negative association with three of the five mental health indicators. In addition, working for pay is associated with lower anxiety and depression. Higher age is related to more symptoms of Somatization, but on Zung Depression, it is the intermediate age category that is the highest. Higher depression is also related to not being married and to having fewer children.

2. On the Housing Index, two of the scales show an association with poor housing: higher somatization and higher depression. Neighborhood Conditions shows the expected association—poorer conditions and greater symptomatology—with four of the five scales.

3. An inspection of the means for the five Study Groups shows the Neighborhood residents to be consistently in best mental health and the Scott Gardens respondents in the worst mental health. The other three groups are intermediate, with Applicants being somewhat closer to Scott Gardens subjects.

4. The two significant interaction effects of the residential parameters and mental health both tell the same story: Within good housing, quality of neighborhood makes little difference, but for residents of bad housing, the negative impact of Neighborhood Conditions is particularly apparent.

5. The Anomia scale shows higher scores among Black respondents and those with lower income. Furthermore, good Neighborhood Conditions are associated with lower Anomia.

Overall, the results in Table 1.4 suggest a modest effect of housing quality and somewhat broader effect of neighborhood conditions. The latter, of course, is a more "subjective" residential parameter, more dependent on the respon-

TABLE 1.5
The Association of Infestation with Indicators of Children's Mental Health, Parenting Behavior, and Respondent's Mental Health

| | Means (in standard scores) by Groups | | | | | | Multivariate | |
	No pests	Cockroaches only	Mice only	Cockroaches and mice	Rats, Rats plus	ANOVA*	Sequential xx	Unique+
N	193	78	17	26	18			
Mother's Report on Child								
Child's Mild Chronic Illnesses	-.09	-.03	.21	.07	.77	<.03	n.s.	n.s.
Anger-Conflict With Parents	-.05	-.23	.53	.14	.82	<.02	<.002	n.s.
Depressed-Resentful Mood	-.20	.12	-.06	.46	.71	<.001	<.001	<.001
Poor School Adjustment	-.21	.12	-.01	.30	.90	<.001	n.s.	n.s.
Peer Conflict-Excitability	-.05	-.06	.27	.15	.26	n.s.	n.s.	n.s.
Mother's Report on Parenting								
Parental Coldness	-.08	-.21	.60	-.08	.96	<.01	<.01	<.04
Parental Punitiveness	-.23	.10	.66	.17	.78	<.001	<.001	<.001
Mother Excitable-Rejecting	-.08	-.02	.18	.31	.21	n.s.	n.s.	n.s.
Parental Inadequacy	-.14	-.06	.62	.16	.71	<.005	<.005	<.01
Respondent's Mental Health (Self-report)								
Aggitated Depression	-.12	.15	.11	.13	.39	n.s.	n.s.	n.s.
Phobic Anxiety	-.12	.20	.07	-.01	.46	<.05	n.s.	n.s.
Somatization	-.17	.17	.17	.06	.88	<.001	<.01	<.05
Anger-Hostility	-.09	.17	-.02	-.02	.28	n.s.	n.s.	n.s.
Zung Depression	-.12	.14	-.21	.34	.45	<.02	<.04	n.s.
Anomia	-.16	.40	-.64	.33	.09	<.05	<.03	<.02

ANOVA: Results of analysis of variance on means.

xxSequential, multivariate: The significance of the contribution of the Infestation variable *after* the following control variables have entered the regression first: age, income, race, years in Waterbury, number of children, marital status, level of education, rent, age of child, persons/room, and Neighborhood Conditions.

+*Unique, multivariate*: The unique variance contributed by Infestation, given the presence of all the above predictors, *plus* Housing Index and Study Group. Represents most rigorous and conservative estimate of effect of infestation.

20

dent's evaluations. The fact that the Study Group variable accounts for the greatest amount of variance on three of the six mental health scales suggests that neither sociodemographic variables nor explicity assessed residential parameters have removed much of the effect due to being in one or another study group. We have already speculated about some of the reasons the Scott Gardens residents may have such poor mental health: a racially more integrated residential setting and, possibly, a less-friendly management. Some of the previous work on residential proximity between the races does suggest adverse effects (Goldman, Warshay, & Biddle, 1962; Kramer, 1951). The classical and well-remembered studies of interracial housing (Deutsch & Collins, 1951; Wilner, Walkley, & Cook, 1955) did show "benefits" of proximity among Whites (i.e., more positive attitudes). However, it does not appear that Blacks were included in those studies and we don't know the effects on them, though there is reason to expect fewer or no benefits for them (Works, 1962). And, in general, the whole "social fit" or "social homogeneity" literature reveals that pathology rates are lower for those whose personal sociodemographic characteristics coincide with the dominant ones for the residential area (see Kasl, 1976, for further references).

Table 1.4 reveals the Neighborhood respondents to be in the best mental health; this is, of course, after removing the contribution of both the sociodemographic and the residential variables. It is a matter for speculation why this group stands out, but self-selection factors are one likely source. This is a residentially stable group that is reasonably satisfied with its housing and has not sought to move out (e.g., by applying to get into Inner City). Additional information suggests that they are particularly satisfied with certain aspects of their housing situation (such as the rent and the size of the dwelling unit), even though the Housing Index reveals them to be quite similar to the Applicants.

At this point we wish to turn to several *exploratory analyses* in order to understand better the basic descriptive findings that have been offered. One area of exploration concerns the notion that various components of the Housing Index may have an unequal impact on the various mental health indicators. A first step in this direction was to examine the intercorrelations among the Housing Index items and to carry out a factor analysis, both for the purpose of creating suitable subscales. However, the results were quite indeterminate, leading to no compelling clustering of items. In order to avoid a fishing expedition that heavily capitalized on chance findings, we selected one dimension for closer scrutiny, *infestation*. This was done because of a recent concern with pest management (Committee on Urban Pest Management, 1980) and because of our belief that this was a sufficiently distinct and important component of housing quality worth additional attention.

The relevant question in the interview asks: "Do you have anything in this apartment such as . . . cockroaches . . . mice . . . rats . . . other insects or pests." The respondent could answer "yes" to any and all of these. The information was combined to create the following, intuitively ordered categories: no pests, cockroaches only, mice only, cockroaches and mice, rats or rats plus. The percent with "no pest" ranged from 44.6% for Applicants to 86.2% for Other Projects, with the other three study groups clustering closely around 54%. Classifying the respondents into the five categories of infestation accounts for 22.5% variance on the Housing Index and 10.4% on Neighborhood Conditions; about ¾ of this between-group variance is attributable to a linear trend.

The basic results of this analysis are summarized in Table 1.5. This table presents a good deal of information in a condensed form. Firstly, for each scale, the unadjusted means for the five groups of respondents, classified by degree of infestation, are presented. The data are in standard scores, to permit comparisons across scales and a quick assessment of the magnitude of differences; for example, a mean of .77 for Symptoms of Mild Illnesses for the group reporting "Rats" means that they are about ¾ of a standard deviation above the mean for all respondents. The column headed ANOVA gives the significance testing based on a simple one-way analysis of variance on means for the five groups, unadjusted for any other variable. The next column, entitled, "Sequential, Multivariate," represents the significance of the contribution of the Infestation Variable after a number of control variables have been entered into the multivariate regression first. They are listed at the bottom of the table. The last column, headed "Unique, Multivariate," represents the significance of the unique variance contributed by the Infestation variable in the presence of all the preceding predictors in the multivariate prediction, *plus* the Housing Index (minus the infestation item) and Study Group. Thus, the major difference between the "Sequential" and "Unique" columns is that in the former the general effect of quality of housing is not explicitly removed from the estimate of the effects due to infestation alone. However, because of the modest association of quality of housing with neighborhood quality and with indices of social status, even the "Sequential" column will have already removed some of the general impact on quality of housing.

The last column in Table 1.5 represents the most conservative estimate of the impact of infestation. It is hard to think of some other potentially relevant sociodemographic or residential variable that could still be included. Moreover, because the causal matrix involving infestation with the other individual quality-of-housing items is poorly understood, the global control for overall housing quality may represent a statistical overcontrolling that leads to an underestimate of the impact of infestation (in the causal sense).

The five scales representing mother's report on the child reveal that two of them, Anger–Conflict with Parents and Depressed–Resentful Mood, show a significant association with degree of infestation even after the effect of sociodemographic and background variables has been removed. Moreover, the latter scale shows a significant association even when the global effect of housing quality and study group is also removed; infestation accounts for 8.5% of the variance in Depressed–Resentful Mood and an inspection of the adjusted means (not shown in Table 1.5) reveals near perfect linear trend.

The mother's report on parenting shows that three of the four scales are related to infestation even under the stringent conditions of the "unique" multivariate analysis. The strongest association is with Parental Punitiveness, and degree of infestation accounts for 11.8% of the variance. The adjusted means, however, do not reveal a linear trend; specifically, the "cockroaches and mice" group has a mean score that is lower than either the "cockroaches only" or the "mice only" group. This, of course, makes little sense and is difficult to interpret. A similar curvilinearity of effect is seen for the other two scales as well.

The respondent's report on her own mental health reveals two scales that are related to infestation when all the other variables, including quality of housing, are introduced as controls first: (1) about 4.3% of variance in somatization is explained by infestation and the effect is reasonably linear; (2) about 5.7% of variance in anomia is explained by infestation, but the nature of the relationship (the "mice only" group being the lowest) defies any sensible explanation.

Overall, the findings in Table 1.5 do suggest that infestation may have an impact that is above and beyond the influence of sociodemographic and general housing and neighborhood variables. The intuitive ordering of groups on degree of infestation was not well-supported, though, generally, the group exposed to rats had the highest values, and, frequently, the group with "no pests" had the lowest values. Infestation thus remains a component of poor quality housing worth further exploration.

The second area of *exploratory* analyses concerns a number of variables that describe the *social setting* and *social relationships* of the respondents. This follows from our introductory comments that dealt with the importance of viewing physical–residential parameters in a wider social context.

One variable chosen for this analysis is a brief four-item scale that we have called *Friendships on Block*. The items deal with perceived friendliness of people in the neighborhood, and the extent to which they know each other, visit, and help each other out. Although this scale does not deal with the primary or most intimate social relations, it is highly relevant here because it comes closest to representing the social context of the residential parameters. The analyses performed were of two types. Firstly, the analyses that form the basis of Tables 1.2–1.4 were repeated with Friendships on Block included in the multiple prediction; this new variable was introduced just ahead of the Housing Index. The results of this analysis were uniformly negative in several different ways: (1) Once the relevant sociodemographic variables were included, Friendships on Block did not show a significant association with any of the dependent variables; (2) introducing this new measure did not alter the previously described contribution of the three residential variables, Housing Index, Neighborhood Conditions, and Study Group. One lone exception was the finding that the variance in Parental punitiveness accounted for by the Housing Index was reduced from 2.1% to 1.1% when *Friendships* was introduced first, thereby rendering it statistically insignificant.

The second type of analysis addressed specifically the issue of statistical interaction between the Friendships scale and the other residential parameters. The three focal variables—Friendships, Housing, and Neighborhood—were dichotomized and introduced into the prediction, as were the three interaction terms reflecting three pairs of variables and one interaction term reflecting triple interaction among these three predictors. The results were again uniformly negative, and the two "significant" interactions observed are of doubtful replicability: (1) On Peer Conflict–Excitability, the influence of Neighborhood Conditions was contingent on friendliness of neighbors: Low conflict was found either in good neighborhood–high friendliness or bad neighborhood–low friendliness cells; (2) on Parental Coldness, a triple interaction was seen: The association between poor housing and parental coldness was primarily seen in one group, the bad neighborhood–high friendliness combination.

The role of social relationships was further explored by constructing five additional scales, which reflect the more intimate and important relations: (1) Disagreements with Spouse or Partner: 7 items reflecting conflict or disagreement over finances, children, leisure, drinking, household chores, etc.; (2) Quality of Relationship: 2 items dealing with perceived happiness and time spent together; (3) Satisfaction with Marriage: 2 items on regrets (doubts) regarding marriage in general and marriage to present spouse in particular; (4) Interaction with Friends and Relatives: 3 items on frequency of getting together; (5) Helpfulness of Friends and Relatives: 3 items on their availability to talk over problems or assist financially. The first three scales show an average intercorrelation of .48, whereas the last two scales correlate .55; clearly, then, two clusters are in evidence.

In order to reduce the number of purely exploratory analyses, the preceding five scales were examined with respect to one specific question: Do they interact with the Housing Index in influencing the mental health of the respondent (Table 1.4 variables only)? The multiple prediction involved: relevant sociodemographic variables, one or another social relations variable and Housing Index (both dichotomies), and Housing by Social Relations interaction term. We only note the significant interaction effects; main effect due to Housing have already been presented, whereas the other main associations (e.g., between Depression or Anger–Hostility and Disagreements with Spouse) are well-described in the general mental health literature.

Overall, six significant interactions with housing were observed: one involving one of the marital scales and five involving the two friends and relatives scales. In all instances, the interaction was of the same kind: (1) when the social variable indicated poorer social relations (e.g., more conflict with spouse, less interaction with friends), then higher levels of symptoms or poor mental health were associated with better housing; (2) when the social variable indicated a better social environment, then more symptoms were found for conditions for poorer housing. The largest interaction effect involved Housing and Disagreements with Spouse or Partner, accounting for 5.8% ($p < .005$) of the variance in Phobic Anxiety. Other interactions accounted for between 1.5 and 2.5% of the variance in Agitated Depression, Phobic Anxiety, Anger–Hostility and Anomia.

The observed interactions are difficult to interpret. The most dominant current framework (LaRocco, House, & French, 1980) treats social support as a buffer and would thus predict a different type of interaction: the adverse effect of poor housing seen only at levels of low social support (i.e., more conflict with spouse, less interaction with friends). The actual interactions we found suggest more complex dynamic processes than a simple buffering effect. For example, respondents in poor housing and in poorer mental health may seek and stimulate higher levels of interaction with and helpfulness from friends and relatives. But respondents in good housing and in poor mental health may, instead, make such interaction with and helpfulness from friends more difficult. This speculation treats the level of social interaction and support as dependent variable, in relation to respondent's mental health, and treats housing as a modifier. This is certainly an uncommon theoretical position.

The previous exploratory analyses involved several variables that characterize the social setting and social relations of the respondents and examined their possible interplay with the residential parameters. The final set of exploratory analyses utilized several additional variables that may be seen as extending the characterization of the broader setting, the wider context, of the respondent's living conditions. Four new scales were utilized: (1) *Satisfaction with Neighborhood Services:* 6 items indicating degree of satisfaction with public schools, police, parks and playgrounds, garbage collection, etc.; (2) *Crime in the Neighborhood:* 3 items dealing with juvenile vandalism, robberies, and attacks on the street; (3) *Management:* 2 items dealing with perceived cooperativeness of the management people and of their readiness to fix or correct housing problems and deficiencies; (4) *Relative Housing Deprivation:* a complex scoring of 6 items in which high deprivation depended on: (a) adverse comparisons of respondent's present housing with that of friends and relatives; and (b) selecting an aspired level of housing (from pictures) where the probability of attaining it was low and the prospective disappointment of not achieving it was high, weighted by personal importance of housing.

The role of these four variables was analyzed in the same manner as the multivariate analysis of Housing Index and Neighborhood Conditions (Tables 1.3–1.4): first the relevant sociodemographic correlates, then the new variable, and then Study Group. The basic question being asked in connection with these analyses is: How do these new "context" variables compare with the Housing

Index and Neighborhood Conditions as sources of variance in Parenting Behavior and Adult Mental Health scales?

Low *Satisfaction with the Neighborhood* was found significantly associated with three scales: high Parental Punitiveness (2.2% of variance), high Anger-Hostility (4.0%), and high Anomia (1.6%). And in all three instances, this represents additional variance, not previously explained by Housing and Neighborhood Conditions. High *Crime in the Neighborhood* was found associated with higher Somatization (1.3%) and higher Anomia (1.4%); the other adult mental health scales accounted for slightly less variance and were of borderline significance. However, none of these associations represents variance explained in addition to the two major residential parameters. Negative evaluation of *Management* was associated with several scales: higher Parental Punitiveness (1.8%), greater Parental Inadequacy (2.3%), greater Anger-Hostility (1.5%), higher (Zung) Depression (1.8%), and higher Anomia (2.6%). These associations reflect variance not accounted for by Housing and Neighborhood Conditions. Higher *Relative Housing Deprivation* was associated with only one scale, higher scores on Mother Excitable-Rejecting (1.9%); it was additional variance, not previously explained.

These results suggest that the area of Management relations is the most promising direction to move in order to enlarge the exploratory variance of Housing Index and Neighborhood Conditions. However, it must be recognized that as one moves away from the primary residential parameters toward more subjective evaluations, such as reported quality of management, one increases the difficulty of interpreting such associations. In particular, traits or response tendencies that determine the self-reports of (or actual levels of) Anger-Hostility or Depression or Anomia can also contribute to the evaluations of quality of management. Thus, the promise of this variable is contingent on our ability to develop "objective" measurement techniques that will help us rule out such possible methodological confounding or "reverse" causation.

SUMMARIZING DISCUSSION

The introductory section of this chapter suggested that the accumulated empirical literature on the residential environment and mental health does not, as yet, lead to any kind of closure. Conclusive and broadly general statements regarding the effects of housing are not possible for diverse reasons, including the fact that many aspects of design methodology and assessment procedures are still changing and evolving, and because of the high probability that the effects are small and richly embedded in a matrix of social-environmental (nonresidential) influences.

The results in this report are offered with the intention of adding to this accumulating literature but without the hope of facilitating the interpretive closure. There are several characteristics of the study design that are sufficiently idiosyncratic so as to forbid facile generalizations and to prevent easy comparisons with results from other studies: (1) The measures of the dependent variables are either new (children's mental health) or as yet infrequently used in the housing studies (SCL-90); (2) the subjects are relatively poor Black and Puerto Rican women living in a moderately sized New England city with its own unique characteristics and history; (3) the purposive selection of the subjects into the five Study Groups catches the respondents at different points in their residential careers: Inner City subjects have experienced a recent move to better housing, Applicants have been temporarily blocked in their intended mobility, Neighborhood subjects are residentially stable, and so on. Furthermore, the five Study Groups represent an open-ended "independent" variable that cannot be fully explicated by reference to some of the other assessed variables, such as social relations, perceived management, or relative housing deprivation.

The effects of the residential parameters on mental health were examined only as if they were explanatory variables that *add on* to the preexisting effects of sociodemographic and background variables. The Housing Index showed several significant associations: Poor housing was related to greater Anger-Conflict with Parents, more Parental Coldness and Punitiveness and Inadequacy, and more symptoms of Somatization and Depression. The amount of variance accounted for was modest, ranging between 1.6 and 3.1%. The Neighborhood Conditions measure showed only one significant association with Child Mental Health or Parenting Behavior (Parental Coldness); however, five of the six adult mental health scales were found related to Neighborhood Conditions. Again, the amount of variance accounted for was quite modest. There were also several suggestions of an interactive effect between Housing and Neighborhood Conditions: In all three instances of such interaction, the adverse effects of one residential variable on mental health were found to be significantly stronger for those respondents whose residential circumstances were worse according to the other variable.

The Study Group variable added explanatory variance to the two residential variables, as much as 12.4% in the case of the Zung Depression scale. In general, Inner City and Neighborhood respondents showed the best mental health and Scott Garden residents, the poorest. These results are not easy to interpret and some speculations were offered earlier regarding the possible role of racial integration, quality of management, and self-selection factors.

The second part of this report dealt with several exploratory analyses. One examined the role of one specific component of the Housing Index, degree of infestation by pests and rodents. The most rigorous and conservative examination of this variable incorporated prior statistical controls for sociodemographic variables, Neighborhood Conditions, Sample, and the remainder of the Housing Index: Infestation was related to Depressed-Resentful Mood of the child, Parental Coldness and Punitiveness and Inadequacy, and to Somatization and Anomia. A large part of this infestation effect was seen in the high scores of the residents who reported rats in their apartment. This analysis showed the promise of attempting to identify the subset of items in the Housing Index that put the residents at greater risk of adverse impact on health.

Another area of exploratory analyses utilized several indices of the social milieu of the residents. Much of the previous literature on the residential environment and a good deal of the theory have emphasized the importance of social-environmental factors as modifiers or as conditioning or intervening variables. To our surprise, the results of these analyses did not particularly agree with such formulations. One measure, Friendships on Block, essentially failed to contribute any explanatory variance, either as a main effect or in interaction with the two residential variables. Three other measures, reflecting the marital (partner) relationship, were equally barren in producing interactive effects with Housing Index. Only the two correlated scales, Interaction with and Helpfulness of Friends and Relatives, showed several significant interactions with housing. However, the specific nature of these interactions was not in agreement with any current notions of the effects of social support and hinted at more obscure dynamics. Overall, the negative results with the social milieu variables could be a function of the idiosyncratic characteristics of our sample and our methods.

The final exploratory analyses looked at several other variables—Satisfaction with Neighborhood Services, Crime in the Neighborhood, Quality of Management, and Relative Housing Deprivation—which might account for additional variance in mental health and thus represent a useful direction in which to enlarge the scope of future enquiry into residential variables. Among those examined, the brief management scale showed the most promise.

Much remains to be done in bringing about a more complete analysis of the data from this study, in particular the results from the second and third years' interviewing, and the data collection based on interviews with the children themselves (now in progress). However, it is clear that we are seeing only modest main effects of the residential environment on mental health. Furthermore, the search for crucial interactive variables, which will reveal a subgroup of respondents particularly vulnerable to the effects of the residential environment, has been only moderately rewarding.

ACKNOWLEDGMENT

Supported by 2R01 MH28370, Effects of Living Space and Locational Variables on Health.

REFERENCES

Altman, I. *The Environment and social behavior*. Monterey, Calif.: Brooks/Cole, 1975.
American Public Health Association. Committee on the Hygiene of Housing. *An appraisal method for measuring the quality of housing*. New York: A.P.H.A., 1950.

Baldassare, M. *Residential crowding in urban America*. Berkeley: University of California Press, 1979.

Booth, A., & Edwards, J. N. Crowding and family relations. *American Sociological Review*, 1976, *42*, 308-321.

Booth, A., Johnson, D. R., & Edwards, J. N. Reply to Gove and Hughes. *American Sociological Review*, 1980, *45*, 870-873. (a)

Booth, A., Johnson, D. R., & Edwards, J. N. In pursuit of pathology: The effects of human crowding. *American Sociological Review*, 1980, *45*, 873-878. (b)

Campbell, A., Converse, P. E., & Rodgers, W. L. *The quality of American life*. New York: Russell Sage Foundation, 1976.

Cantril, A. H., & Roll, C. W., Jr. *Hopes and fears of the American people*. New York: Universe Books, 1971.

Committee on Urban Pest Management. *Urban Pest Management*. Washington, D. C.: National Academy Press, 1980.

Derogatis, L. R., Lipman, R. S., & Covi, L. SCL-90: An outpatient psychiatric scale: Preliminary report. *Psychopharmacology Bulletin*, 1973, 9, 13-27.

Derogatis, L. R., Lipman, R. S., Rickels, K., Uhlenhuth, E. H., & Covi, L. The Hopkins Symptom Checklist (HSCL): A self-report symptom inventory. *Behavioral Science*, 1974, *19*, 1-15.

Deutsch, M., & Collins, M. E. *Interracial housing: A psychological evaluation of a social experiment*. Minneapolis: University of Minnesota Press, 1951.

Downs, A. *Opening up the suburb*. New Haven: Yale University Press, 1973.

Gersten, J. C. Measures of family functioning. In G. D. Grave & I. B. Pless (Eds), *Chronic childhood illness*. Washington, D.C.: DHEW Publication (NIH) 76-877, 1976, 193-201.

Gilbertson, W. E., & Mood, E. W. Housing, the residential environment, and health—A reevaluation. *American Journal of Public Health* 1964, *54*, 2009-2113.

Goldman, M., Warshay, L. H., & Biddle, E. H. Residential and personal social distance toward Negroes and non-Negroes. *Psychological Reports*, 1962, *10*, 421-422.

Gove, W. R., & Hughes, M. In pursuit of preconceptions: A reply to the claim of Booth and his colleagues that household crowding is not an important variable. *American Sociological Review*, 1980, *45*, 878-886. (a)

Gove, W. R., & Hughes, M. The effects of crowding found in the Toronto study: Some methodological and empirical questions. *American Sociological Review*, 1980, *45*, 864-870. (b)

Gove, W. R., Hughes, M., & Galle, O. R. Overcrowding in the home: An empirical investigation of its possible pathological consequences. *American Sociological Review*, 1979, *44*, 59-80.

Hinkle, L. E., Jr., & Loring, W. C. (Eds.). *The Effect of the Man-Made Environment on Health and Behavior*. Washington, D.C.: DHEW Publication No. (CDC) 77-8318, 1977.

Kasl, S. V. Work and mental health, In J. O'Toole (Ed.), *Work and the quality of life*. Cambridge, Mass.: The MIT Press, 1974.

Kasl, S. V. Effects of housing on mental and physical health. In *Housing in the Seventies, Working Papers 1*. Washington, D. C.: U. S. Department of Housing and Urban Development, 1976, 286-304.

Kasl, S. V. The effects of the residential environment on health and behavior: A review. In L. E. Hinkle, Jr. & W. C. Loring (Eds.), *The Effect of the Man-Made Environment on Health and Behavior*. Washington, D. C.: DHEW Publication No. (CDC) 77-8318, 1977, 65-127.

Kasl, S. V. Epidemiological contributions to the study of work stress. In C. L. Cooper & R. Payne (Eds.), *Stress at work*. New York: Wiley, 1978.

Kasl, S. V., & Rosenfield, S. The residential environment and its impact on the mental health of the aged. In J. E. Birren & R. B. Sloane (Eds.), *Handbook of mental health and aging*. Englewood Cliffs, N. J.: Prentice-Hall, 1980.

Kramer, B. M. *Residential contact as a determinant of attitudes toward Negroes*. Cambridge: Harvard University, unpublished dissertation, 1951.

Kriesberg, L. *Mothers in poverty*. Chicago: Aldine, 1970.

Langner, T. S., Gersten, J. C., & Eisenberg, J. G. *Subscales composing screening inventory and scoring codes for pathological responses.* New York: Columbia University, unpublished manuscript, 1973.

Langner, T. S., Gersten, J. C., McCarthy, E. D., Eisenberg, J. G., Greene, E. L., Herson, J. H., & Jameson, J. D. A screening inventory for assessing psychiatric impairment in children 6 to 18. *Journal of Consulting and Clinical Psychology,* 1976, *44,* 286–296.

LaRocco, J. M., House, J. S., & French, J. R. P., Jr. Social support, occupational stress, and health. *Journal of Health and Social Behavior,* 1980, *21,* 202–218.

Pynoos, J., Schafer, R., & Hartman, C. W. (Eds.). *Housing urban America.* Chicago: Aldine, 1973.

Report of the President's Committee on Urban Housing. *A Decent Home.* Washington, D.C.: U. S. Government Printing Office, 1969.

Rosow, I. The social effects of the physical environment. *Journal of the American Institute of Planners,* 1961, *27,* 127–133.

SAS Institute. *SAS User's Guide.* Raleigh, N. C.: SAS Institute, 1979.

Schorr, A. L. *Slums and Social Insecurity.* Washington, D. C.: Social Security Administration Research Report No. 1, 1963.

Srole, L. Social integration and certain corollaries: An exploratory study. *American Sociological Review,* 1956, *21,* 709–716.

Stokols, D. A social psychological model of human crowding phenomena. *Journal of the American Institute of Planners,* 1972, *38,* 72–83.

Stokols, D. Environmental psychology. *Annual Review of Psychology,* 1978, *29,* 253–295.

U. S. Department of Commerce, Bureau of Census. *Annual Housing Survey: 1973, Part B, Indicators of Housing and Neighborhood Quality for the U. S. and Regions.* Washington, D. C.: U. S. Government Printing Office, Current Housing Reports, Series H-150-73-B, 1975.

Wilner, D. M., Walkley, R. P., & Cook, S. W. *Human relations in interracial housing.* Minneapolis: University of Minnesota Press, 1955.

Wilner, D. M., Walkley, R. P., Pinkerton, T. C., & Tayback, M. *The housing environment and family life.* Baltimore: The Johns Hopkins Press, 1962.

Works, E. Residence in integrated and segregated housing and improvement in self-concept of Negroes. *Sociology and Social Research,* 1962, *46,* 294–301.

Zung, W. W. K. A self-rating depression scale. *Archives of General Psychiatry.* 1965, *12,* 63–70.

2 Built Space, The Mystery Variable in Health and Aging

Sandra C. Howell
Massachusetts Institute of Technology

Both age and physical health intervene in transactions between person and environment. As individuals age, their relationships to particular environments become more habituated, making it more difficult than at younger ages to modify either their environment or their behavior. As well, a concomittant of aging frequently is disease-based physical frailty, which creates problems of function for the individual, producing tenuous relationships to the environment (Byerts, Howell & Pastalan, 1979).

The complexity of interactions among age, health, and environment stimulated something of a conceptual crisis for theoreticians and researchers who wished to understand the psychodynamics of this interaction. Pure life-crisis formulations of adaptation to aging are in a state of empirical modification (Palmore, Cleveland, Nowlin, Ramm & Siegler, 1979). Several theoretical models have been proposed, none of which is adequately explanatory (Windley & Scheidt, 1980). The most prominent of the theoretical structures in current vogue is an *adaptation* model (Lawton & Nahemow, 1973). According to this model, the individual, consciously or unconsciously, processes information about her/his health status and the surrounding environment and modifies behaviors so that there is the least stress between the perceived self and the perceived environment. Within this theory, behavioral accommodations are made in accordance with a Maslow-like hierarchy of needs.

Kahana (1975) proposed a *congruence* model of person–environment (P-E) fit as a basis for studying the dynamics of adjustment of older people to particular residential or therapeutic environments and attempted to make the concept of person–environment fit operational in a recently reported empirical study (Kahana, Liang, & Felton, 1980). In this study ''stringent'' statistical analysis showed predictive value of P-E fit on morale.

Kahana's model is especially sensitive to dimensions of environment most likely to be influential to the older individual's self-perceived needs. However, the dimensions being developed are dominantly concerned with psychosocial and organizational attributes of environments, thus where spatial or architectural attributes are suggested by a single dimension (e.g., privacy), they are not really yet stated in operational form.

Researchers who do not have ready access to the conceptual material in this literature may wish to review the original dimensional descriptions in the model (Table 2.1). Because Kahana's suggested psychosocial issues are consistent with the growing work of others (Moos, 1974), it would be valuable to attempt to elaborate some of the architectural implications of these dimensions. For example, within the *segregate* area, the dimension of "continuity or similarity with previous environment of resident" might, in fact, overlap architecturally with the dimension of "privacy" in the *congregate* area and include such items as: (1) range of spaces available for resident display and placement of personal objects and furnishings; (2) character of direct to indirect access from private space to

TABLE 2.1
Dimensions of Congruence

1. Segregate Dimension	
Environment	*Individual*
A. Homogeneity of composition of environment. Segregation based on similarity of resident characteristics (sex, age, physical functioning and mental status).	A. Preference for homogeneity, i.e., for associating with like individuals. Being with people similar to yourself.
B. Change vs. sameness. Presence of daily and other routines, frequency of changes in staff and other environmental characteristics.	B. Preference for change vs. sameness in daily routines, activities.
C. Continuity or similarity with previous environment of resident.	C. Need for continuity with the past.

2. Congregate Dimension	
Environment	*Individual*
A. Extent to which privacy is available in setting.	A. Need for privacy.
B. Collective vs. individual treatment. The extent to which residents are treated alike. Availability of choices in food, clothing, etc. Opportunity to express unique individual characteristics.	B. Need for individual expression and idiosyncracy. Choosing individualized treatment whether that treatment is socially defined as "good" treatment or not.
C. The extent to which residents do things alone or with others.	C. Preference for doing things alone vs. with others.

(continued)

TABLE 2.1 (*Continued*)

3. Institutional Control

Environment	*Individual*
A. Control over behavior and resources. The extent to which staff exercise control over resources.	A. Preference for (individual) autonomy vs. for being controlled.
B. Amount of deviance tolerated. Sanctions for deviance.	B. Need to conform.
C. Degree to which dependency is encouraged and dependency needs are met.	C. Dependence on others. Seek-support, nurturance vs. feeling self-sufficient.

4. Structure

Environment	*Individual*
A. Ambiguity vs. specification of expectations. Role ambiguity or role clarity, e.g., rules learned from other residents.	A. Tolerance of ambiguity vs. need for structure.
B. Order vs. disorder.	B. Need for order and organization.

5. Stimulation - Engagement

Environment	*Individual*
A. Environment input (stimulus properties of physical and social environment); (not only availability of stimulation even to which that is directed to resident).	A. Tolerances and preference for environmental stimulation.
B. The extent to which resident is actually stimulated and encouraged to be active. (Jackson)	B. Preference for activities vs. disengagement.

6. Affect

Environment	*Individual*
A. Tolerance for or encouragement of affective expression. Provision of ritualized show of emotion (e.g., funerals).	A. Need for emotional expression-display of feelings, whether positive or negative.
B. Amount of affective stimulation. Excitement vs. peacefulness in environment.	B. Intensity of affect, e.g., need for vs. avoidance of conflict and excitement (shallow affect).

7. Impulse Control

Environment	*Individual*
A. Acceptance of impulse life vs. sanctions against it. The extent to which the environment gratifies needs immediately vs. postponed need	A. Ability to delay need gratification. Preference for immediate vs. delayed reward. Degree of impulse need.

(*continued*)

TABLE 2.1 (*Continued*)

gratification. Gratification/deprivation ratio.

B. Tolerance of motor expression—restlessness, walking around in activities or at night.

B. Motor control; psychomotor inhibition.

C. Premium placed by environment on levelheadedness and deliberation.

C. Impulsive closure vs. deliberate closure.

*Kahana, E., "A Congruence Model of Person-Environment Interaction", In P. G. Windley, T. O. Byerts and F. G. Ernst (eds.) *Theory Development and Aging*, Washington, DC: The Gerontological Society, 1975.

outdoors. On the other hand, an architectural issue that may represent discontinuity with prior residential environment might also include "scale of building," which not only requires specification of: (1) similarity of size of residential structure with those structures in the proximate neighborhood; but (2) number of enclosed, private residential units (or rooms) in present, compared with those of past setting and even perceived normative residential structure (i.e., what some writers might refer to as building density, but on a more architectural basis).

Rowles (1978) has produced a unique theoretical interpretation of the relationship between age and environment. Based upon in-depth psychoenvironmental

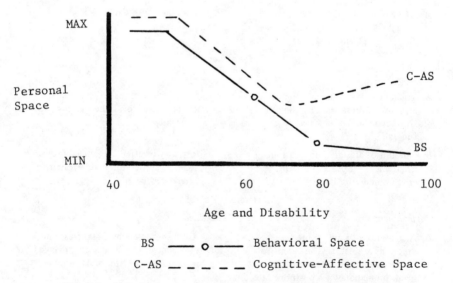

FIG. 2.1.   Behavioral and cognitive space as a function of age and disability.

explorations with an admittedly small sample, Rowles hypothesizes that as behavioral space is constricted (by illness, reduced mobility, and loss of social networks), cognitive space (affect-laden, remembered ventures in space) assume prominence. Figure 2.1 suggests Rowles' hypothesis.

MEASURES OF HEALTH

Virtually all studies of aging and environmental effects show health as a significant intervening variable. Behavior, attitude, morale, and satisfaction are all affected by indices of poor health, whether objectively measured by medical records, special scales and tests, or subjectively reported by respondents.

It was on the basis of this replicated research that Lawton and Nahemow (1973) proposed their competence hypothesis that asserts that as functional capacity diminishes environmental effects (Press) are more pronounced. The implications of this hypothesis to interventions in residential treatment environments for the aging person are discussed later.

For the psychologist, it is important to know that older individuals evidence reliable self-perceptions of their global health status, compared both to their own prior health condition and to others their age (Maddox & Douglas, 1973). However, not all health-status issues may be equivalently appropriate to research in environment and behavior. Clear problems of environmental mastery are presented for individuals with sensory or musculoskeletal disabilities, which reduce a previously mobile individual residing on a third-floor walkup to isolation and progressive depression. Although seen from an alternative environmental mastery perspective, the presence of an optional stairway in a sheltered setting might positively challenge the competence of a generally or mentally frail elder, and its twice-per-week use (instead of the elevator) reinforce mastery and high morale.

So-called objective health-status measures range from codifiable medical diagnoses to broad-spectrum activity of daily living (functional assessment) scales. Diagnoses are so distant from good operational variables in Environment–Behavior research that they are virtually useless. For purposes of data convergence, most gerontology researchers recommend the use of Activity of Daily Living (ADL) scales, as they appear in the Duke University OARS assessment instrument (Table 2.2). In environment-specific studies, these can always be augmented by the researchers and respondents. A cautionary note is appropriate to those conducting postoccupancy evaluations, however, in that questions of the form: "Can you (e.g., wash your windows)?" require, for the elderly, supplementary queries: "Do you (wash your windows)?", with opportunity for respondent to indicate why not, if not, or particular problems encountered, if act performed. It may not be health that restricts environmental activity but: (1) psychological fear of height because of resident floor location; or (2) others have usurped the activity.

TABLE 2.2
Activities of Daily Living Item from Oars Interview Schedule

41.   I'm going to read you a list of things that people usually have to do during the
day. After I read each one, please tell me if you can do it or not.

(READ LIST)	Can do it? No	Yes	(If "Yes") When do you do it, does someone help you or do you use a mechanical aid?* Yes, someone	Yes, mechanical aid	No aid required
Dressing and putting on shoes	58-1	-2	59-1	-2	-3
Bathing	60-1	-2	61-1	-2	-3
Cutting Toenails	62-1	-2	63-1	-2	-3
Reading	64-1	-2	65-1	-2	-3
Preparing meals	66-1	-2	67-1	-2	-3
Going on walks outside	68-1	-2	69-1	-2	-3
Climbing stairs	70-1	-2	71-1	-2	-3
Cleaning the house	72-1	-2	73-1	-2	-3
Hearing over the telephone	74-1	-2	75-1	-2	-3
Going grocery shopping	76-1	-2	77-1	-2	-3
Riding a bus	78-1	-2	79-1	-2	-3
Driving a car	8-1	-2	9-1	-2	-3

*Cane, crutches, walkerette, walker, wheelchair, brace, hearing aid, glasses.
"Used with permission from Duke Center, The OARS Methodology: A Manual, Second Edition.
Durham University Center for the Study of Aging and Human Development, 1978."

In addition to physical disease and disability, approximately 3–10% of older
persons may have some mental disability. Those over the age of 80 estimated to
have moderate to severe dementia may reach as high as 20%. Jarvik (1980) has
reviewed organic brain diseases prevalent among the aged. The outstanding issue
of relevance to environmental researchers, which she reaffirms, is the difficulty
of cleanly disentangling social and environmental from organic etiology. Because organic brain diseases (senile dementias) among the aged are predominantly diagnosed through behavioral measures, "inappropriate" behaviors of
older people are too often stereotypically misdiagnosed as organic. States of
confusion, disorientation, depression, and other cognitive, affective, and social
signs may, according to Jarvik and her colleagues, be brought on by malnutri-

tion, complex drug therapy, social isolation, relocation, or sensory loss (particularly partial deafness). For the most part, neither etiologic evaluation nor levels of interaction between organic decrement and etiology are entered into the choice of experimental or control subjects in current environment behavior research (Howell, 1978).

Two important issues for environmental research emerge as a result of the difficulties of assessing the mental health status, particularly of the older and frailer elderly person:

1. Base-line behavioral measures that are used to match experimental and control groups may provide a distorted estimate of the expected effects of the intervention. For example, if the assumption is that depressive symptoms are organic in origin and the interventions are institutionally oriented behavioral modifications (e.g., reinforcements of time—place awareness), the absence of significant effects or the slippages in effect may not be due to organicity, but to perceived loss of: (1) familiar milieu; (2) personal control; or (c) social networks. Holding the relearned behavior may simply have little intrapsychic salience to the Subject.

2. The physical environment itself may contribute to the base-line assessment of behaviors and to the outcome measures in unrealized ways. For example, in many institutional (and housing) environments, long, undifferentiated corridors with highly reflective surfaces, which separate patient (tenant) private space from group spaces, may produce confusion and disorientation in subjects who have visual disabilities or anxiety about their mental, physical, or social state.

Experimental paradigms that systematically test these issues do not appear in the literature, although many authors in gerontology now refer to the consequences.

STIMULATION IN THE ENVIRONMENT OF BRAIN DAMAGE

Pfeiffer (1977) has defined adverse brain conditions of aging as follows:

The constellation of symptoms pathognomic of organic brain disease are a variety of disturbances of intellectual and cognitive function. These specifically include *impairments of ability to remain oriented to one's environment,* or short- and long-term memory, of visual motor coordination, of *learning and retaining spatial arrangements,* of ability to abstract, to change sets, and to assimilte new information, and of ability to carry out sequential tasks (such as serial mathematical tasks or the correct sequencing of events in the individual's personal history) [emphasis mine] [p. 660].

In the face of a too-simplistic interpretation of deficits as reconstitutable behaviors, according to rules of conditioning, Howell (1978) has proposed that the use of interactive sensory stimulation within the context of routinized therapeutic environments should be explored. The argument presents a case for the primacy of neurological *attention* over social adaptation and engages the subject in recreating her/his own levels of awareness and control in the environment.

Current intervention research and therapy tends to *impose* rather than to *elicit* behavioral choices. Howell's hypothesis suggests that the perception of stimulus control, by the subject, must precede more social-environmental relearning. In a most creative effort, Reid, Haas, and Hawkins (1977) developed an instrument that combined the issue of *perceived control* with that of the *desire for control* of those aspects of the social and physical environment that are characteristic of homes for the aged. These authors argue that the value a subject places on the expected reinforcement (be it primary or secondary) will determine the extent to which control is applied and that, further, the application of control is situationally specific, which is what we should expect in accordance with the newer theories of the role of social learning in personality development (Baltes & Schaie, 1973). Reid, Haas, and Hawkins incorporated such environmental control factors as: (1) daily activity decisions (which might have been more finely specified in terms of waking time, meal time and place, movement around setting, open or closed doors, windows, etc.); (2) placement of possessions, and (3) provision for privacy.

An interesting research result, with particular implications for institutional populations that are dominantly male, was that the desire to control the sociophysical environment was significantly more highly correlated with self-concept in the men (n = 30) than in the women (n = 30) studied. Preliminary explorations of men and women in congregate and independent community settings suggest that the reinforcers for desired and expected control in these situations may also be different for men and women (Howell, 1980c). It is also suggestive that women exposed to 5 months of intensive Reality Orientation (RO) had significant return of verbal and social behaviors without concomitant return of self-care (ADL) skills (Harris & Ivory, 1976).

In the case of the more severely impaired male, then, we might hypothesize that areas of environmental-social responsiveness within which vestiges of control may be evoked would be more directly as operatives than as interactors. To put it more simply, a major social learning experience of the male in our society is to manipulate objects. When brain damage prevents the utilization of those sensory-motor and cognitive skills that reinforce manipulative capacities, the incentives to perform verbal or social functions may fall very low in the hierarchy of responses. Measures of intervention that tap behavioral change only in social self-care behaviors may therefore be deceptive.

DESCRIPTORS OF ENVIRONMENT

Researchers concerned with environment and behaviors generally have had great difficulty in enumerating the attributes of the built environment that are expected to constitute the independent variable side of deductive equations (Windley & Scheidt, 1980). In part, this is due to the social scientists' lack of familiarity with observation and description of built space. Thus, in research on "privacy" within nursing (institutional) settings, the independent variable may contain a range of social densities (1-4 versus 5-10-person rooms) and varying sets of organizational rules (e.g., open versus closed doors) but will rarely include such operational attributes of the physical environment as: (1) physical proximity of subject's bed to window, own storage cupboard, or door to corridor or toilet; (2) visual sightlines from subjects' bed to control-relevant environment (e.g., can subject see out open room door and how far down corridor to such activity spaces as nursing station?); (3) linear distance of resident's room to nursing station or dayroom.

The absence of such explicit design-behavior variables from our paradigms may indeed distort the behavioral results we now report. For example, Nehrke, Morganti, Willrich and Hulicka (1979), in a paper titled *Health Status, Room Size and Activity Level*, mean by "room size" the number of residents per sleeping space, not either the size nor the physical configurations of the room variable. Because their study settings are Veterans Administration domiciles, 1-2-person rooms are excluded from the sample and a 40-bed "room" (sic) is included. The finding that activity level is high in lowest and highest density settings may here imply quite different Environment-Behavior transactions. Similarly, when comparative studies of the effects of different residential densities on behaviors are conducted, the attributes of buildings, per se, are rarely defined (e.g., building height, number of residential units/floor, single versus double-loaded corridor, etc.) (Howell, 1980a; Nahemow, Lawton, & Howell, 1977).

There are two principal ways in which presumably relevant physical attributes of the environment can (and must) be entered into research in aging, health, and behavior. Firstly, the experimental and control subjects might be sampled proportionally and purposively relative to the representativeness of their private physical setting within the studied environment (Friedman, 1966). Thus, in an eight-story building, 15 units per floor, hypotheses about social activity level would require secondary sampling at low and high floors and of units proximate and distal from vertical circulation (i.e., elevator). Although primary sampling might have been by age, marital status, and functional health, these independent variables are insufficient to test environmental effects.

The second way environmental attributes can be entered is in the initial selection of the to-be-studied environments. Thus, nursing homes may be conceived of as describable laboratories and explicitly selected for those physical characteristics anticipated to be appropriate independent variables (e.g., presence or absence of a nursing station at a particular central location relative to room distribution, central versus peripheral location of "dayroom" or resident lounge, etc.). Lawton and Simon (1968), in their study of floor lounges in elderly housing, attempted this type of experimental design, and Howell (1980a) explicitly chose three housing projects where the physical relationship between building entry and social space varied in measureable (operational) ways, for a comparative study of social attitudes and behaviors of tenants.

DESCRIBING HEALTH ENVIRONMENTS

Categories appropriate to describing environments of aging have some peculiar characteristics. Because of the high prevalence of chronic diseases among older people (with or without continuous and intrusive disability), every environment in which an older person resides could be classified on some scale of promoting healthy function. At a recent conference of specialists in psychology of aging (San Diego, November 1980), participants did, in fact, argue that the only basis for evaluating the healthiness of an environment for an older person was the individual case work-up. The implication of this conclusion is that we still do not know enough about the predictable transactions between aging and environment to make aggregate statements based on diagnostic category and facility type. It is usual, however, to characterize health environments in terms of their therapeutic or treatment qualities. The descriptions to be used in research on age, health, and environment depend on the objectives of the study and the manner in which hypotheses are formulated.

Studies of environmental quality in which the primary independent variables include facility ownership characteristics (i.e., proprietary, religious group, or public) appear to this writer to be purely political in motivation. If the objective of a study is to determine the effects of environmental control on the behaviors and psychological states of moderately mentally impaired aged, then architectural attributes of environment (e.g., presence of optional stairways, alternative common spaces, and location of staff settings) as well as the organizational rules within the setting (locked exists, forbidden areas, allowable eating times and locations, allowable behaviors in private and public spaces) are relevant to the study and could and do occur across ownership types.

In accordance with architectural and organizational classifications, a major set of intervening variables becomes the number and types of active treatment programs conducted within the setting, and the staff and organizational rules that accompany such programs. The so-called long-term care facility varies, in treatment dimensions, from primarily medical-custodial through active rehabilitation to dominantly residential with available health and social service staff supports. Although the latter setting is not formally referred to as "long-term care," Lawton, Greenbaum & Liebowitz (1980) show that all age-concentrated settings possess this inevitability.

Probably the most complete attempt to organize a taxonomy of treatment settings is that being developed by Moos (1974). In the early development of an instrument by which the psychosical environment of settings might be assessed with some reliability and validity across a very wide range of setting types, Moos focused entirely on "social climate" variables without regard for the architectural design features that might be involved. Recently, however, a Physical and Architectural Features Checklist (PAF) has been developed and tested in a large number of sheltered care settings for elderly (Moos & Lemke, 1980). The nine dimensions, each supported by a set of dominantly yes–no or size measurement responses, are purported to represent a common collection of environmental resources supportive of human functioning in any type of facility for this age group (Table 2.3).

Unfortunately, there are two rather strong counter-intuitive faults with this experimental instrument. Firstly, its application results in the physically larger and more complex architectural environments being adjudged superior and thus perpetuates a residential form that, for the mentally and socially frailer elderly, may be highly discrepant with past living (Howell, 1980 b, c, Ullman, 1981). A second problem with the instrument about which the authors are sensitive is that each item receives the same weight in scoring. Relative to behavioral goals, the presence of certain supportive features may reinforce dependency rather than enhance independence.

Given the known patterns of health and aging and the residential environments that have been created in the United States ostensibly for the well aged and/or to minimize institutionalization, Lawton, Greenbaum and Liebowitz (1980) present a very interesting dynamic that will now be required for environmental descriptors. Whereas an architectural structure may remain constant over time, its characteristics as a context for behavior will tend to change as a result of the aging (and enfrailing) of its residents and its management policy (whether "accommodating" to frailer tenants or maintained "constant" by relocating frail tenants) Figure 2.2 proposes the intervention implications for each of Lawton's alternatives.

An issue of policy-planning relevance to the aging (i.e., all of us) relates to segregation versus integration of residential environments by age, economic status, or health status. Limited research on these issues suggest that original formulations have perhaps been biased by prevailing agency pressures and current programs, and that researchers need to apply much more refined conditions and constructs in the furtherance of this research (Harel & Harel, 1978; Lawton, 1980).

TABLE 2.3

Physical and Architectural Features Checklist (PAF)*
Subscale Descriptions and Item Examples

1. Physical Amenities	measures the presence of physical features which add convenience, attractiveness, and special comfort. (Is the main entrance sheltered from sun or rain? Are the halls decorated?)
2. Social-Recreational Aids	assesses the presence of features which foster social behavior and recreational activities. (Is the lounge by the entry furnished for resting and casual conversation? Is there a pool or billiard table?)
3. Prosthetic Aids	assesses the extent to which the facility provides a barrier free environment as well as aids to physical independence and mobility. (Can one enter the building without having to use stairs? Are there handrails in the halls?)
4. Orientational Aids	measures the extent to which the setting provides visual cues to orient the resident. (Is each floor color coded or numbered? Is a map with local resources marked on it available in a convenient public location?)
5. Safety Features	assesses the extent to which the facility provides features for monitoring communal areas and for preventing accidents. (Is the outside walk and entrance visible from the office or station of an employee? Are there call buttons in the bathrooms?)
6. Architectural Choice	reflects the flexibility of the physical environment and the extent to which it allows residents options in performing necessary functions. (Does each resident have access to both a bathtub and a shower? Are there individual heating controls?)
7. Space Availability	measures the number and size of communal areas in relation to the number of residents, as well as size allowances for personal space. (How many special activity areas are there? How large are these areas altogether? What size is the smallest per person closet area?)
8. Staff Facilities	assesses the presence of facilities which aid the staff and make it pleasant to maintain and manage the setting. (Are the offices free of distractions from adjacent activities? Is there a staff lounge?)
9. Community Accessibility	measures the extent to which the community and its services are convenient and accessible to the facility. (Is there a grocery store within easy walking distance? Is there a public transportation stop within walking distance?)

*Source: (Moos & Lemke, 1981, p. 573)

FIG. 2.2
MODELS FOR PLANNING AND MANAGEMENT

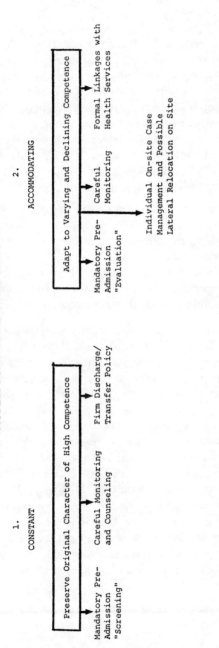

FIG. 2.2. Graphic reinterpretation of models proposed by Lawton, Greenbaum & Liebowitz (1980b).

CONSEQUENCES OF INTERVENTIONS

The traditional paradigms of psychology involve structuring the experimental context, labeling independent and dependent variables, and controlling, via sampling, treatment procedures, or base-line behavioral measures, potentially distorting intervening variables. In the case of aging subjects, such paradigms appear highly questionable, even were it possible to match experimental and control groups on the basis of health status, because they imply a linearity that probably has no place in environment—behavior transactional analysis.

Studies of the consequences of residential relocation are a good case in point (Borup & Gallego, 1981; Boureston & Pastalan, 1981; Schultz & Brenner, 1977). The studies adopt a set of assumptions about relevant variables that have not themselves been verified. These assumptions include at least the following:

1. That all subjects attach the same meanings to the initial pre-relocation setting;
2. That the rate of health deterioration is consistent and predictable across individuals in experimental and control groups;
3. That perceived salience of the move, to the self, is consistent with the labels by which the experimenter has defined the dependent variables and is, further, common across individuals and constant over time.

Scheidt and Schaie (1978) have attempted to rectify some of the errors contributed by these assumptions. They constructed a base-line instrument that presumably elicits, for each subject, a set of contextual saliences. Howell (1980c) proposes that researchers go beyond this level of immediate saliency and seek cues from psychoenvironmental histories as to consistency and change in salience.

The automatic ways in which we have been labeling demographic variables in descriptive and analytic environment–behavior research become particularly problematic when health is an added concern. Lawton (1981) presented a convincing argument that *marital status,* in the case of persons over 65, is salient both as an antecedent and a consequence in the ecology of aging. Using National Health Survey and Annual Housing Survey data, he finds, for example, that the single never-married man is in far greater jeopardy in terms of residential environment, social network support, and health maintenance than the never-married woman or widowed counterparts. If this is true, then studies of adaptation to institutional environments need to account for these antecedent factors among the sample and controls.

NORMS OF BEHAVIOR

Because very little is known about life-span transactions between the individual and the built environment and because interindividual variability is known to be high among populations of elderly, it becomes very difficult to establish or validate sets of behavioral norms for "old people." As a consequence, much of the published research on environments and aging adopts norms based upon expected behaviors applicable to younger adult age groups. Thus, for example, it is expected that grouping age peers within a single residential setting will result in certain forms of social interaction, and that the absence of such social interactions (e.g., visiting, participating in formal and informal activities on site) is indicative of deviation from normative behavior. This is all the more surprising given the replicated descriptive fact that fewer than one-third of residents in age-concentrated housing settings engage in on-site social activities (Howell, 1980a; Lawton, 1980).

Norms of interaction, a heavily used intervening variable, contain still other operational problems. It turns out that it does, in fact, make a significant difference to theory how a researcher measures interpersonal contact. Conner, Powers, and Bultena (1979) have stated:

> It seems that it is not "how often" or with "how many" one interacts, but rather under what circumstances, for what purposes, with what degree of intimacy and caring the interaction takes place that will have its impact on morale. As in other areas of life, we have been working from the assumption that "more is better". In the case of social involvement, we find that abundance is not necessarily associated with the more positive life adjustment of older people. Although some older persons may find happiness in a crowd, others seek the solitude of isolation with equally positive results. Morale, adjustment and life satisfaction imply an expression of the quality, or meaning of the life experience. We suggest that it is in the quality of the interactional experience that a broader understanding of adjustment to the process of aging will ultimately be found. (p. 120–121)

Expectations of outcome of environmental interventions are often expressed in terms of return to "pre-morbid function," improved scores on standardized instruments (MSQ, ADL, morale scale), or higher frequency of observed behaviors accepted as adaptive "norms" within the environment. Depending on how one chooses to view and value institutional environments, so-called successful outcomes might be seen as a "Catch-22" adaptation. Some portion of the frustration expressed by researcher-practitioners using Reality Orientation (RO) probably results from their own non-acceptance that competent function, in activities of daily living, is perceived by residents as antithetical to living in a medically oriented institutional environment, where dependency is a way of acting out the sick role (Zepelin, Wolfe and Kleinplatz, 1981).

According to Tobin and Lieberman (1976), outcomes of an environmental intervention, particularly a relocation or institutionalization, are strongly influenced by the *discrepancies,* to the individual, between old and new environment. They also see in their research evidence that a selection process operates in who, among the aged, enter institutions such that comparisons between institutionalized and non institutionalized (matched controls) may not truly represent comparable potential behaviors or adaptive characteristics. The same problem of selection applies in comparing the well-being of community-based to congregately housed older residents (Lawton, Brody & Turner-Massey, 1978).

It seems easy enough to identify discrepancies in daily living activities between community residences and nursing care institutions (e.g., uniformity of meals, scheduled activities, rules of dress). It is much more difficult to identify the personal salience of discrepancies in the built environment, and probably these are not in themselves important without accounting for the relationship between the building design characteristics and the activities that these enable or constrain, in relation to the individual's past activities.

SOCIALIZATION TO ENVIRONMENTS OF AGING

Whereas a relocation (voluntary or involuntary) is a clear example of an intervention requiring psychological and social adjustment for an older person, the nature of the to-be-adjusted-to environment in terms of norms at variance with past experiences has received little attention. The role of self-perceived and imposed social norms is critical to an understanding of environment–aging transactions. Rosow (1974) has best presented the issue of socialization to old age in a way that may permit the built environment to be used to test parts of theory. For example, role rehearsal, an integral part of childhood socialization to adult environments, is essentially absent for age-concentrated, long-term care environments. If women of current old age cohorts have been socialized to domestic pursuits, and if, in old age, the role of nurturant domestic is withdrawn either through environment (removal of kitchen), health, or loss of nurturing objects (spouse and relatives), then the environment–behavior symbioses that had been constructed over a lifetime may be expected to break down. It was interesting to note in this connection a preference for an eat-in kitchen by a national sample of elderly women in subsidized housing (Howell, 1980a). Rosow (1974) asserts:

> Two basic psychological conditions seem necessary to a given role. First, the person must see the role [its context] and its associated values as legitimate in a system to which he belongs or aspires to belong. Secondly, he must personally identify with the role [and context] so that his access to it seems proper to him [parentheses mine] (p. 34).

There are many unprobed issues in resocialization to the environment of aging that are still to be studied. We know very little about the environmental expectations of currently aging Americans, except that they tend to: (1) reject nursing homes; (2) prefer not to live with adult children; and (3) dominantly stay in their *owned* homes, even in the face of widowhood and health pressures.

Just as early socialization involved the child's learning of the rules of the society, so, too, the later stages of life must involve adopting or creating *new* sets of rules to the transactions with environments of built space.

REFERENCES

Baltes, P. B. & Schaie, K. W. *Life Span Developmental Psychology*. New York: Academic Press, 1973.

Borup, J. H. & Gallego, D. T. Mortality as affected by interinstitutional relocation: update and assessment. *Gerontologist*, 1981, *21*, 8–16.

Boureston, N. & Pastalan, L. The effects of relocation on the elderly: a reply to Borup, Gallego and Heffernan. *Gerontologist*, 1981, *21*, 4–7.

Byerts, T. O., Howell, S. C. & Pastalan, L. A. *Environmental Context of Aging*, New York: Garland Press, 1979.

Conner, K. A., Powers, E. A .& Bultena, G. L. Social interaction and life satisfaction: An empirical assessment of late-life patterns. *Journal of Gerontology*, 1979, *34*, 116–121.

Duke Center, *The OARS Methodology: A Manual*, Second Edition. Durham University Center for the Study of Aging and Human Development, 1978.

Friedman, E. P. Spatial proximity and social interaction in a home for the aged. *Journal of Gerontology*, 1966, *21*, 566–574.

Harel, Z. & Harel, B. B. On-site coordinated services in age-segregated and age-integrated public housing. *Gerontologist*, 1978, 153–158.

Harris, C. S. & Ivory, P. B. C. B. An outcome evaluation of reality orientation therapy with geriatric patients in a state mental hospital. *Gerontologist*, 1976, *16*, 496–503.

Howell, S. C. *Designing for aging: patterns of use*. Cambridge, MASS: MIT Press, 1980(a).

Howell, S. C. Environments and aging. In C. Eisdorfer (ed.), *Annual review of Gerontology and Geriatrics*. New York: Springer, 1980(b).

Howell, S. C. Environments as hypotheses in human aging research. In L. W. Poon (Ed.), *Aging in the 1980s*. Washington, D.C. American Psychological Association, 1980(c).

Howell, S. C. *Environmental stimulation and the brain-damaged person*. Paper presented at a Conference sponsored by the U.S. Veterans Administration and N. A. S. A., Minneapolis, 1978.

Jarvik, L. E. Diagnosis of dementia in the elderly: A 1980 perspective. In C. Eisdorfer (ed.) *Annual Review of Gerontology and Geriatrics*. New York: Springer, 1980.

Kahana, E. A congruence model of person-environment interaction. in P. G. Windley, T. O. Byerts & F. G. Ernst (eds.), *Theory development in environment and aging*. Washington, D. C.: The Gerontological Society, 1975.

Kahana, E., Liang, J. & Felton, B. J. Alternative models of person-environment fit: Prediction of morale in three homes for the aged. *Journal of Gerontology*, 1980, *35*, 584–595.

Lawton, M. P. An ecological view of living arrangements. *Gerontologist*, 1981, *21*, 59–66.

Lawton, M. P. *Environment and aging*. Monterey, Calif.: Brooks-Cole, 1980.

Lawton, M. P., Greenbaum, M. & Liebowits, B. The lifespan of housing environments for the aging. *Gerontologist*, 1980, *20*, 56–64.

Lawton, M. P. & Nahemow, L. Ecology and the aging process. in C. Eisdorfer & M. P. Lawton (eds.), *The psychology of adult development and aging*. Washington, D.C.: American Psychological Association, 1973.

Lawton, M. P., Brody, E. M. & Turner-Massey, P. The relationship of environmental factors to change in well-being. *Gerontologist*, 1978, *18*, 133–137.

Lawton, M. P. & Simon, B. The ecology of social relationships in housing for the elderly. *Gerontologist*, 1968, *8*, 108-115.

Maddox, G. L. & Douglas, E. B. Self-assessment of health: A longitudinal study of elderly subjects. *Journal of Health and Social Behavior*, 1973, *14*, 87-93.

Moos, R. H. *Evaluating treatment environments*. New York: Wiley, 1974.

Moos, R. H. & Lemke, S. Assessing the physical and architectural features of sheltered care settings. *Journal of Gerontology*, 1980, *35*, 571-583.

Nahemow, L., Lawton, M. P. & Howell, S. C. Elderly people in tall buildings, In D. Conway (ed.), *Human responses to tall buildings*. Stroudsburg, P.A.: Dowden, Hutchinson & Ross, 1977.

Nehrke, M. F., Morganti, J. B., Willrich, R. & Hulicka, I. M. Health status, room size and activity level: Research in an institutional setting. *Environment and Behavior*, 1979, *11*, 451-463.

Palmore, E., Cleveland, W. P., Nowlin, J. B., Ramm, D. & Siegler, I. C. Stress and adaptation in later life. *Journal of Gerontology*, 1979, *34*, 841-850.

Pfeiffer, E. Psychopathology and social pathology. In J. Birren & K. W. Schaie (eds.) *Handbook of the psychology of aging*. New York: Van Nostrand, 1977.

Reid, D. W., Haas, G. & Hawkins, D. Locus of desired control and positive self-concept of the elderly. *Journal of Gerontology*, 1977, *32*, 441-450.

Rosow, I. *Socialization to old age*. Berkeley: University of California Press, 1974.

Rowles, G. D. *Prisoners of space? Exploring the geographical experiences of older people*. Boulder, Colo.: Westview Press, 1978.

Scheidt, R. J. & Schaie, K. W. A taxonomy of situations for an elderly population: Generating situational criteria. *Journal of Gerontology*, 1978, *33*, 848-857.

Schultz, R. & Brenner, G. Relocation of the aged: A review and theoretical analysis. *Journal of Gerontology*, 1977, *32*, 323-333.

Tobin, S. & Lieberman, M. A. *Last home for the aged*. San Francisco: Jossey-Bass, 1976.

Ullman, S. Assessment of facility quality and its relationship to facility size in the long-term care industry. *The Gerontologist*, 1981, *21*, 91-97.

Windley, P. G. & Scheidt, R. J. Person-environment dialectics: Implications for competent functioning in old age. In L. W. Poon (ed.), *Aging in the 1980s*. Washington, D.C.: American Psychological Association, 1980, 407-423.

Zepelin, H., Wolfe, C. C. & Kleinplatz, F. Evaluation of a year-long reality orientation program. *Journal of Gerontology*, 1981, *36*, 70-77.

3 Development of a Methodology for Assessing Daily Experiences

Arthur A. Stone
Long Island Research Institute

John M. Neale
Department of Psychology
State University of New York at Stony Brook

ABSTRACT

Serious shortcomings in existing instruments for assessing life events coupled with the inadequacy of retrospective designs in evaluating hypotheses concerning the causal impact of experience led to the development of a new methodology for assessing daily occurrences. Firstly, a sample supplied a pool of events using diary recordings. These events were then categorized, arranged in outline form, and linked to a set of dimensions used to rate psychological reactions to the events that were experienced. This initial instrument was pilot tested for 2 weeks with husbands (targets) reporting their own experiences and their wives completing the form as observers. The instrument allowed husbands to adequately record their daily experiences, and several predictions were confirmed (e.g., desirable events related directly to "positive" moods). Nonetheless, husband–wife concordance was low and prompted an additional study. Several revisions based on participants' comments and our own experience with the initial form were made, and more extensive training was provided to the participants. Additionally, some subjects received phone calls on selected days to allow us to better understand the reasons for low husband–wife concordance. The major source of discordance was that information known to the target was unavailable to the observer. Thus, the instrument appears to be a convenient way of collecting accurate data on daily experience.

Explorations of the association between environmental events and illness mushroomed following the development of Holmes and Rahe's (1967) method of

49

quantifying life stress. They compiled a list of 43 events, the Social Readjustment Rating Scale (SRRS), which subjects rated using Steven's (1974) magnitude estimation technique. Each event was rated according to the amount of "social readjustment" necessary to accomodate to it compared with the amount of readjustment inherent in getting married (the scaling modulus). The readjustment coefficients were then used to weight scores on the Schedule of Recent Events (SRE), a paper and pencil measure parallel in form to the SRRS, on which subjects indicate which of the 43 events they have experienced. The sum of the SRE, called the Life Change Unit (LCU), was used to predict various measures of psychiatric functioning and physical illness.

Psychiatric, psychological, and sociological journals are currently replete with studies using the SRRS/SRE method, and the conditions studied range from myocardial infarction to severe depression. Although its success as measured by popularity may be impressive, criticism of the substance and methods of the SRRS/SRE has been plentiful (for example, Andrews & Tennant, 1978; Brown & Harris, 1978; Cline & Chosy, 1972; Dohrenwend & Dohrenwend, 1974; Wershow & Reinhard, 1974).

The sample of events found in the SRRS was not chosen with any particular sampling strategy, other than "common sense," and as such has been criticized on several accounts. Most of the events are undesirable and severe; thus, they are not representative of the events most people experience (Dohrenwend, 1974). Also, a large number of life experiences of potential etiological significance remain unrecorded. The partial overlap between event and symptom measures (e.g., treating "frequent minor illnesses" as an event when somatic dysfunction is the outcome) has been an often cited confound; not unexpectedly, removal of these redundent items lowers the relationship between events and illness (Lehman, 1978; Stone & Neale, 1981).

Event-weighting dimensions or qualities deserve careful attention as they define investigators' notions of stress, but there is no agreed-upon set of dimensions or qualities that define stress. Holmes and Rahe used "social readjustment," a concept closely linked to Selye's theoretical position that environmental change defines stress (Selye, 1956). In more recent years, many other qualities of events have been used by life-events researchers: desirability (Gersten, Langner, Eisenberg, & Orzeck, 1974); upsettingness (Theorell, 1974); exit versus entrance (Paykel, 1974); degree of control over event occurrence (Brown, Sklair, Harris, & Birley, 1973); life area (Chiriboga & Dean, 1978); threat (Brown & Harris, 1978); and stressfulness (Stone & Neale, 1978). The strength of association between a dimension and a criterion appears to depend on which criterion is being predicted. For example, the gain–loss dimension is associated with the onset of depression (Paykel, 1978), yet, is more weakly related to other psychiatric conditions. Thus, an important consideration in the assessment of the environment is which dimensions are to be used to rate experience. It is unlikely that any single dimension exhaustively indexes the concept of stress.

Another issue is the manner in which ratings of experience are obtained. Holmes and Rahe chose to use SRRS ratings from one group of subjects to weight the SRE scores of others. Although there is evidence that SRRS ratings are fairly uniform across various ethnically defined samples (Miller, Bentz, Aponte, & Brogan, 1974), there is substantial variation about the mean ratings indicating individual differences within the samples (Wershow & Reinhart, 1974). Moreover, there are instances when individuals' subjective ratings of experiences were more strongly related to outcome than those obtained from the normative samples (Theorell, 1974; Vinokur & Selzer, 1975). But these individual ratings of events were collected after the outcome was known and could have been subject to retrospective distortion, possibly in a way that would result in stronger correlations (Dohrenwend, Krasnoff, Askenasy, & Dohrenwend, 1978). This issue is not simply a methodological one but raises the larger question of whether life-event inventories are trying to measure "objective" stress that impacts on most people in the same way, or "subjective" stress defined by the meaning of the event to the individual. Unfortunately, this distinction has not yet received much attention, but it is crucial to the kinds of questions that studies in the field can answer (Stone, in press).

The stability of data gathered by event checklists is also a concern. Rabkin and Struening (1976) report that very few studies have examined reliability, and those that have report generally low test–retest coefficients, within the range of .26 to .90 (Rahe, 1974). Factors affecting the statistics were the testing interval, education of subjects, period during which events were recorded, wording and format of questionnaire, and the associations among life events. Recent studies have shown that recall or major events declines in frequency approximately 5% for each retrospectively recalled month (Jenkins, Hurst, & Rose, 1979; Uhlenhuth, Balter, Lipman, & Haberman, 1977).

Finally, the associative relationships found in life-events research are difficult to interpret causally (Brown, 1974). Most of the studies have used either purely retrospective designs or partially prospective designs (in which illness is prospectively assessed, but life events are rated for the period prior to the data collection). The retrospective nature of these designs clearly opens the door to the possibility of serious contamination of the data. Although truly experimental studies are almost impossible to conduct in the natural environment, nonexperimental, prospective research has the potential to untangle the temporal sequence of events and illness.

In response to some of these criticisms, at least two new checklists loosely following the SRRS/SRE method have appeared in the literature. Sarason, Johnson, and Siegel's Life Experiences Survey (1978) includes subjects' ratings of a combined desirability—impact scale for events experienced within the past several months. Thus, they abandoned the group approach to event weightings in favor of an individual, subjective approach. On the other hand, the Psychiatric Epidemiological Research Interview developed by Dohrenwend, Krasnoff, Askenasy, and Dohrenwend (1978) was based on a sampling of recent major events for several carefully defined demographically homogeneous groups. The events and those on a previously prepared event checklist were scaled by a group of subjects according to the amount of change they required. The authors used a complex scheme to categorize events according to whether they were stable across groups, within groups, or neither. Furthermore, all events were classified by four judges on several dimensions (probability of occurrence; whether it was a gain, loss, or ambiguous; if it was likely to be a consequence of a psychological condition, physical illness, or independent of both conditions; and, if the subject was the central figure in the event).

Both of these inventories incorporate significant changes compared to the original SRRS/SRE method. Nonetheless, the basic retrospective method of collecting event data remains unchanged: Subjects still are required to recall their experiences for the past several months. This approach is limiting not only for the reasons discussed earlier (namely, potential biases inherent in the retrospective method) but also because the interplay between individuals and their environment over time is completely ignored. For researchers concerned about the linkage between psychosocial stress and health, the data are as enlightening as describing an entire motion picture by presenting the contents of a single frame.

An alternative to the static model of current life-events assessment methods has been proposed by Lazarus and his colleagues (Folkman, Schaefer, & Lazarus, 1979; Lazarus, 1966; Lazarus & Cohen, 1977; Lazarus, Cohen, Folkman, Kanner, & Schaefer, 1979). Their transactional model is similar in spirit to an interactive approach, where nonadditivity of effects is the rule, yet is extended to include a time dimension. Dynamic models such as this are a step closer to allowing more complex processes, perhaps even including reciprocal effects across time (Coyne, 1976), to emerge. In its complete form, a transactional approach allows for a redefining of stimuli based on immediately prior experiences. A single assessment of the individuals' event ratings is inadequate within this model. Transactional investigations study behaviors over many points in time, and their data analyses call for procedures such as time series and path analysis rather than more traditional methods designed for cross-sectionally collected data (e.g., analysis of variance).

In this chapter we describe the development of a new questionnaire, the Assessment of Daily Experience (ADE), which is designed to allow individuals to record and rate their daily experiences in prospective investigations. The rationale for developing another "life-event" assessment is founded on both criticisms of the life-event inventories we have previously described and a desire to explore the temporal, interactional processes among life experiences and outcomes. We chose days as the unit of analysis because we felt that a thorough characterization of a 24-hour period was possible without major retrospective-recall bias. With days as the unit of analysis, the specific life events to be rated must include more mundane happenings than are found in previous life-event inventories. Yet, the inventory would not exclude major events that have been retrospectively reported in other inventories: They can still be recorded, probably with greater reliability. Furthermore, there is theoretical and clinical support for the idea that minor daily events are related to illness. These minor, daily events may be *subjectively* important to individuals for reasons not addressed by the researcher. The meaning of events may be linked to past experience with similar events (many failures with it, for example), to more general personality characteristics (an anxious individual faced with a public speaking engagement), or to the cultural–religious background of the individual (divorce for a strict Catholic).

Several prominent researchers have commented on the impact of daily experiences on health. Lazarus had discussed the etiological significance of environmental stresses ranging from large-scale catastrophes to more personal daily "hassles" (Lazarus & Cohen, 1977). Wolff has offered clinical support for the effects of "minor" events on somatic health (Wolff, Wolf, & Hare, 1950), as have several Soviet researchers (Kurstin, 1976). Thus, we chose to assess daily experiences because they are not subject to the methodological shortcomings of previous life-event work and would allow us to examine the life-events–illness relationship over time.

There is a small history of the study of daily experience. In monograph remarkable for its detail, Barker and Wright (1951) reported the minute by minute activities of a day in a young boy's life. The observers, armed with pad and pencil, followed the boy throughout an entire day in half-hour shifts. Although extraordinarily complete, collecting data in this manner is clearly impractical for most investigations. Diaries are another method that has been used. Wolff often instructed his patients to record, in diary format, significant daily happenings, feelings, and health changes. Although associations between emotionally arousing reports and exacerbation of various symptoms were observed (Wolff, Wolf, & Hare, 1950), quantification of the degree of daily stress was not attempted. More recently, Rehm (1978) had college students note significant pleasant and unpleasant events in a diary for 14 consecutive days. A count of the number of recorded pleasant and unpleasant events served as the environmental measure. Similarly, Roghmann and Haggerty (1973), in a study of health service utilization, had mothers in 200 families use a diary format to log significant happenings of all family members. Each day was characterized by the researchers on a five-point stress scale. Finally, Holmes and Holmes (1970) had a sample (predominantly medical students) chronicle their daily experience. These free-format responses were translated into the SRE items, enabling the authors to assign daily LCU scores based on SRRS ratings.

A major problem with these diary assessments is that the reliability and validity of the data are unknown. A checklist, wherein a constant set of event stimuli are presented over days, offers several advantages. The difference between diary and checklist methods may be likened to that between recall and recognition. Because recognition is a more sensitive measure of retention than recall, presentation of an event checklist will likely increase accuracy compared to the free recall format of a diary. The greater structure of a checklist method may also minimize the effects that daily fluctuations in mood, health, etc. might have on event reporting with less-structured recall methods. A checklist approach also allows experiences to be readily rated on several dimensions. Finally, the checklist method is more convenient for subjects, an important consideration in longitudinal research where they will complete the form daily over weeks or even months.

Several checklists assessing particular aspects of daily experiences have been developed in the last decade. Two major research groups, Lewinsohn's at Oregon and Lazarus's at Berkeley, try to assess the previous month's daily events with a single administration of their checklists. Lewinsohn's Pleasant Events Schedule (PES; MacPhillamy & Lewinsohn, 1971) and Unpleasant Events Schedule (UES; Lewinsohn, 1975) are each checklists of 320 minor daily events. Subjects rate the frequency of each item's occurrence during the past month on a three-point scale as well as its enjoyability (PES) or aversiveness (UES). A summation of the products of frequency and enjoyability/aversiveness is used to characterize the past month and is assumed to measure the amount of response-contingent reinforcement or punishment experienced by an individual.

Lazarus's research group has also developed two monthly checklists for assessing daily experience: the Hassles and Uplifts scales consisting of 117 and 135 items, respectively. Like the UES and PES, these items are also rated on two three-point scales, severity and persistence for hassles and "how strongly" and "how often" for uplifts. A count of the number of items checked, a sum of their ratings, and the average item rating are used to index the magnitude of hassles and uplifts for the previous month.

Although both sets of questionnaires attempt to accurately measure daily events, they may well fall prey to the same sorts of methodological pitfalls that we discussed earlier for SRE/SRRS type checklists. Retrospective distortion of recall for minor daily events over a 1-month period is certainly plausible. In Lazarus's work, the finding that "how often" and "how strongly" correlate .95, a result that is contradictory to major life events where intensity is inversely related to frequency, suggests that an overall impression of the month, and not the particular event occurrences, is what is remembered and reported.

In addition to his monthly assessment, Lewinsohn has developed a 160-item version of the PES, which is completed on a daily basis (Lewinsohn & Graf, 1973; Lewinsohn & Libet, 1972). It is not a standardized inventory of a particular set of items but is compiled to suit each subject: The individualized PES contains only those items that had a high frequency on the subject's full PES. Subjects are instructed to rate each item on a three-point scale of pleasantness. In Lewinsohn's studies depressives and control subjects have been followed for up to 30 consecutive days with daily recordings of both events and mood.

Another assessment of a specific aspect of daily experience was developed by Wills, Weiss, and Patterson (1974). The Spouse Observation Checklist (SOC) contains 105 events that could occur in a marriage. (There are other versions of the SOC containing up to 409 events.) With the original version of the SOC, subjects indicated how many times an event had occurred during a day and rated it on a seven-point pleasingness–displeasingness scale. The frequency of all occurrences and the sum of the products of each item's frequency times its pleasingness rating were used to predict marital satisfaction.

Our objective in these studies was to construct a checklist of daily events that would characterize an individual's experience. These events would then be rated on several dimensions to assess individuals' psychological reactions to them. Unlike Lewinsohn and Wills, Weiss, and Patterson, we were interested not in a single aspect of daily functioning, such as the reinforcing value of unpleasant events or marital events, but in the activities of an entire day. Several considerations directed our efforts: (1) Because we intended to have people use the checklists for lengthy periods, the list had to be of reasonable length. A burdensome task, such as a checklist of several hundred items, could result in high attrition rates and/or haphazard reporting; (2) we wanted to representatively sample daily experience and not be limited to any particular class of events such as negative experiences. Adequate sampling of event content would enable us to test hypotheses concerning the effects of composite indices of daily experiences, for example, the ratio of positive to negative events; (3) because self-reports could be biased, especially for events that cast an unfavorable light on the subject, we developed a protocol for daily recording incorporating both self-report and the ratings of another person to increase report validity; (4) as no single quality of the environment has been agreed upon as defining "stress," we designed the form such that checked items could be rated on several dimensions relating to the stress concept; (5) finally, because some psychological theories of stress regard anticipated experiences as similar to actual occurrences in that they may exert an effect on health (Lazarus, 1966), we allowed for these expected experiences to be recorded.

A series of three studies was conducted, and all drew upon a pool of subjects selected several months prior to the first study. Only married couples were accepted into the pool, so we would have a convenient source of information from a significant other with whom the target individual had daily contact. Couples were solicited from local communities with mailings to addresses randomly selected from the county telephone directory and advertisements in local newspapers. Payment of 20–$80, depending on which of the three studies the couples participated in, was offered. Participants were geographically limited to nearby communities as we planned interviews with subsamples of the pool. A variety of questionnaires, including demographic questions, a life-event inventory, and health history, were sent to couples expressing interest, and those who returned completed questionnaires entered the subject pool. It is impossible to accurately gauge the response rate given that letters were sent to ineligible households (not married, separated), and we have no idea how many eligible couples read the advertisement. However, we may be certain that the selection was not truly random. Subsequently, we report the attrition rates in each of the specific studies.

Rather than separately present the demographic characteristics of the parts of the subject pool used in each of the three studies, we present a description of the entire pool in Table 3.1. The sample was almost entirely white, largely middle class, well-educated, and predominantly Catholic. Mean ages for husbands and wives were 38.8 and 36.0, respectively. Although the acquisition of subjects

TABLE 3.1
Demographic Characteristics of Subject Pool

	Sex of Respondent	
	Male	*Female*
Age		
Mean	38.8	36.0
Standard Deviation	10.6	9.3
Race		
White	99%	96%
Hispanic	0%	1%
Black	0%	0%
Other	1%	3%
Education		
1st - 6th grade	1%	1%
7th - 9th grade	6%	5%
10th - 12th grade	27%	44%
Some college	37%	33%
B.A. or equivalent	16%	6%
M.A.	10%	10%
Ph.D., M.D., etc.	4%	0%
Social Class[1]		
I (highest)	12%	
II	22%	
III	30%	
IV	33%	
V	4%	
Religion		
Catholic	47%	51%
Protestant	14%	16%
Jewish	27%	29%
Other	5%	4%
None	6%	0%

[1]Social class computed per family based on husband's status

depended on voluntary selection, the statistics presented in Table 3.1 correspond reasonbaly well to census characteristics of the area from which they came.

STUDY 1

Our first goal was to obtain a sample of daily activities by having participants record their experiences, in diary form, over a 2-week period. It was neither desirable nor practical to have couples record everything that they experienced during a day, so we chose to limit the content of their recording. Two concepts—importance and emotion-inducing—were chosen, which we felt would not unduly restrict content variety. Our rationale was that subjectively minor happenings would not influence later health, at least not through psychological processes. Each concept is applicable to both "positive" and "negative" experiences, "gains" and "losses," "upsettingness," and many other qualities related to stress. Thus, the initial selection criterion would not exclude experiences qualitatively similar to those previously investigated and opened up the possibility of obtaining experiences that had not been included in other life-event assessments. In the second part of this study, we reduced the reported experiences into a set of more general categories to produce a manageable checklist. A checklist format was necessary for accurate and quick recording and provides other advantages that were discussed earlier.

Method

Subjects.   Thirty-two couples were selected from the subject pool. Seven couples (22%) did not properly complete the forms or dropped out of the study.

Materials and Procedure.   Couples were randomly assigned to the cells of a 2 × 2 factorial design. One factor was recording content (RC), the types of experiences subjects were to record. Half the subjects received instructions that they should record experiences that "are, in some way, important," whereas the remaining subjects were to record experiences "about which your feelings are stronger than usual, stronger in the sense that you feel more joy, more aggravation, more sorrow, more anger, more compassion, etc., than you usually do." The second factor was the amount of space available for recording experiences. Daily recording forms were printed on legal-size sheets; 11 horizontal lines defined 10 time periods and intersected with vertical lines that formed small rectangles, where subjects were to briefly describe experiences. Half the subjects had three boxes for each time slot, whereas the remaining half had six boxes. This allowed us to explore how this method factor, number of recording spaces (NRS), affected the frequency of event reporting.

Couples in all conditions were mailed 28 daily recording forms and 14 stamped return envelopes. Accompanying these materials were instructions informing both husbands and wives to each complete a form, preferably before bed, on each of 14 consecutive days. Completed forms were to be returned to us on the following day.

Results

An average of 12.1 days were recorded by each person, with a range of 6 to 14 days. A total of 1848 experiences were logged on 604 completed forms. The average number of experiences recorded per person–day, 3.06, did not differ for husbands and wives. An analysis of variance of number of daily experiences using sex of respondent, RC, and NRS as factors did not yield significant main effects or interactions.

Most of the events reported were relatively minor occurrences such as "started a new sewing project," "fishing trip was good," "went to Mass," "tense meal at in-laws," and "stopped at friend's home for a drink." We were, however, surprised at the number of major experiences this group of 25 couples reported during only 2 weeks of recording: for example, "father very ill," followed a few days later with "father died," "friend's wife may have cancer," "coworker had heart attack," "death of son's friend," "worried about ill sister," "saw accident on expressway," and "aunt in critical condition."

We next proceeded to summarize the content of the 1848 items. Two research assistants familiarized themselves with the items, and each was instructed to produce a list of content categories arranged in outline form. The instructions did not specify either the themes to be used in organizing the items or the number of categories and outline levels. However, the assistants knew that the purpose of their work was to produce an event checklist for daily use. Following initial outline construction, they were instructed to use their outlines to classify a sample of the raw experiences as a means of checking the adequacy of their categories.

Although major differences in the two outlines were observed at the heading and subheading level, many of the categories were similar. To produce a single checklist, the two assistants and one of the authors (A.S.) met and worked out a new list that incorporated features of both the originals. This task differed in one important respect from the original content summarization procedure. Because the checklist items would be rated on several dimensions, which are described later, some of the items could be worded more generally than was the case in the two original outlines. For example, there would be no need to include the two separate items "pleasant family visit" and "unpleasant family visit," because the pleasantness attribute would be rated later by the subject. Therefore, only the generic item "family visit" was required. The resulting checklist included four major headings and 16 subheadings: Work Related Activities (concerning your boss, supervisor, upper management, etc., concerning coworkers and/or employees, general happenings concerning self at work), Leisure (physical, social with friends, vacation, family outings, personal, financial), Family and Friends (concerning spouse, concerning children, concerning relatives, concerning friends and neighbors, family duties), and Other Happenings and Activities (personal, other). Sixty-six individual items were distributed across the 16 sub-headings. These items themselves were often brief, having been partially described by the two levels of headings, although examples were included in parentheses for some of them.

At this point, it was not clear if the checklist was readily understandable or if experiences could be properly coded with it. As a preliminary check, two additional teams of two research assistants each used the checklist to classify two separate sets of approximately 400 of the original experiences with the intent of locating problematical categories. We found that none of outline categories were particularly difficult to understand, and the interrater disagreements did not aggregate in any single or small set of categories. A stronger test of the adequacy of the checklist was performed in the next study.

Discussion

There are several aspects of ADE that distinquish it from other checklists. Items were derived by sampling a wide variety of daily experiences, as opposed to some subset of content based on an investigator's particular needs. Experiences were arranged in an outline structure to make completing the form easier. The items are considerably different than those on other event lists, as they are often nonspecific with regard to the qualities that will later be rated by participants. For example, Holmes and Rahe (1967) include the items "Mortgage under $10,000" and "Mortgage over $10,000," presumably because they thought the larger mortgage would be more meaningful than the smaller one. By linking rating dimensions to the event checklist, participants can rate an item on just how meaningful it is. Thus, our single item "loans" covers the psychological impact of both large and small loans according to its rating. Some items, however, are more specific than this example. Within the category of job-related experiences, for example, there are 16 items tapping much specific content. Thus, we can distinquish among various *kinds* of work-related experiences, such as "under a lot of pressure at work" versus "criticized for inadequate work, lateness, etc."

An item by item comparison of the SRE with our daily-experience list revealed several overlapping content areas, yet many of the major events found on the SRE were not included in the daily list. Death of spouse, divorce, marital separation, and jail term, for example, are not found in ADE and would have to be written in by the participant (a feature we have built into ADE). Other major events, though, such as death of family member, fired at work, pregnancy, and change in financial state, are covered by ADE. Furthermore, the ADE is much more thorough with regard to less-catastrophic experiences. Another difference between the two lists concerns the SRE's "change" items, such as "change in number of arguments with spouse" or "change in recreation." Items worded in this manner imply an unspecified change over time, presumably over days, and as such, are not applicable to the daily list. Because ADE includes an ongoing measure of daily events, a direct and probably more valid measure of "change" is available.

STUDY 2

With the initial checklist in hand, we next laid out the questionnaire with the items and their rating dimensions and developed a protocol for completing the form. The form was piloted with a sample of community couples with the intent of assessing the practicality of its daily use and of testing several hypotheses concerning its validity.

The dimensions on which daily experiences were rated were taken from a factor-analytic study reported by Redfield and Stone (1979). In that investigation, 94 rather major life events were rated by college students on six bipolar scales suggested by previous life-event studies. The original scales were reduced to three factors labeled desirability, change, and meaningfulness. Although these dimensions emerged from a sample of major events rated by college students, we retained them, as the alternative was an uninformed selection of dimensions, and these factors appeared to adequately represent the qualities used in previous studies. Two of the dimensions were bipolar, change–stability and desirable–undesirable, whereas the meaningfulness dimension was unipolar. In addition to events that have actually occurred, we allowed items to be checked and rated if they were anticipated as occurring in the near future. In accord with Lazarus' (1966) theory, this step was taken to allow the possible psychological impact of anticipations to be assessed. Items checked as anticipations should not be considered "events" as there is no objective stimulus; however, we included them because their psychological impact may be as great as that of real events (Lazarus, 1966).

Several ways of rating experiences on these dimensions were explored, but two considerations led to our choice of adjective anchored, 14-(bipolar) or 7-(unipolar) point scales. Daily recording of event qualities with the psychophysical techniques of magnitude estimation or production (Stevens, 1974) was rejected because it would be too time consuming. Category scales were of interest because they are easy to complete, and anchored categories would be comparable from day to day. The drawback of the category method is that the intervals between categories are not equal as is usually assumed (Stevens, 1974). Although we do not present the data here, the adjectives used to anchor the numerical values on the three dimensions were scaled with magnitude production techniques, thus providing metric information from category-like scales. The conjunction of magnitude scaling techniques and category scales provides a satisfactory rating system for our needs.

Couples used the form in the following way. One member of the couple served as the "target" and completed the form about himself/herself. The other person served as an "observer," whose task was to complete the form about the target based on his/her direct knowledge of the target's day. Because we did not want to reduce the power of our statistical tests by analyzing the data for effect of sex of respondent in these studies, husbands served as targets and wives as observers. Observers completed the form independently of targets in this study and based their responses only on what they observed; therefore, they had less information about the target's daily activities than did the targets themselves. A good example of this is in the area of work-related items; observers clearly knew much less about what went on at the target's work site because they were not there.

Some of the validity hypotheses tested in this study used what we call concordance rates as the dependent measure. Concordance rates reflect the agreement between targets' and observers' report of the targets' daily experience and were computed using the familiar formula of agreements divided by agreements plus disagreements. The difference between concordance and interrater reliability is not computational, as both use the same formula, but is based on the amount of information the raters have at their disposal. For interrater reliability, both raters observe the same phenomenon and thus have the same amount of information about it; however, for concordance, the targets have more information about their daily activities compared to the other raters, the observers. Given the differential amounts of information raters have in the two instances, we expected concordance to be considerably lower than results from usual interrater reliability assessments.

Our hypotheses were based on several assumptions we made about how concordance rates should interface with various other features of the recording task. If these hypotheses were not supported, we would have less confidence in the way that participants were using the materials. This is in some ways parallel to the usual construct validation procedure, in the sense that a measure is expected to covary with different measures in predicted ways.

The first hypothesis was that the importance of individual experiences, as defined by the husband's rating of meaningfulness, would directly covary with target–observer concordance. We expected higher concordance with the more meaningful experiences because important experiences should generally be more public and more readily available to observers. Secondly, concordance rates should be higher on weekends because spouses would likely spend more time with one another. Thirdly, events checked as anticipated would have lower concordances compared to those checked as occurring during the day because these anticipated experiences would be less accessible to the observer. Finally, by collecting daily mood ratings, using the brief version of the Nowlis Mood

Adjective Checklist (Nowlis, 1965), we examined the relationship between life events and affect. The validity of ADE would be supported if we replicated previous findings, that unpleasant events are associated with "negative" affective states (e.g., depression) and pleasant events with "positive" emotions (Rehm, 1978).

A second major purpose of this study was to locate difficulties people had using the form and assess their hypotheses about the purpose of the research. This was accomplished by telephone interviews conducted after the daily recording was completed.

Method

Subjects.   Thirty-two couples were selected from the subject pool, 12 of whom had also participated in the first study (several months passed between the two studies). Five couples (16%) did not complete the materials yielding a final *N* of 27.

Materials.   Daily-experience checklists were printed on both sides of legal-size sheets. Spaces were available at the top of the sheet for name, date, day, and sex of the respondent. Immediately below these spaces were the three event-rating dimensions (desirability, meaningfulness, and change) with a one-sentence description of each scale and either seven or 14 adjectives (Immeasurably, Extremely, Quite, Very, Moderately, Somewhat, Slightly) modifying the dimension (the adjectives were repeated in reverse order for each pole of the bipolar scales). Just to the right of each adjective-dimension combination was a number ranging from 1-7 for meaningfulness and from 1-14 for desirability and change. A fourth scale was used for the events that were anticipated. Subjects indicated the probability that the anticipated experience would actually happen with a scale ranging from a 1 in 10 to a 9 in 10 chance of occurrence.

Just below the rating keys was the event checklist. In addition to the 66 items, three blank lines were appended at the end of the list to allow items to be written in. The write-in category allowed us to gather further data concerning whether people adequately recorded their daily experiences with the checklist and also provided a means for people to note major but low-frequency events such as those on the SRE. Written-in items were rated in the same manner as the original 66 items. Subjects were instructed to place a check in a circle located to the left of each item, if the event was experienced by the target or an "A" for anticipated happenings. To the right of the item there were four sets of open parentheses that were in alignment with four column headings: one for each of the three rating dimensions and one for the anticipation rating. Whenever an item was marked with a check or an "A," subjects were to rate the event on each of the three dimensions. As a reminder to participants of their target–observer status, the sentence "Wives: Be sure to rate your husbands, not yourselves" was placed at the top of each form.

Procedure. Couples were mailed packets containing a detailed letter explaining the recording procedure, 28 blank daily recording forms (14 per individual) and 14 stamped return envelopes. Instructions stated that the forms should be completed independently at the end of each of 14 consecutive days, preferably just before bed, starting on a specified date (the same for all couples). After completion, both spouses' forms were to be placed into an envelope and mailed the following morning.

Results

Before examining the hypotheses, we report some data on how the forms were used. The average number of days for which couples completed the forms was 13.2. On the 704 completed forms returned, 3700 actual experiences were checked, or 5.26 per form. Husbands and wives reported similar numbers of experiences, 1856 and 1844, respectively. Anticipated experiences were reported less frequently: 848 were reported, or 1.20 per day.

The optional blank space for recording experiences not on the list was used 106 times (2% of all checked items). Many of the write-ins received low ratings on meaningfulness and for the most part could have been coded with one of the 66 items. Those that we felt were not covered by the list deserve attention, as they suggested modification in checklist content. There were four such experiences, accounting for 20 write-ins: visits to health-care professionals; witnessed an unusual happening; death of friend or acquaintance; and psychiatric difficulties. Besides providing useful information for the next version of the checklist, the finding supported our continued use of the write-in procedure.

As for the dimensional ratings of daily experiences, we briefly discuss the frequency distributions of each of them. Change–stability approximated a normal distribution, though the slope was steeper on the change side with a modal value of "slightly changing." The shape of the desirability distribution was skewed toward the undesirable pole and had a modal value of "very desirable." Except for the two extreme endpoints, "immeasurably" and "extremely," the distribution of meaningfulness was rectilinear. There were markedly fewer responses on "extremely" and even fewer at "immeasurably." The three dimensions were moderately intercorrelated, desirability with change, −.33, desirability with meaningfulness, .50, and change and meaningfulness, −.06.

In total, 883 events were reported as occurring on the same days by both spouses, 973 were reported by husbands alone, and 961 were reported by wives alone, yielding an overall concordance rate of .31. Generally, the outline heading with the lowest item concordances was Work-Related, whereas Leisure activities generally had the highest concordances. Family and Friends' items yielded great variability in concordance rates.

The first hypothesis, that experiences defined as meaningful by husbands would have higher concordances than those rated as less meaningful, was tested by examining the concordance rate at each of the seven levels of meaningfulness. A significant positive correlation among meaningfulness descriptors and concordances supports the hypotheses, whereas a negative or nonsignificant correlation does not. The product-moment correlation was $+.76$ ($df = 5$, $p < .02$), supporting the hypothesis.

Examination of differences in concordance rates on each day of the week tested the second hypotheses. Visual inspection of the rate, and an examination of the rate broken down further by husband-rated meaningfulness, revealed no increases in concordance rates on weekends. No statistical testing was performed on the basis of the visual inspection.

The third hypothesis, that the concordance rate based on anticipated experiences would be lower than the rate based on those experiences that occurred, required comparing the concordance rates for events that had occurred or were anticipated. Computed across all families, the concordance rate for anticipated events was .13, and for the actually experienced events it was .31. Using variability estimates in the rates among couples, a correlated t test between the two was highly significant ($t(25) = 6.98$, $p < .001$), lending support to the hypothesis.

Finally, using the targets' ratings, events were classified as desirable or undesirable and correlated with the Nowlis Mood Scales across days. In general, the number of desirable experiences was directly related to the positive mood scales (elation, $r = +.28$, vigor, $r = +.25$, social affection, $r = +.20$, all $p < .01$) and inversely related to the negative scales (anxiety, $r = -.16$, skepticism, $r = -.17$, both $p < .05$). Undesirable events showed the reverse pattern (anxiety, $r = +.26$, sadness, $r = +.20$, surgency, $r = -.23$, all $p < .05$). Correlations of *spouses'* ratings of their husbands' mood with husband-reported events revealed the same pattern of relationships that husband-reported mood and events produced (Stone, 1981). Thus, the relationship between events and mood, as reported by targets, did not appear to have been spuriously inflated.

Within 9 days of completing the last daily recording form, couples were contacted and responded to a set of questions read to them by the interviewer. In all but one case targets (husbands) were interviewed. Most participants thought that the purpose of the study had something to do with marital communication given the protocol of wives rating their husbands and not themselves. Initially, in open-ended questions, none of the husbands guessed the actual purpose of the study, yet, when asked directly if it concerned stress, many thought that it might. Participants were also asked about their use of the 7- and 14- point scales: Most said they referred to the adjective key when filling out the form, whereas the small remaining portion of the sample reported that they had memorized the response keys and had not needed to constantly refer to them. As for daily completion, participants reported that they varied from a nightly routine on the average of once during the 2-week period. The time needed to complete the form was about 12 minutes.

An open-ended section of the interview requested that participants discuss difficulties they had using the form. Many critical comments were made about the Change–Stability scale. According to the subjects, it was somewhat difficult to understand and was not always relevant because it only seemed to apply to "major" events. The Anticipation scale elicited similar, though fewer, comments. Several respondents expressed a need for a not-applicable or zero point on the scaling keys. Three husbands said there were too many numbers (adjectives) on the scales. As for the event outline itself, there were no comments; however, some participants said that some outline categories did not apply to them, that more "child categories" were needed, and that a category for working around the house would be useful.

Discussion

Our first attempt at an assessment of daily experience yielded a large number of checked events recorded over 352 person days. Based on the low frequency of write-in events and the postrecording interviews, the checklist appeared to allow respondents to adequately describe the events of these days. An important point was that participants generally enjoyed completing the form, as attrition rates in studies using the form for longer periods would probably be high if subjects disliked the task. The amount of time needed to complete the form, on the average 12 minutes, appeared reasonable. Three of the four hypotheses tested concerning concordance were supported. More meaningful experiences had higher husband-wife concordances compared to less-meaningful ones, anticipated experiences had lower concordances than those that actually happened, and mood was reliably related to events in the directions suggested by previous research. The hypotheses that concordance rates would increase on weekends because of more spouse contact was not supported. Perhaps our assumption of more contact on weekends is not justified (the weekend fisherman could be such a case). Further information on validity was provided by the fact that the correlation between self-rated events and self-rated mood was replicated by the spouse-rated mood and event correlations.

A major issue was posed by the relatively low husband–wife concordances. A recent study by Jacobson and Moore (in press) using a long version of the SOC has one spouse rate his/her own or the remaining spouse's behavior. This data gave them the opportunity to examine self- versus spouse-report of detailed marital events. Overall, spouses agreed roughly half the time, and when these figures were corrected for chance agreements (with kappa), the agreement figures were considerably attenuated. Their agreement percentage, although somewhat higher than the ones achieved in our studies, focused solely on behaviors that both spouses had equal access to. Thus, although the concordance figures are similar to those obtained in studies of the accuracy of self-monitoring (also see Nelson, 1977, for a review), we felt that concordances could be increased by increasing the clarity of the form itself and by providing more training to participants.

A revision of ADE incorporated the participants' comments and several additional changes that we felt were needed to increase the form's clarity and ease of completion. The number of items was reduced from 66 to 61 by collapsing a few items into expanded single ones, often with examples. The item "under close scrutiny by boss, supervisors, etc.," for example, was subsumed by "under a lot of pressure at work," with close scrutiny as an example. A "not applicable" option was added to each of the rating scales to accommodate those times when a scale did not seem to apply to an experience.

The format of the checklist was changed as well. A permanent booklet with the items, detailed instructions, and a description of how to classify experiences replaced the separate instruction/answer sheet arrangement of the previous study. Answer sheets were designed to be placed into the booklet during use; thus, they could be mailed back with relatively low postage expense. Finally, the theoretically interesting dimension of "control over an event's occurrence" was added to the rating dimension section of the checklist (Averill, 1973).

In the next study, couples were also visited in their homes and given training in using the revised form to be sure that it was being completed properly. Some couples were also contacted while they were completing the forms to explore the reasons for the husband–wife disagreements.

STUDY 3

This study had two purposes: exploring the origins of the low husband–wife concordance rates observed in the previous study and piloting the revised checklist and training procedure. Specifically, our concerns centered around the origin of husband–wife "errors" in recording, especially instances where the wives reported events that their husbands did not report, as these implied that either husbands were not recording their experiences completely or that the form was being improperly used.

Method

Subjects.   Ten couples were selected from the subject pool, eight of whom had participated in Study 1. Couples were selected for participation only if they had an extension telephone in their home, so that we could interview husbands and wives simultaneously. All participants completed this study.

Procedure. Couples were randomly assigned to either the call group or no-call group, such that there were five in each group. Prior to daily recording, each couple was visited by a research assistant and received detailed instructions on how to complete the form. The entire form was reviewed, and, as a practice exercise, subjects coded the previous 2 days using the instrument and received immediate feedback about their recording. Visits averaged approximately 2.5 hours. The call group received several late-evening telephone calls after the day's forms were completed during the course of the 2-week recording period. All items on the checklist were reviewed, and any disagreements were discussed during these calls and recorded by the interviewer. The no-call group was included so that the effects of the phone-call procedure on concordance could be assessed. This group simply completed the form for 2 weeks.

Results

Six couples reported for 14 days, whereas the remaining four couples reported for 15 days (the latter couples completed the two extra forms we routinely left). During the 288 person-reporting days, 985 experiences were checked or 3.42 per day, and 113 anticipated experiences were noted, or .39 per day. Unlike Study 2, husbands reported considerably more events, 3.93 per day, than wives did about their husbands, 2.91 per day. The overall concordance figure, .34, was only slightly higher than the one obtained in the previous study. The average concordance rate of the call group was higher than that of the no-call group, .39 versus .31, respectively, but this difference was not significant ($t(8) = -.91$).

Of the nonconcordant responses, 65% resulted from the wife not reporting an event recorded by the husband. Surprisingly, though, 35% were due to the wife reporting an event that the husband did not record. The subjects who received telephone calls allowed us to better understand the sources of disagreement.

Couples in the call group received a total of 23 telephone calls, an average of 4.6 per couple. During those 23 days a total of 173 events, 146 actual and 27 anticipated, were checked by husbands and wives; of the actual events, 72 were concordant and 74 were nonconcordant, whereas only 7 anticipated events were concordant and 20 were nonconcordant. Thus, the concordance rate for days on which phone calls were made was 46%. Sources of disagreements, as determined from the interviews, are presented in Table 3.2.

Nine events (12% of the total errors) were coded by both husband and wife, but with different categories. The majority (72%) of events coded only by husbands were those that the wife did not observe. Of the remainder, the wife forgot six events (13%) and judged another six as too minor to be coded. Of the events coded only by wives, five (38%) were viewed by the husbands as too minor to code. In three instances (23%), the husband had forgotten the event and in another three, the husband was unaware of the event's occurrence. (In these latter cases, typically found in the Family and Friends section, the wife had presumed

TABLE 3.2
Sources of Nonconcordance*

A. Both husband and wife coded the experience but used different categories - N = 9.
B. Target (husband) coded experience, wife did not

Reason for disagreement	N of occurrences
Forgot	6
Unaware of event	33
Thought it too minor to code	6
Other	1

C. Wife (observer) coded experience, husband did not

Reason for disagreement	N of occurrences
Forgot	3
Unaware of event	3
Thought it too minor to code	5
Thought it was not codeable	1
Other	1

*The errors do not sum to 74 because of instances where husband and wife differed in coding an experience as one event or as several.

that the husband was aware of some occurrence such as a child's special achievement.)

Discussion

The revised forms and more detailed training did produce a slight, but nonsignificant, increase in the overall concordance figure. More importantly, however, the data from the telephone call revealed that many instances of discordance were not actually "errors." The observer was often unaware of many husband-reported events. And in some instances, the husband had forgotten an event reported by the wife. These two categories comprised about half the discordant responses of the group that received telephone calls. Recalculating an overall concordance figure, with these categories not counted as disagreements, yields a value of 67%.

These data provide support for our original position that concordance should be viewed as conceptually distinct from standard measures of reliability. The telephone calls revealed that most of the reporting disagreements, at least during the days we sampled, came about because the observer had less information than the target concerning the target's daily activities. Nonetheless, there was room for recording improvement as evidenced by the occasional use of different categories for recording the same event and by the times the target did not record events that had occurred yet were recorded by the observer.

FINAL REVISION

Based on the comments solicited from participants in this study, two additional items were added to the checklist: hobbies, readings, letter writing, and daily routine getting to you. Table 3.3 presents the final version of ADE including major and minor outline headings, the experiences themselves, and any parenthetical elaborations or clarifications of the experiences.

A major change in the way the form is completed grew out of the data from the previous study. In an effort to increase the form's validity, the daily recording procedure was modified to incorporate observers' knowledge into targets' report of their daily experiences.[1] Having an additional source of information would approach the ideal situation in which all people who had any contact during the day with the target would also record his/her experiences. This is, we believe, what is usually meant by declaring that something is objective; namely, that it meets some agreed-upon consensual criterion.

The ADE's procedure now includes three steps. In the first, target and observer work separately filling out a section of the checklist called the "workspace." The target checks those items that occurred throughout the day or that were anticipated as happening in the near future. The observer completes the form in the same way, although about the target. Question marks and other notations may also be used in this step, as these are only the first impressions. In the second step, target and observer discuss all the items they marked in the previous step with the goal of coming to some mutually agreed-upon set of experiences representing the target's day. Given the target's more intimate knowledge of the experiences, disagreements are resolved by the target. The set of experiences produced in this step are recorded in either occurred or anticipated boxes on both target's and observer's ADEs. In the last step, target and observer work separately rating the checked experiences on the four dimensions.

The first and second steps are intended to maximize accurate characterization of the target's daily experience. By having participants independently arrive at an approximation of the target's day, the procedure avoids a situation in which either the target or observer may become too dominant. Thus, ADE's experience assessment becomes more objective as it is based on the reports of two people. On the other hand, perception of experience qualities are rated separately, as here we are interested in the more personal, psychological impact of events, and this demands subjectively.

We have recently completed a major study using this revised procedure. Couples were to complete ADE, the Nowlis Mood Adjective Checklist, and a

---

[1]ADE could, of course, be used without gathering data from observers, as the results of Study 3 indicate that the target's reports are generally accurate. However, the multiple recording procedure does appear to offer some incremental validity.

TABLE 3.3

Major headings, secondary headings and items appearing on ADE

MAJOR HEADING	SECONDARY HEADING		EXPERIENCE	ELABORATION
Work Related Activities	Concerning boss, supervisor, upper management, etc.	(1)	Praised for a job well done	a specific task or job, or general
		(2)	Criticized for inadequate work, lateness, etc.	
	Concerning co-workers, employees, and/or clients	(3)	Employees not working well	
		(4)	Emotional interactions with co-workers, employees, clients	arguments, personality conflicts, pleasant interactions
		(5)	Firing or disciplining (by Target)	
		(6)	Socializing with staff, co-workers, clients	lunch, work parties, etc.
	General happenings concerning target at work	(7)	Promotion, raise	
		(8)	Fired, quit, resigned	
		(9)	Some change in job	
		(10)	Under a lot of pressure at work	deadlines, close scrutiny by boss, extra work, etc.
Leisure Activities	Physical	(11)	Done alone, primarily non-competitive	jogging, joga, etc.
		(12)	Social leisure activities primarily competitive	tennis, bowling, etc.
	Non-physical activities	(13)	Out alone	movies by oneself, bar, etc.
		(14)	Dining or entertaining at home or out	
		(15)	Club or group meeting	Elks, community group, etc.
		(16)	Out with friends	bar, dance, get together, play, concert, movie
	Vacation	(17)	Spent at home	
		(18)	Spent away from home	
	Outings	(19)	Beach, park, picnic, fishing, museums, auto show, ball games, etc.	

Personal	(20) Self improvement	high school or college courses, craft classes, etc.
	(21) Hobbies, reading, letter writing	
Financial Activities	(22) Loans	
	(23) Investing	
	(24) Major selling	car, boat, house, etc.
	(25) Major buying	car, boat, house, etc.
	(26) Inheritance or windfall	
	(27) Financial problems	trouble making ends meet
Family and Friend Activities	(28) Close interaction with spouse	special sharing, etc.
	(29) Sexual interaction	within last 24 hours
	(30) Not getting along well with spouse	but no specific argument or problem
	(31) Arguments or reprimands from spouse	
	(32) Praise from spouse	
	(33) Spouse away	business, vacation, etc.
	(34) Pregnancy or birth in family	daily reaction
Concerning children	(35) Disciplinary problems	children fighting among themselves or peers
	(36) Children getting along well together or with peers	
	(37) Children have some special achievement	Academic, athletic, etc.
	(38) Children have disappointment or failure	
	(39) Problems at school	
	(40) Children away from home	at relatives, camp, etc.
	(41) You are getting along well with children	
	(42) Children sick or injured	

(continued)

TABLE 3.3 (*Continued*)

Major headings, secondary headings and items appearing on ADE

MAJOR HEADING	SECONDARY HEADING	EXPERIENCE	ELABORATION
	Concerning relatives	(43) General contact with relatives	telephone calls, etc.
		(44) Relatives sick or death of relative	
		(45) Visit with relatives	
		(46) Problems getting along with relatives	
	Concerning friends and neighbors	(47) Death of friend, neighbor or acquaintance	
		(48) Helping a friend, neighbor or acquaintance	
		(49) Problems with friend, neighbor or acquaintance	
		(50) Especially good interactions with friend, neighbor or acquaintance	
	Family duties	(51) General housework	painting, gardening, cleaning, putting in storm windows, etc.
		(52) Other family-related duties away from home	special shopping, errands, servicing car, dry cleaning, etc.

Other Activities and Happenings	Concerning target		
		(53) Not meeting up to self-expectations	not a previously checked item
		(54) Accomplishing goals or meeting self-expectations	not a previously checked item
		(55) Minor personal problem or frustration	burned breakfast, scratch on car, etc.
		(56) Major personal problem or frustration, but not a previously checked item	auto accident, law suit, etc.
		(57) Illness or injury to self	
		(58) Visit to health care worker for bodily complaint	
		(59) Visit to health care worker for psychological complaint	including pastoral advice, etc.
		(60) Weather getting to you	
		(61) Daily routine getting to you	e.g., work, household, social
		(62) Traveling problems	unusual traffic, ticket, missed plane, etc.
		(63) Witnessed something unusual	hold-up, etc.

TABLE 3.4
Means, Standard Deviations, and Ns of Ratings Dimensions for Each Event

	Desirable Undesirable			Changing Stabilizing			Meaningfulness			Control		
	M	sd	N	M	sd	N	M	sd	N	M	sd	N
WORK RELATED ACTIVITIES												
Concerning Boss, Supervisor, Upper Management, Etc.												
1. Praised for a job well done	4.5	1.4	243	7.8	2.3	188	5.0	1.7	224	3.0	1.1	237
2. Criticized for inadequate work, lateness, etc.	11.1	1.4	51	5.9	1.4	34	5.6	1.3	45	3.6	1.0	52
3. Employees not working well	10.4	1.9	85	5.4	1.4	54	4.7	1.2	72	3.9	.9	86
4. Emotional interactions with	6.2	2.3	775	7.3	2.3	469	5.3	1.4	689	3.0	.9	778
5. Firing or disciplining (by T)	9.1	2.1	17	6.4	2.0	9	5.7	1.2	15	1.8	.9	17
6. Socializing with staff, co-workers, clients	5.8	1.3	700	7.5	1.8	382	6.0	1.2	616	2.6	.9	700
General Happenings Concerning Target at Work												
7. Promotion, raise	3.1	1.4	17	7.4	2.7	16	4.3	1.6	17	2.5	1.0	17
8. Fired, quit, resigned	7.0	2.0	3	3.7	2.9	3	2.7	.6	3	2.3	1.5	3
9. Some change in job	5.9	2.5	209	6.1	2.0	178	5.1	1.7	159	3.1	1.1	211
10. Under a lot of pressure at work	8.9	2.1	541	6.1	1.4	309	5.6	1.4	403	3.6	1.1	542
LEISURE ACTIVITIES												
Physical												
11. Done alone, primarily non-competitive	4.5	1.4	599	8.4	1.7	471	4.7	1.5	556	1.3	.7	601
12. Social leisure activities, primarily competitive	4.2	1.5	350	8.4	2.4	261	4.7	1.4	307	2.1	.9	349
Non-Physical												
13. Out alone	5.1	2.6	47	7.6	2.5	21	4.5	1.9	39	2.1	1.3	48
14. Dining or entertaining at home or out	4.4	1.5	867	8.3	2.4	537	4.7	1.5	787	2.7	1.0	869

#	Activity												
15.	Club or group meeting	4.5	1.4	201	9.5	2.2	163	4.5	1.3	187	3.1	1.0	200
16.	Out with friends	4.4	1.5	389	8.1	2.5	271	4.8	1.5	352	2.6	.9	388
	Vacation												
17.	Spent at home	4.4	1.6	241	9.1	2.5	145	4.1	1.5	158	1.9	1.1	242
18.	Spent away from home	3.4	2.0	169	7.4	4.0	145	3.5	1.8	156	2.2	.9	168
	Outings												
19.	Beach, park, picnic, fishing, museums, auto show, ball game, etc.	4.1	1.7	195	8.3	2.9	137	4.3	1.7	167	2.3	1.0	196
	Personal												
20.	Self improvement	5.3	1.9	195	7.7	2.3	168	5.2	1.5	183	2.5	1.2	194
21.	Hobbies, reading, letter writing	5.1	1.5	1256	8.6	1.6	945	5.3	1.5	1073	1.7	.9	1258
	FINANCIAL ACTIVITIES												
22.	Loans	6.6	3.5	28	6.9	3.2	20	3.9	1.6	24	2.9	1.4	30
23.	Investing	5.6	1.3	51	6.9	1.5	16	5.4	1.5	20	1.3	.6	63
24.	Major selling	3.9	1.4	12	6.3	2.2	9	5.6	1.0	10	1.8	.6	12
25.	Major buying	5.1	2.1	52	6.4	3.1	38	4.8	1.9	38	2.5	1.0	51
26.	Inheritance or windfall	3.1	1.8	17	6.3	3.6	18	3.5	2.0	16	3.3	1.4	17
27.	Financial problems	10.1	2.0	132	6.2	1.2	116	5.5	1.6	112	3.8	.9	131
	FAMILY AND FRIEND ACTIVITIES												
	Concerning Target and Spouse												
28.	Close interaction with spouse	3.8	1.5	2137	9.1	2.5	1807	3.9	1.4	2125	2.7	.8	2118
29.	Sexual interaction	2.9	1.3	777	9.4	3.1	584	3.2	1.4	744	2.3	.8	765
30.	Not getting along well with spouse	10.6	2.0	164	5.4	1.9	122	4.5	1.7	139	3.5	.8	161
31.	Arguments or reprimands from spouse	10.4	2.0	310	5.7	1.8	218	5.0	1.7	250	3.4	.9	303
32.	Praise from spouse	3.9	1.2	349	9.4	2.0	284	4.2	1.3	343	3.7	1.2	336
33.	Spouse away	7.2	3.3	67	7.8	2.8	58	4.4	1.7	62	3.4	1.1	66
34.	Pregnancy or birth in family (daily reaction)	4.8	1.7	84	6.7	3.2	84	3.3	1.3	84	4.3	.8	78

(continued)

TABLE 3.4 (Continued)

	Desirable Undesirable			Changing Stabilizing			Meaningfulness			Control		
	M	sd	N	M	sd	N	M	sd	N	M	sd	N
Concerning Children												
35. Disciplinary problems	10.0	1.8	201	5.9	1.5	133	5.1	1.6	145	3.4	1.0	200
36. Children getting along well together or with peers	3.7	1.3	1044	10.0	1.9	861	3.9	1.4	1016	3.8	1.1	991
37. Children have some special achievement	3.9	1.5	248	8.6	2.4	203	4.2	1.6	242	4.3	.9	237
38. Children have disappointment or failure	9.9	1.6	59	6.4	1.5	38	5.2	1.7	47	4.3	.9	60
39. Problems at school	9.9	1.7	39	5.9	1.9	27	5.2	1.6	29	4.3	1.0	38
40. Children away from home	5.8	2.2	231	8.0	2.5	181	4.6	2.0	212	2.5	1.3	231
41. You are getting along well with children	3.7	1.4	1641	9.8	2.5	1384	3.8	1.4	1632	2.8	.8	1635
42. Children sick or injured	10.0	2.2	215	6.5	1.8	125	4.8	1.6	132	4.8	.5	198
Concerning Relatives												
43. General contact with relatives	5.5	1.8	1034	8.2	2.0	626	5.0	1.5	904	3.0	1.4	1054
44. Relatives sick or death of relative	10.0	3.3	269	5.3	1.5	239	5.0	1.4	248	4.2	1.0	258
45. Visit with relatives	5.0	1.6	685	7.9	2.4	505	4.9	1.5	615	2.8	1.1	686
46. Problems getting along with relatives	10.8	2.0	33	5.6	2.2	23	4.7	1.6	30	3.7	1.1	33
Concerning Friends and Neighbors												
47. Death of friend, neighbor or acquaintance	11.4	1.9	23	6.2	1.1	11	4.7	1.7	19	5.0	.0	20
48. Helping a friend, neighbor or acquaintance	5.3	1.5	270	8.7	2.0	174	5.1	1.3	242	2.5	1.0	280
49. Problems with friend, neighbor or acquaintance	10.8	2.0	22	5.8	1.7	12	4.9	1.6	14	3.7	1.6	19
50. Especially good interactions with friend, neighbor or acquaintance	4.3	1.3	578	8.6	2.5	445	4.6	1.4	561	2.7	.9	579

Family Duties													
51. General Housework	6.4	1.9	1148	8.0	2.0	666	5.5	1.4	825	2.0	1.1	1206
52. Other family-related duties away from home	6.4	1.8	1117	8.1	1.9	614	5.6	1.4	829	2.2	1.0	1202
OTHER ACTIVITIES AND HAPPENINGS												
Concerning Target												
53. Not meeting up to self-expectations, but not a previously checked item	10.9	2.3	95	6.2	1.3	69	4.8	1.6	91	2.7	1.1	95
54. Accomplishing goals or meeting self-expectations	4.4	1.6	415	8.6	2.6	380	4.6	1.5	399	2.5	1.1	415
55. Minor personal problem, or frustration	10.0	2.1	297	6.0	1.4	188	5.2	1.6	201	3.8	1.1	299
56. Major personal problem, but not a previously checked item	11.4	2.1	57	4.9	2.7	50	3.6	1.6	49	4.3	1.1	56
57. Illness or injury to yourself	11.4	2.0	121	4.7	2.0	80	3.8	2.1	70	4.2	1.3	117
58. Visit to health care worker for bodily complaint	7.3	3.6	33	6.1	2.7	28	4.1	1.3	29	2.2	1.4	36
59. Visit to health care worker for psychological complaint	5.4	1.5	19	6.4	1.8	19	5.4	1.2	19	3.4	1.0	19
60. Weather getting to you	10.5	1.8	262	5.5	1.7	161	5.6	1.5	138	4.6	.7	253
61. Daily routine getting to you	9.9	1.9	137	5.3	1.3	63	4.9	1.4	77	4.0	1.0	132
62. Traveling problems	10.1	2.2	148	5.4	1.6	70	5.6	1.5	92	4.5	.8	145
63. Witnessed something unusual	8.6	3.4	34	6.9	2.0	21	5.0	1.6	33	4.5	.9	39
64. Write In	5.6	3.2	364	7.9	3.2	308	4.4	1.5	315	2.7	1.6	361
65. Write In	4.6	3.2	31	7.9	3.2	26	3.6	1.1	28	2.7	1.4	29
66. Write In	3.8	1.6	6	5.5	3.1	4	4.2	1.8	6	3.8	1.9	4

Note: For the bipolar scales, desirable/undesirable and changing/stablizing, the left hand concept (desirable or changing) was modified as follows: 1 = immeasurably, 2 = extremely, 3 = quite, 4 = very, 5 = moderately, 6 = somewhat, and 7 = slightly; and the right hand concept (undesirable or stablizing) was modified as follows: 8 = slightly, 9 = somewhat, 10 = moderately, 11 = very, 12 = quite, 13 = extremely, and 14 = immeasurably. Meaningfulness was modified by adjectives 1 through 7. Control had a different set of adjectives: 1 = complete, 2 = quite a lot, 3 = some, 4 = slight, and 5 = none.

checklist of daily physical symptoms and conditions for 90 consecutive days. Although we are now only in the midst of analyzing the data collected in this study, some information about the utility of ADE in a longer-term investigation can be provided. Seventy-nine couples participated in the training interview. Thirteen declined further participation after the interview. Of the remainder, 16 completed less than 40 days of recording, whereas the other 50 completed an average of 86 days. Thus, over 70% of the subjects who began the study completed a satisfactory number of recording days for analytic purposes. Furthermore, the 90-day recording period did not have a major impact on number of events reported, which was 5.26 per day, a figure comparable to ones we obtained in the brief studies already described. Therefore, the revised ADE does appear suitable for more extensive longitudinal investigations.

In Table 3.4 we present some data on the frequencies and dimensional ratings of the 22,745 events that the 50 subjects marked as actually occurring. There is a large amount of variation in the item frequencies, ranging from a low of 3 for "quit or fired" to a high of over 2000 for "close interaction with spouse." Rating-dimension means represent the average perception the subjects had of each event, whereas the standard deviations indicate the degree of variability of these perceptions. (The table caption describes the meaning of the numbers.) We present this information only to point out the range both in the mean ratings and in the variability; there may well be individual differences in these ratings and differences due to the context in which they were made, for example, day of week.

GENERAL DISCUSSION

Based on the data reported in the three studies, we believe that we have developed an instrument that can be used in the prospective, longitudinal study of the relationship between life events and illness. Important features of ADE include the following: (1) The sample of events was based on an empirically generated pool that was then reduced to a manageable number of items. The low frequency of unique write-ins in our study demonstrated that the categories were indeed adequate for the task of allowing participants to record their daily experiences; yet we retain the write-in option for the few times when events cannot be otherwise recorded; (2) the checklist method minimizes the effects of daily fluctuations in mood and health that might seriously contaminate diary methods; (3) subjective reactions to the events are rated on four dimensions (three of them empirically derived), rather than the unidimensional approaches of past efforts. To our knowledge, this is the only life-event instrument that includes ratings of the perception of anticipated events; (4) ratings are obtained from individuals on adjective-anchored 7- or 14- point scales that can be scaled using magnitude production; (5) the form takes only 10–15 minutes to complete, thus reducing the likelihood of substantial attrition in longitudinal studies; (6) the determination of event occurrence is a joint process, wherein the subject is aided in recalling and defining events by a person with some knowledge of their day.

The issue of reliability was addressed by examining target–observer concordance in event reporting. Overall concordance figures were .31 (Study 2) and .34 (Study 3). But our concordance figures are not the same as a traditional interobserver estimate of reliability. As revealed by the telephone-call part of Study 3, a substantial proportion of discordance was due to observers not being aware of events reported by the targets.

Our current procedure, having the forms completed by both target and observer, is designed to maximize the accuracy of the report of a day's events. Several possible sources of error are reduced by having the target and observer first fill out ADE independently and then reconvene to go over each other's checklists. Firstly, in instances of target-alone reports, the target is forced to corroborate the occurrence of those events that the observer was not able to witness. Secondly, in the case of observer-alone reports, the observer's checklist functions as stimulus for the target's recall. Thirdly, the couple is forced to agree on the category in which to code an event, thus minimizing the use of inappropriate categories. Finally, the procedure brings the recordings of both target and observer under each other's scrutiny, which may increase accuracy by minimizing haphazard reporting and simple errors.

Validity was addressed by examining predicted differences in concordance rates and by relating data from ADE to daily reports of mood. As expected, concordance was higher for more meaningful experiences and higher for actual than for anticipated events. Also as anticipated, the number of desirable events was directly related to scores on positive mood scales, and the number of undesirable events was directly related to scores on negative mood scales.

In conducting prospective work, investigators using ADE must continue to be aware of the admonitions of Dohrenwend (1974) about groups of events defined by their possible linkages to psychiatric and somatic states. For example, when studying physical illness, the investigator should be particularly careful not to include items "Illness to self" and "Visit to health-care worker" and must be cautious in interpreting the meaning of any other items that might bring the target in contact with illness (namely, children, wife, or relative sick). Furthermore, we have taken the view that both objective and subjective assessments are important, and these are reflected in the event occurrence and event ratings. However, two items concerning self-expectations and goals were included, because they tap important psychological experiences that are precipitated by "objective" environmental events but are not themselves objective. We recognize that some investigators may not wish to include these items in a purely "environmental score."

We hope that ADE will also prove useful in research areas where daily events are of theoretical significance. Recent work in daily physiological changes has shown that catecholamine and corticosteroid peaks precede illness onset by a few days (Gruchow, 1979; Mason, Buescher, Belfer, Artenstein, & Mougey, 1979). Considering that increases in these substances have been broadly linked to the occurrence of psychosocial stimuli (Mason, 1968; Ursin, Baade, & Levine, 1978), this work suggests that an instrument such as ADE be included to provide a potential predictor of these physiological changes.

With regard to psychiatric dysfunction, current theories of depression (Brown & Harris, 1978; Lewinsohn, 1974; Seligman, 1974) emphasize the relationship among events, perception of events, and depressed mood. These theories can best be evaluated in prospective studies employing an adequate means of assessing daily experience and subjective reactions to it. A major issue here is whether depression is related to the objective occurrence of many undesirable events, or whether people who become depressed have subjectively more intense reactions to events. By comparing data on event occurrence versus event ratings, ADE could address this issue. Similarly, daily experiences (particularly "stressful" ones) are commonly invoked as explanations, either by themselves or in interaction with diatheses, of many forms of psychopathology (Davison & Neale, 1978). But the research on which these claims have been made is seriously flawed, resting principally on retrospectively obtained information. ADE could be particularly valuable in studying vulnerable populations or in following discharged patients to observe the possible association between life events and clinical remission.

ACKNOWLEDGMENTS

The authors thank Susan Hedges, Eileen McKearney, Bruce Reed, and Willo White for their assistance. This research was supported in part by the Office of Naval Research.

REFERENCES

Andrews, G., & Tennant, C. Being upset and becoming ill: An appraisal of the relation between life events and physical illness. *The Medical Journal of Australia*, 1978, *1*, 324–327.

Averill, J. R. Personal control over aversive stimuli and its relationship to stress. *Psychological Bulletin*, 1973, *80*, 286–303.

Barker, R. G., & Wright, H. F. *One boy's day*. New York: Harper & Row, 1951.

Brown, G. W. Meaning, measurement, and stress of life events. In B. S. Dohrenwend & B. P. Dohrenwend (Eds.), *Stressful life events: Their nature and effects*. New York: Wiley, 1974.

Brown, G. W., & Harris, T. *Social origins of depression*. New York: Free Press, 1978.

Brown, G. W., Sklair, F., Harris, T. O., & Birley, J. L. T. Life-events and psychiatric disorders (Part I): Some methodological issues. *Psychological Medicine*, 1973, *3*, 74–87.

Chiriboga, D. A., & Dean, H. Dimensions of stress: Perspectives from a longitudinal study. *Journal of Psychosomatic Research*, 1978, *22*, 47–55.

Cline, D. W., & Chosy, J. J. A prospective study of life changes and subsequent health changes. *Archives of General Psychiatry*, 1972, *27*, 51–53.

Coyne, J. C. Depression and the response of others. *Journal of Abnormal Psychology*, 1976, *82*, 186–193.

Davison, G. C., & Neale, J. M. *Abnormal psychology: An experimental clinical approach* (2nd ed.) New York: Wiley, 1978.

Dohrenwend, B. P. Problems in defining and sampling the relevant population of stressful life events. In B. S. Dohrenwend & B. P. Dohrenwend (Eds.), *Stressful life events: Their nature and effects*. New York: Wiley, 1974.

Dohrenwend, B. S., & Dohrenwend, B. P. Overview and prospects for research on stressful life events. In B. S. Dohrenwend & B. P. Dohrenwend (Eds.), *Stressful life events: Their nature and effects*. New York: Wiley, 1974.

Dohrenwend, B. S., Krasnoff, L., Askenasy, A. R., & Dohrenwend, B. P. Exemplification of a method for scaling life events: The PERI life events scale. *Journal of Health and Social Behavior*, 1978, *19*, 205–229.

Folkman, S., Schaefer, C., & Lazarus, R. S. Cognitive processes as mediators of stress and coping. In V. Hamilton & D. M. Warburton (Eds.), *Human stress and cognition: An information-processing approach*. London: Wiley, 1979.

Gersten, J. C., Langner, T. S., Eisenberg, J. G., & Orzeck, L. Child behavior and life events: Undesirable change or change per se? In B. S. Dohrenwend & B. P. Dohrenwend (Eds.), *Stressful life events: Their nature and effects*. New York: Wiley, 1974.

Gruchow, H. W. Catecholamine activity and infectious disease episodes. *Journal of Human Stress*, 1979, *5*, 11–17.

Holmes, T. S., & Holmes, T. H. Short-term intrusions into the life style routine. *Journal of Psychosomatic Research*, 1970, *14*, 121–132.

Holmes, T. H., & Rahe, R. H. The social readjustment rating scale. *Journal of Psychosomatic Research*, 1967, *11*, 213–218.

Jacobson, N. S. & Moore, D. Spouses as observers of the events in their relationship. *Journal of Consulting and Clinical Psychology*, 1981, *49*, 269–277.

Jenkins, C. D., Hurst, M. W., & Rose, R. M. Life changes. Do people really remember? *Archives of General Psychiatry*, 1979, *36*, 379–384.

Kurstin, I. T. *Theoretical principles of psychosomatic medicine*. New York: Wiley, 1976.

Lazarus, R. S. *Psychological stress and the coping process*. New York: McGraw-Hill, 1966.

Lazarus, R. S., & Cohen, J. B. Environmental stress. In I. Altman & J. F. Wohwill (Eds.), *Human behavior and the environment: Current theory and research*. New York: Plenum Press, 1977.

Lazarus, R. S., Cohen, J. B., Folkman, S., Kanner, A., & Schaefer, C. Psychological stress and adaptation: Some unresolved issues. In H. Selye (Ed.), *Guide to stress research*. New York: Van Nostrand Reinhold, 1979.

Lehman, R. E. Symptom contamination of the schedule of recent events. *Journal of Consulting and Clinical Psychology*, 1978, *46*, 1564–1565.

Lewinsohn, P. M. A behavioral approach to depression. In R. M. Friedman & M. M. Katz (Eds.), *The Psychology of depression: Contemporary theory and research*. Washington, D. C.: Winston-Wiley, 1974.

Lewinsohn, P. M. *The Unpleasant Events Schedule*. University of Oregon, 1975 (Mimeo).

Lewinsohn, P. M., & Libet, J. Pleasant events, activity schedules, and depressions. *Journal of Abnormal Psychology*, 1972, *79*, 291–295.

Lewinsohn, P. M., & Graf, M. Pleasant activities and depression. *Journal of Consulting and Clinical Psychology*, 1973, *41*, 261–268.

MacPhillamy, D., & Lewinsohn, P. M. *The Pleasant Events Schedule*. University of Oregon, 1971 (Mimeo).

Mason, J. W. A review of psychoendocrine research on the pituitary-adrenal cortical system. *Psychosomatic Medicine*, 1968, *8*, 576–607.

Mason, J. W., Buescher, E. L., Belfer, M. L., Artenstein, M., & Mougey, E. H. A prospective study of corticosteroid and catecholamine levels in relation to viral respiratory illness. *Journal of Human Stress*, 1979, *5*, 18-28.

Miller, F. T., Bentz, W. K., Aponte, J. F., & Brogan, D. R. Perception of life crisis events: A comparative study of rural and urban samples. In B. S. Dohrenwend & B. P. Dohrenwend (Eds.), *Stressful life events: Their nature and effects*. New York: Wiley, 1974.

Nelson, R. O. Methodological issues in assessment via self-monitoring. In J. D. Cone & R. P. Hawkins (Eds.), *Behavioral assessment: New directions in clinical psychology*. New York: Brunner-Mazel, 1977.

Nowlis, V. Research with the mood adjective checklist. In S. S. Tompkins & C. E. Izard (Eds.), *Affect, cognition, and personality*. New York: Springer, 1965.

Paykel, E. S. Life stress and psychiatric disorder: Applications of the clinical approach. In B. S. Dohrenwend & B. P. Dohrenwend (Eds.), *Stressful life events: Their nature and effects*. New York: Wiley, 1974.

Paykel, E. S. Contribution of life events to causation of psychiatric illness. *Psychological Medicine*, 1978, *8*, 245-253.

Rabkin, J. G., & Struening, E. L. Life events, stress, and illness. *Science*, 1976, *194*, 1013-1020.

Rahe, R. H. The pathway between subjects' recent life changes and their near-future illness reports: Representative results and methodological issues. In B. S. Dohrenwend & B. P. Dohrenwend (Eds.), *Stressful life events: Their nature and effects*. New York: Wiley, 1974.

Redfield, J., & Stone, A. Individual viewpoints of stressful life events. *Journal of Consulting and Clinical Psychology*, 1979, *47*, 147-154.

Rehm, L. P. Mood, pleasant events, and unpleasant events: Two pilot studies. *Journal of Consulting and Clinical Psychology*, 1978, *46*, 854-859.

Roghmann, K. J., & Haggerty, R. J. Daily stress, illness, and use of health services in young families. *Pediatric Research*, 1973, *7*, 520-526.

Sarason, I. G., Johnson, J. H., & Siegel, J. M. Assessing the impact of life changes: Development of the life experiences survey. *Journal of Consulting and Clinical Psychology*, 1978, *46*, 932-946.

Seligman, M. E. P. Depression and learned helplessness. In R. J. Friedman & M. M. Katz (Eds.), *The psychology of depression: Contemporary theory and research*. Washington, D. C.: Winston-Wiley, 1974.

Selye, H. *The stress of life*. New York: McGraw-Hill, 1956.

Stevens, S. S. *Psychophysics: Introduction of its perceptual, neural and social prospects*. New York: Wiley, 1974.

Stone, A. A. *The objectivity and subjectivity of life events. Journal of Clinical Psychology*, in press.

Stone, A. A. The association between perceptions of daily experiences and self- and spouse-rated mood. *Journal of Research in Personality*, 1981.

Stone, A. A., & Neale, J. M. Life event scales: Psychophysical training and rating dimension effects on event weighting coefficients. *Journal of Consulting and Clinical Psychology*, 1978, *46*, 849-853.

Stone, A. A., & Neale, J. M. Hypochondriasis and tendency to adopt the sick role as moderators of the relationship between life-events and somatic symptomatology. *British Journal of Medical Psychology*, 1981, *54*, 75-81.

Theorell, T. Life events before and after the onset of a premature myocardial infarction. In B. S. Dohrenwend & B. P. Dohrenwend (Eds.), *Stressful life events: Their nature and effects*. New York: Wiley, 1974.

Ursin, H., Baade, E., & Levine, S. *Psychology of stress: A study of coping men*. New York: Academic Press, 1978.

Uhlenhuth, E., Balter, M., Lipman, R. S., & Haberman, S. J. Remembering life events. In J. S. Strauss, H. M. Babigian, & M. Roff (Eds), *The origins and course of psychopathology: Methods of longitudinal research.* New York: Plenum, 1977.

Vinokur, A., & Selzer, M. L. Desirable versus undesirable life events: The relationship to stress and mental distress. *Journal of Personality and Social Psychology,* 1975, *32,* 329-337.

Wershow, H. J., & Reinhart, G. Life change and hospitalization-A heretical view. *Journal of Psychosomatic Research,* 1974, *18,* 393-401.

Wills, T. A., Weiss, R. L., & Patterson, G. R. A behavioral analysis of the determinants of marital satisfaction. *Journal of Consulting and Clinical Psychology,* 1974, *42,* 802-811.

Wolff, H. G., Wolf, S., & Hare, C. C. *Life stress and bodily disease.* Baltimore, Md.: Williams & Wilkins, 1950.

4

Feelings of Threat and Private Views of Illness: Factors in Dehumanization in the Medical Care System

Howard Leventhal, David R. Nerenz, Elaine Leventhal
University of Wisconsin–Madison

The atrocities of World War II, particularly the barbarisms that took place in Nazi concentration camps, raised profound questions with respect to the moral and social control of behavior. What factors produced an environment in which guards arbitrarily confined human beings to pens, deprived them of their clothes and control of excretory function, and played with and destroyed life in capricious games of chance (Bettleheim, 1943; Cohen, 1953)? How did prisoners respond to these deprivations: the removal of control, the absence of attention to and concern with their physical needs and emotional response to their environments? How did they respond to the removal of traditional social support networks?

Observers of these horrors too readily ascribed them to attributes of the perpetrators, such as national character or personality. But revelations about Chinese prisoner of war camps (Lifton, 1961; Schein, 1956), Russian gulags (Solzhenitsyn, 1974), and reigns of terror and destruction in Vietnam, Cambodia, Jamestown, Guyana, and Iran make clear that the Nazi atrocities were not unique to the German character or to advanced, decadent industrialized society. The presence of an authority giving orders, the willingness to accept commands, and a belief in the justness of the orders interact in generating these behaviors (Milgram, 1974). Indeed, it appears that dehumanizing behaviors, albeit in less extreme form, also appear in settings supposedly designed to promote people's welfare. Medical-care institutions are one such example; many articles have been written expressing concern about the occurrence of dehumanizing expreiences in these settings (Howard & Strauss, 1975; Leventhal, 1975; Reiser, 1978; Snow, 1973). If dehumanization can occur in supposedly benign as well as blatantly malevolent institutions, it seems worthwhile to raise the following two questions:

(1) "What processes are at work when people experience dehumanization, and what are the basic features of the experience?"; and (2) "How do environments lead people to act as dehumanizing agents when they do not intend to do so?." We address these questions using observations from medical-care settings, though we draw on data from other sources as well.

WHAT IS DEHUMANIZATION?

We can experience considerable difficulty when trying to define terms such as dehumanization, control, self, and emotion. These concepts lable fuzzy sets defined by multiple and substitutable criteria with vague boundaries (Oden & Massaro, 1978). Some definition of dehumanization is essential, however, to bring the content or substance of our task into focus. The dictionary provides two points of departure: "(1) To deprive of human qualities or attributes; (2) To render mechanical and routine" (Morris, 1969). Both components of the definition emphasize a process: Something is happening to or being done to a human being. There is an active agent doing the dehumanizing, and there is a target person who presumably feels dehumanized. Labeling an act or an environment as dehumanizing must be based either on characterisitcs of the act or in the response of the target person. The two kinds of criteria for labeling need not be congruent: Acts that would be labeled as dehumanizing by outside observers may not produce such feelings in a target person, and people may feel dehumanized in situations where neither observers nor active agent would have predicted (or intended) that feeling. Both criteria can be used to identify dehumanizing experiences. Either an actor or an abserver can identify when a "deprivation of human qualities or attributes" has taken place. But what human qualities must be destroyed in order to feel dehumanization? We believe that depends in part on the nature of the specific situation, the expectations seen to be appropriate for that environment, and whether and how these expectations are blocked. Because the focus of this chapter is on the medical-care system, we concentrate on three areas of human concern that are related to dehumanization in that system: (1) actual or threatened changes to physical appearance and competence; (2) the inability to make decisions or to act on the basis of one's interpretations and feelings (i.e., loss of control); and (3) inattention, deliberate or unintended, to the individual's inner, psychological life.

Conditions for Dehumanization

Potential or Actual Physical Change.   Breast loss in the female cancer patient (Ringler, 1981; Weisman, 1976), loss of control of excretory functions in colon cancer, and pain and tiredness in patients undergoing cancer chemotherapy (Nerenz, 1979) destroy and mutilate the body, result in loss of body functions, disrupt economic and social roles, and threaten death. They also stimulate fears of social and sexual rejections, fears that are frequently realistic. These threatened or actual alterations of the self represent fundamental changes in the human condition. However, change alone is not sufficient to produce feelings of dehumanization. Dehumanization appears to arise as one reflects upon or observes these changes; it is an interpretation, an imposition of meaning on objective change.

Loss of Control.   Medical treatment often involves extensive loss of control over the details of daily life. Hospitalized patients who are capable of walking may be taken to their rooms in a wheelchair. They find their clothes replaced with strange hospital gowns. Their time of waking is controlled by nurses making rounds with medications. Their time of eating is regulated by others. Treatment is carried out by strangers: An unkonwn anesthesiologist may put them to sleep and an unknown surgeon cut their bodies to remove and/or repair internal damage.

Experiences in an outpatient clinic may be less dramatic but also entail some loss of control. Can a patient feel in control of his/her treatment when he/she does not understand the bulk of what is said (Ley, 1977)? Can a patient feel in control when he/she does not understand the nature of his/her disorder or the rationale for treatment (Leventhal, Meyer, & Nerenz, 1980)? Can individuals perceive themselves in control when instructed to perform behaviors (quitting smoking, losing weight) that they do not desire to do and that they have failed to do on past attempts?

Lack of understanding, lack of skills, absence of adequate social supports, and unrealistic expectations of cure all set limits on the degree to which the individual feels able to control his or her fate. These feelings are likely to be a regular part of medical-care experiences, unless the individual has an unusual level of understanding and behavioral preparation for dealing with difficult settings.

Inattention to Inner Psychological Life.   In the past decade, numerous articles have commented on the tendency of physicians to focus on the measurable, technical, and disease component of the patient and to ignore the patient's subjective or personal view of the illness. It is no surprise that practitioners, particularly physicians, ignore the inner life. Medical training focuses on the biochemistry, physiology, and anatomy of the body. Enormous amounts of technical information and prescriptive rules must be learned in a short time. There is little time for supplemental reading. Indeed, patients appear to want the technically proficient and perfect physician; they fear less. Yet they may complain bitterly when that is all they receive.

They physician lacks the necessary theoretical training to sensitize him or herself to ways in which communications may be misunderstood and lead to counterproductive behaviors. Moreover, physicians may omit important details in prescribing treatment routines, be inconsistent in their recommendations about treatment, fail to monitor patient understanding and patient compliance with prescriptions, and neither correct incorrect reactions nor reward correct ones (Svarstad, 1976).

Inattention to patient interpretations, skills, and feelings is not solely the fault of the physician. Patients may fail to communicate when asked. They expect the doctor to discover the problem and provide miraculous cures without participation or effort on their part. They may refuse to disclose information because they fear criticism or anticipate ridicule for holding foolish ideas (Meyer, Leventhal, & Gutmann, in press). Communication may be disrupted because patients do not know what to report. They have so much information, much of it novel, that they may be unable to distinguish the relevant from the irrelevant or to describe their experience, be unsure whom to inform, be embarrassed by what they wish to say, and be distressed by their uncertainty and insecurity (Leventhal, 1975).

The Experience of Dehumanization

Our brief discussion of the three basic kinds of events leading to dehumanization in medical settings did not address the subjective aspect of dehumanization because it will differ across situations. However, there are eight relatively distinct aspects of the subjective experience that we have distilled from previous work in the area as well as from our own recent research.

1. Separation of the Physical and Psychological Self.   The fact of illness and the appearance of bodily sensations and symptoms focus attention on the self and lead to the experience of the self as a physical object or thing. Leventhal (1975) has said: "In extreme cases a patient seems to report a complete separation of the conscious psychological self from the physical self [p. 121]." This experience seems to be the basis for depersonalization: a subjective state that may be important for, but is not identical to, that of dehumanization.

2. Alteration and Loss of Parts of the Physical Self.   Illness poses the threat of actual or imagined losses of parts of the physical self, making one feel "less complete," less one's self, and less human. The magnitude of feared change may greatly exceed the realistic threat. Nevertheless, behavior is affected by anticipations and fears.

3. Emotional Distress, Hopelessness, and Despair.   Negative emotions, such as fear, terror, and depression, and the experience of pain and distress are common components of a dehumanizing experience. These emotions are provoked by injury, pain, and threat of harm and death; they feed back into and alter the perception of the eliciting conditions. Emotional arousal can intensify pain experiences (Beecher, 1959; Leventhal & Everhart, 1979; Sternbach, 1974), enhance the perceived magnitude of threat (Johnson, 1975; Leventhal et al., 1980; Nisbett & Schachter, 1966), and stimulate feelings of hopelessness and inability to cope (Abramson, 1980). Because negative emotions can intensify pain and exacerbate perceived threat, they can be seen as "evidence" that one is unable to manage life situations (Bandura, 1977; Rosen, Terry, & Leventhal, in press).

4. Perceived Strangeness of the Environment. The novelty of the medical-care settings (i.e., the presence of equipment that has a complex and frightening appearance, the intrusion of unknown persons, both staff and patient) fosters a sense of strangeness that may increase feelings of threat and vulnerability and stimulate fear (Janis, 1951, 1958; Jarvinen, 1955; Urrutia, 1975; Weiss, 1972). That unknown people have access to one's body and personal functions can enhance the sense of strangeness and lack of control over one's immediate environment, as well as introduce a sense of breakdown of personal privacy and integrity.

5. Uncertainty and Cyclic Thought. Confusion as to how one is to behave will appear when an individual encounters internal (e.g., pains and other symptoms) and external events (e.g., diagnostic tests, strange persons, and new clothes) that are novel, inadequately labeled, and poorly understood. Indeed, patients have a need to know what causes an event, when it will occur, what its outcome will be, and what effect their reactions will have on it. Without this information, they may become uncertain about whether their experience is valid (i.e., external and verifiable by others) or purely subjective. Repetitive reviewing and rehearsal of mental images and coping intentions are likely to accompany these states (Horowitz, 1970).

6. Sense of Isolation. The isolation of one's conscious, psychological self from other conscious, psychological selves seems to be a major factor in the experience of dehumanization. The feeling appears to arise from the practitioner's inattention to an individual patient's interpretations and feelings about his/her condition: The practitioner is focused on the illness, the diseased organ, not on the patient's belief about the organ, or his/her private beliefs about his/her symptoms.

But focusing on the patients as a collection of physical and physiological processes is only one part of the sense of isolation. Another is the strangeness and incomprehensibility of the language used by practitioners (Ley, 1977). Practitioners may pronounce diagnoses and prescriptions for behavior in abbreviated, technical language, leaving patients very much aware of their ignorance and separateness.

7. Sense of Inability to Communicate. Isolation, the uncertainty about body symptoms, or the novelty of the setting may combine to generate a strong sense that one cannot communicate ideas or feelings to others. The experience of barriers to communication rests on both cognitive and motivational grounds. Cognitive factors may be important when we see individuals unable to categorize and describe their experience. The complexity of internal physical sensations and the endless cycle of self-stimulating fantasies and fluctuating shades of negative emotion may well defy description. In addition, the strangeness and apparent abnormality of these experiences may provoke anxiety about one's mental stability. It may lead to guarded and defensive behavior to avoid the criticism and negative self-appraisal that are expected to follow the expression of such thoughts and feelings. Motivational barriers may also be based on the conviction that others are totally disinterested in one's peculiar mental states.

8. Planlessness and Loss of Competency. We see at least four major ways in which medical care can induce a sense of planlessness and loss of competency. First, the illness may diminish one's physical competency; one is less complete and no longer able to perform particular tasks. Second, the illness may threaten or diminish one's ability to fulfill a variety of work and social roles. Third, the illness may threaten or reduce one's ability to control basic body functions (e.g., urination or defecation may no longer be voluntary acts). Finally, the technical demands of treating illness and the effort required for rehabilitation from illness may exceed the patient's actual or perceived competence.

The sense of incompetence and loss of control can also be generated by the role changes demanded of the patient in the medical-care system. To become a patient (i.e., to step out of ongoing life roles and be hospitalized) has been conceptualized as a shift from everyday social roles to sick-role behavior (Mechanic, 1972; Parsons, 1975). This change may be comforting to some but it is distressing to most. The shift back to self-regulation demanded when the individual enters a rehabilitation program or is discharged requires another difficult change in self-concept.

Unfortunately, there is no empirical evidence to determine whether this list of eight attributes gives an exhaustive description of dehumanization; there may be more, there may be fewer attributes than those listed. Moreover, the degree to which the eight are interrelated is unknown. Whether empirically correlated or not, we believe these features of dehumanized experience can be identified and can be varied, either singly or in combinations, by selectively changing environmental circumstances. However, whereas factors from one or more of the three categories (threat to physical self, loss of control, and inattention) may be necessary to provoke features of dehumanizing experience, we do not believe they are sufficient to create that subjective state. Something must be added to the mix.

The Moral Context for Humanizing and Dehumanizing Interactions

For physical change, loss of control, and inattention to inner pyschological life to generate feelings of dehumanization, the cultural and moral context in which they occur must define their *opposites* as crucial components of humaneness. Threats of or actual experience of physical injury can be experienced as exciting and glorifying in a cultural context that makes human life subservient to the external goals of sports or politics. In a culture where subservience is taught from childhood and obedience is an important part of self-definition, loss of control is unlikely to generate feelings of dehumanization. Where inner events are universally agreed to be private and of concern only to the individual, inattention by doctors to idiosyncratic interpretations and subjective feelings are unlikely to generate feelings of dehumanization. In short, where the cultural morality defines physical risk, loss of control, and inattention to psychological states as necessary conditions for sensible integration into the matrix of social and cultural life, reflection on one's human condition is unlikely to generate perceptions and feelings of dehumanization (Antonovsky, 1979).

A point we wish to emphasize is that perceptions and feelings of dehumanization arise from self-reflection (i.e., observing oneself in a particular way at a given point in time in relation to past and future times within a cultural context, Scheier & Carver, 1977). Thus, we are assuming a hierarchical system where the experience of physical loss, of loss of control, or inattention to psychological states is processed at one level, then reflected upon, interpreted, and felt as dehumanizing in relation to another, higher level of processing involving comparison to moral values.

The dehumanization experience is thus a cognitive-emotional complex of component parts (e.g., loss of control, feelings of distress, fear, and anger, and the awareness that these perceptions and affects do not fit a sensible, culturally prescribed definition of self). Not all elements of the experience need to be present in any single episode; fractional experiences of dehumanization are clearly possible. Our recent research has focused on the cognitive processes through which patients understand and cope with medical threats. We feel that study of these processes can provide a deeper understanding of the dehumanization experience and provide fruitful suggestions for intervention.

The next section of our chapter provides a brief discussion of what we have learned about the operation of the processing mechanism from studies in the medical-care setting. After presenting specific characteristics of the processing system, we discuss how they generate dehumanizing outcomes in the medical-care system. We then move on to discuss how both the medical-care system and the culture at large provide environmental supports for dehumanizing behaviors.

THE INFORMATION-PROCESSING SYSTEM AND THE CREATION OF DEHUMANIZING EXPERIENCES

Our view of information processing combines two quite different traditions: one that emphasizes categorization, interpretation, or labeling of events, and a second that emphasizes extracting information from the continually available textural features of the environment—a perspective that is continuous with the traditions of gestalt psychology and the theoretical approach of J. J. Gibson (1966). It is this latter aspect that makes our analytic efforts of particular relevance to the environmental psychologist.

An Overview of the Processing Mechanism

We view patients as active problem solvers. Our model proposes that adjustment (or problem solving) depends on the presence of a set of mediating processes that include at the minimum an image or goal, coping or response skills, and a mechanism for monitoring output against specific evaluative criteria. All three components are essential for the workings of a self-regulatory system. In this respect, our model is similar to feedback models developed by Carver (1979), Kanfer (1977), Lazarus (1966), Miller, Galanter, and Pribram (1960), and others. Our model thus presents three stages in the processing of a health threat: (1) the initial *representation* phase, the way in which the patient develops a personal view of the illness episode; (2) the *planning–action* phase, the way in which the patient develops coping alternatives based on the representation; and (3) an *appraisal* or *feedback* phase, the way in which coping outcomes are evaluated and revised. This stepwise feature is the first, important characteristic of our model.

A second feature of the model is the postulate that separable, parallel processing mechanisms generate objective representations or images of one's health problem and affective reactions to these representations (fear, grief, etc.) (Leventhal, 1970, 1980; Zajonc, 1980). These mechanisms are described as *separable* because operations can be devised to demonstrate their independence, though they typically function together. Their independence, however, allows for the combination of a variety of emotions with otherwise similar objective representations of health threats. Both the reality-oriented image of the health problem and the affective reaction direct subsequent coping behaviors and influence the selection of appraisal criteria and the outcomes of the appraisal processes.

The third major feature of the model is its emphasis on hierarchical processing mechanisms. Feedback or control systems exist at multiple levels. Those at higher levels must include key features of lower-level processes to regulate lower-level functioning (Powers, 1973). Self-reflection, discussed earlier, involves an interaction between processing levels. The synthesis of affective and reality-oriented processing is also likely to be dependent on higher levels directing attention to and integrating perceptions and emotional experiences generated by lower-level systems.

The Representation of the Health Threat

The way a health threat is represented (i.e., the information used and the way it is assembled into a representation of the illness episode) is central to the dehumanization experience. Because the representation is the patient's view of the problem and the basis for coping and appraisal activities, it forms the groundwork for his/her communications about the episode. When this groundwork is ignored, in error, not shared by practitioners, or discrepant with reality (i.e., with the actual mechanisms underlying the illness), patients are likely to experience loss of control, inattention to their inner interpretations and emotional states, and a heightened sense of threat of potential or actual physical loss.

Prior models of health behavior have dealt with illness representations and coping in a decision theory framework (i.e., they postulate that individuals see themselves as vulnerable to an illness of a specific magnitude of severity or threat and as having access to coping responses effective in warding off the threat, Becker & Maiman, 1975; Ben–Sira, 1977a, b; Rogers, 1975; Rosenstock, 1974). These models are normative, and the variables appear to be defined from a shared cultural perspective. Thus, although they provided an adequate basis for the initial exploration of illness behavior, they did not capture the processes involved in the *construction* of the illness representation nor did they capture the details of content that form the basis for generating representations (Leventhal, Safer, & Panagis, in press).

Our perspective begins with the individual's experience of his or her body. The everyday experience of the body forms the familiar texture or ground of the physical self. Departures from these sensory features (i.e., the appearance of sensations or symptoms) attract attention and stimulate processing (Leventhal, 1975; Mechanic, 1972; Pennebaker & Skelton, 1980). Many departures are themselves "familiar" or readily explained in terms of daily life experiences (i.e., the end of day tiredness that is experienced after hard physical labor, Robinson, 1971). Other sensory experiences are given illness labels (e.g., flu, gastric upset from spicy food). Present experience (e.g., information from friends and relations, Safer, Tharps, Jackson, & Leventhal, 1979) and past history or past schemata of illness experience (Leventhal, Meyer, & Nerenz, 1980; Pennebaker & Skelton, 1980) integrate these sensory experiences and illness labels into a representation of the individual's present illness episode. A number of key processes are prominent in this constructive process.

The Representation is Abstract and Concrete. Patients define illness in terms of both abstract concepts (e.g., cancer, heart disease, flu, diabetes) and signs and symptoms (pain, masses, heart beating, warmth and flushing of face, coughing or dizziness). When a person experiences symptoms, he or she seeks to define or label them. When given a label, the patient will seek to define it by finding concrete manifestations or symptoms.

The Representation Includes Perceived Causes and Temporal Expectations. Both hypertensives (Meyer, 1980) and cancer patients (Nerenz, 1979; Ringler, 1981) identify a variety of etiologies and time courses for their disease. The co-occurrence of specific environmental events (e.g., stresses, foods eaten) with symptom onset plays a critical role in generating specific causal attributions, and many attributions occur because culturally established beliefs direct attention to events that are likely to confirm these expectations. For example, if a person is told his blood pressure is elevated and subscribes to a cultural belief that stress causes high blood pressure, his stress model will direct his attention to search for stress episodes prior to his diagnosis.

The temporal features of illness representations are also critical, as every illness and every treatment has a time line. The most common notion of time is the *acute* disease model. The problem (cancer, high blood pressure) is usually attributed to some external, antecedent agent; the symptoms indicate the presence of the disease; the treatment is applied for a finite period of time; and the symptoms and disease disappear in some finite period of time. The majority of hypertensives, either newly discovered at screening sites or new to treatment (51 and 40%, respectively), conceptualize hypertension as an acute disorder (i.e., curable within a finite period of time). And 57.7% of the newly treated patients behaved accordingly by dropping out of treatment either when their symptoms disappeared, presumably believing that they were "cured," or because their symptoms did not change, presumably believing the treatment ineffective. In comparison, only 28.6% of those patients with cyclic or chronic models left treatment.

Coping (Action Plans), Appraisal, and the Health Threat

Action plans and appraisal, the two final stages of the self-regulatory system, are best discussed together, as appraisal of coping is necessarily closely related to the nature of the coping response. The very first point we wish to make about action plans and appraisal, however, is that both are linked or directed by the representation of the health problem. The concrete signs that define the presence of the illness, the perceived nature of the causal agent and its routes of attack, and the temporal expectations of the illness duration define the illness problem and direct the selection, execution, and evaluation of coping responses (Leventhal, Meyer, & Nerenz, 1980). Thus, whereas the stages are "independent" (i.e., affected by different variables and structured at different points in time), the three stages work together in generating self-regulating reactions.

Critical Features of Planning and Action.   The very first question for planning and action is the selection of an appropriate coping response. What response is chosen? How does it relate to the problem? Is it an attempt to block exposure to disease agents?; an attempt to destroy the agent?; An attempt to minimize symptoms with no concern for impact on the agent? (This latter choice could reflect a focus on *affect* control rather than control of *threat* or *danger,* Leventhal, 1970).

The perceived cause of an illness can influence response selection. A patient convinced that stress is the major determinant of his malignant lymphoma may sharply reduce his work commitments or cut back on other stress-inducing activities (Nerenz, 1979). Additions (e.g., taking vitamins, body building exercises) and subtractions (e.g., cutting back on work) to life activities are often based on causal interpretations of illness (Hayes–Bautista, 1976; Leventhal, Meyer, & Nerenz, 1980).

The patient's use of additive treatments (stress management) as substitutes for medical prescriptions can have two serious consequences. First, these behaviors may place the individual at increased risk. For example, if a hypertensive patient begins to treat his/her headaches, taking more medication when headaches are present and skipping medication when they are absent, his/her blood pressure may be controlled for only brief periods of time. If the physician's measurements confirm that blood pressure control is poor, he/she is very likely to change and to increase the recommended antihypertensive medication. These changes and the physician's worried comments may suddenly persuade the patient that her self-medicating procedures are inappropriate and frighten her to closely adhere to treatment.

Because the prescribed treatment has been so intensified, this abrupt "improvement" in adherence may actually lead to severe drug reactions. The patient's surprise and distress at these responses may persuade him/her that the treatment is inappropriate and that the physician does not know how to cure hypertension, leading him/her to drop out of treatment. This outcome would lead to maximal risk.

Second, the patient's awareness of his/her deviation from protocol may stimulate secretiveness. Whereas defying the doctor's orders may be routine, it is far from open, and the patient will become unwilling to communicate for fear of discovery and the stress of embarrassment, disapproval, and abandonment for acting badly and disagreeing with authority (Garrity, 1980; Meyer, 1980; Svarstad, 1976). Fully 64% of Meyer's (1980) actively treated hypertensives spontaneously asked the interviewer not to communicate information about medication taking, self-monitoring of symptoms, etc. to their physician. Whether the figure would be as high in other settings is irrelevant. The key issue is that self-monitoring, causal analysis, and self-treatment can stimulate anxiety about discovery and rejection and, therefore, disrupt communication between practitioner and patient.

The temporal feature of the illness representation will also influence the selection of specific responses and the choice of response strategy. Perhaps the most important of these is the individual's commitment to short-term rather than to long-term coping regimens. Continuing coping with smoking reduction, weight control, and regenerating motor and speech skills subsequent to major injuries requires a long-term perspective of the underlying problem. Commitment to specific actions, which may establish the time perspective for the entire treatment, are typically short-term. If the perspective is too long, a person may continue a coping pattern (e.g., the sick role) after it should be discarded. If the time perspective is too brief, he or she will not give the response a chance to work (e.g., weight loss for blood pressure control, Haynes, Taylor, & Sackett, 1979).

Finally, the responses selected may be more or less familiar, more or less practiced, and more or less automatic. Modeling and response rehearsal (Bandura, 1977) will be critical in performing complex, unfamiliar actions. These behaviors make greater demands on attentional capacity, and their performance can generate stress and strain for individuals facing complex, crisis situations.

Critical Features of Appraisal and Attribution.   Representation plays an important role in determining criteria for appraisal and for subsequent attributions. If coping is focused on the minimization of concrete sumptoms, the appraisal and interpretation of outcomes will be symptom oriented. For example, a patient in chemotherapy treatment for cancer who is monitoring size of tumors and expects a "complete, 100% cure, nothing less" will interpret the disappearance of the tumors as cure and see anything less than total disappearance as treatment failure. If the tumors do in fact disappear, it may be difficult for this patient to accept continued stressful treatments (Nerenz, 1979). The criteria, tumor disappearance, is concrete and the time line used is appropriate only to a typical, acute, infectious disease.

This focus on symptoms may well encourage appraisal to follow an acute disease model, because the prototypic history of symptom experience is typical of infectious illness. Moreover, current symptom experience is characterized by constant fluctuation due not only to change in the underlying illness but to shifts in attention, changes in coping (Pennebaker & Skelton, 1978), and increases and decreases in emotional distress (Mechanic, 1972; Zborowski, 1952; Zola, 1963). This variation in ongoing experience encourages the expectation that symptoms will disappear and the illness be cured.

The choice of criteria also affects the attributions made after coping outcomes (i.e., is the success or failure of the coping response seen to be a function of: [1] the patient's underlying competence or skill in coping; [2] the physician's skills; [3] the adequacy of the therapeutic agent; [4] the characteristics of the disease (e.g., a responsive type of tumor, a mistake in diagnosis); or [5] unexpected bad or good fortune? Attributions in the typical medical settings are to the skills of the practitioner and the power of the therapeutic agent with the practitioner as the active diagnostic and treating agent, the patient as a passive recipient of disease and treatment benefits (Brickman, Karuza, Cohn, Rabinowtiz, Coates, & Kidder, 1980). This orientation is inappropriate, however, to sustain and evaluate the ongoing treatment of chronic risks or chronic illness such as hypertension and diabetes or the active rehabilitation necessary after extensive coronary surgery. By seeking 100% cures, the patient is led to set short-term, rigid criteria rather than both short- and long-term criteria that are graded for evaluating coping and treatment outcomes. With chronic conditions the consequence of the former is likely to be disconfirmation of expectations, the arousal of emotional distress, the attribution of failure or lack of effectiveness to the treatment or to oneself, belief in the overwhelming power of the disease agent, and the discontinuance of treatment or coping efforts (Garrity, 1980; Marlatt & Gordon, 1980).

An important factor in making attributions about the effectiveness of treatment and the cause of the underlying illness is whether concrete symptoms are attributed to disease or to treatment. Our interviews with patients in chemotherapy treatment for cancer and hypertension suggest that people devise a variety of strategies for determining whether concrete symptomatic cues are due to one or the other. Judging the temporal contingency between the treatment and the symptom seems to be the most important strategy. Symptoms that begin immediately after treatment are not attributed to illness or other nontreatment changes. The specificity or diffuseness of the symptom is a second factor affecting this differentiation. Diffuse, vague symptoms such as fatigue and distress are much more likely to be attributed to underlying changes in disease state than to be seen as side effects of treatment, while specific effects such as nausea and vomiting or loss of sexual potency are often attributed to treatment. Overlap with prior illness symptoms is also important: Pain is likely to attributed to illness, but novel symptoms stem from treatment. Finally, preparatory information has a major impact on attributions: Patients are told about hair loss, nausea, and vomiting before cancer chemotherapy and are sometimes forewarned about hypotensive dizziness when standing, sexual impotence, etc., when in treatment for high blood pressure. The preparatory information may be given by practitioners, learned from other patients, or simply reflect hearsay.

Patients also seem to develop complex expectations about the impact of specific treatments that are based on their representations of the illness. For example, magnitude or dose-dependent rules generate important expectations about treatment outcomes. One such notion is that the more severe the illness, the more severe the treatments. Thus, one expects and is willing to tolerate more severe treatments for more severe and threatening diseases. A second notion is that treatments that replace earlier unsuccessful treatments will produce a greater number of side effects and more intense symptoms. Finally, there appears to be a decline in optimism about outcomes with successive treatments. This is visible in cancer patients and in patients treated for chronic pain (Sternbach, 1974).

How Does Processing Illness Information Dehumanize?

The Representation and Dehumanization.   How does patients' processing of their representation of the illness help generate critical components of the experience of dehumanization? The first step to dehumanization appears to arise from focusing on symptoms: The act of attending to a symptom objectifies the self and may lead to separation of the symptom and the body from the psychological self and/or to intense feelings of threat upon realizing that the physical signs could mean self-destruction (Leventhal, 1975).

The patient's symptomatic focus is also a cause for breakdown in communication. Although symptoms provide clues to diagnosis, the physical examination and x-rays and chemical tests are the physician's primary guides to diagnosis (Reiser, 1978). Hence, the physician's attention is at least divided, if not entirely drawn, to various readings and information usually outside the patient's purview: The physician does not seem attentive to the patient's feelings. The incompleteness of diagnosis interviews attests to this (Platt & McMath, 1979). The possibility for dehumanization is further enhanced because the patients recognize the "validity" of the physician's technical instruments and feel they should adopt the practitioner's instrumented definition of their problems and accept the treatment and appraisal strategies that accompany them. Yet, this technical view is incomplete and partial. At the least, it pays little attention to symptoms. And if symptoms are persistent (painful and disruptive, etc.), little affected by treatment, and associated (in the patient's mind) with the disease, it is difficult to be a "good" patient and follow the orders based on the technical diagnosis of the problem.

These are not false issues. Patients are concerned about symptoms, and the stonger the symptom the stronger their concern (Zborowski, 1952; Zola, 1963). This concern is not necessarily shared by the doctor. From the physician's expert perspective, the severe pain, gasping, and rapid breathing represent an anxiety attack rather than a coronary incident, the painful, inflamed node is a minor disturbance, but the silent, enlarged node indicates "real" trouble. The symptom most important to the illness hypothesis of the patient is not necessarily the most salient and most important to the illness hypothesis of the practitioner.

Patients are not only faced with communication problems based on their overevaluation of intense, salient symptoms; they may also be subjected to uncertainties that arise when the physician's testing instruments and procedures detect and treat disease of which they were unaware. What can produce more uncertainty about one's environment than to discover one has high blood pressure or a malignant tumor, when one was asymptomatic and felt great! There are no warnings, no way of predicting exacerbations. Mineka and Kihlstrom (1978) suggest that the key to learned helplessness is the occurrence of threat in the absence of warning (Mandler, 1975; Seligman, 1975).

Conditions such as the aforementioned are likely to be a prime stimulus to uncertainty and cyclic thought and depression. Examples abound. Gutmann (1981) has interviewed coronary bypass patients before and after surgery and finds that those who are asymptomatic before surgery cope with initial, post-operative pains and stress extremely well; the pain and distress clearly *belong* to the surgery. But as the wounds of surgery heal and pain and distress vanish, the individual is again asymptomatic and lacks cues for danger. Moreover, the subjective experience is the same as the preoperative state: Could he/she still be ill? There is no way of knowing. Depression becomes a common outcome for these patients.

Nerenz (1979) interviewed patients in chemotherapy for malignant lymphoma and compared distress levels for patients monitoring concerous nodes that disappeared, either suddenly or gradually. To his surprise, but consistent with Gutmann's findings, levels of distress were substantially greater when a patient's tumors disappeared suddenly. The medical conceptualization of the disease demanded continued treatment, but this no longer made sense from the patient perspective. If he/she is cured (tumors are gone), why be treated? If not cured, then where inside him/her were the tumors spreading? What might have seemed a joyous outcome was associated with high levels of uncertainty, threat, and emotional distress.

Physicians are notoriously lax about reviewing family history and life situations immediately surrounding problem and symptom onset, though they may refer to various life events when discussing illness symptoms. Allusions to the causal nature of these events can stimulate patients to think back and to attend to the relationship between life stress and symptoms. Because stress is likely to intensify symptomatology, the search procedure will verify the patient's hypothesis that stress causes illness. It is not surprising, then, that people in treatment for hypertension vary their medication dose in association with symptoms and life events. Indeed, some patients take medication preventively! How much vitamin taking is reinforced by such mechanisms is unknown. Given that placebos stimulate endorphin production for anxious people, taking inert pills during stressful life episodes may play a crucial role in attenuating symptomatology.

Thus, much of practitioner behavior appears to strengthen the illusion of a correlation between symptoms, life events, and disease labels. Symptoms appear under a wide variety of circumstances; indeed, the body is a rather "noisy" substrate providing a rich array of aches, pains, inflammations, and conditions of the eyes, nose, and throat that are usually ignored (Pennebaker & Skelton, 1978). It is easy, then, for patients to locate "symptoms" to confirm the physician's diagnosis, especially when this is further reinforced by questions about particular body sensations. The questions need not *produce* the symptoms (they are not consequences of suggestion); the symptoms are there to be found. It is not necessary for the practitioner to link them to illness labels; the patient will do that by him or herself! However, the tendency to focus on positive instances may lead the physician to encourage such illusory formulations. For example, when a patient asks, "Do you think my headache is due to high blood pressure?," it is likely that the physician will respond, "Maybe. Why not take your pressure when you have a headache?." The advice overlooks the fact that the chronically hypertensive patient will have high readings whether he/she has a headache or not and fails to test the no headache–blood pressure link. As a consequence, the patient may take medication only when he/she has headaches and be fairly certain that he/she is taking the appropriate precautions, even though he/she is unlikely to discuss his/her actions with his/her physician. Isolation, uncertainty in the relationship, inability to communicate underlying strategies, etc. emerge, and all are conditions for dehumanization.

Coping, Appraisal, and Dehumanization.   There are so many obvious ways in which normal coping activity is disrupted by illness and the patient role that it seems unnecessary to mention more than a few. Most important, of course, is the passive nature of the patient role. Illness is "visited on us" (Brickman et al., 1980; Herzlich, 1973), and given that we are not responsible for its occurrence, we are also not held responsible for its cure. The expert diagnoses, treats, and prescribes for us. Our activity is passive, except for following orders. The reward is temporary exemption from normal role demands (Mechanic, 1972; Parsons, 1975).

It is important to repeat that the components of dehumanization experience will be further intensified by the likelihood of conflict between the plans and actions demanded and suggested by pain and distress and the patient's common-sense view of illness. Symptoms demand redress; there is a need for medication to relieve pain and for therapy to cure the sensory experiences that the patient sees as part of the disease, a disease that could be more serious than the doctors are willing to admit. Indeed, considerable anguish, feeling of isolation, unwillingness to communicate, and even some degree of paranoia can appear because of discrepancies between the treatments offered by the practitioners and the treatments imagined to be effective by the patients. If symptoms are diffuse and severe, wouldn't it make sense to look for a more deadly general disorder such as cancer or heart disease than to suggest a disorder of a particular organ? This process may underlie the behavior of the "worried well," people who appear at every available health-screening site and are more likely to return to screening or treatment, even when given negative test results, than people whose test findings are positive and are in need of treatment (Garfield, 1970).

Discrepancies can also occur between a known, severe disease when treatment seems too innocuous. Ringler (1981) interviewed several women receiving chemotherapy for breast cancer who, for unknown reasons, were "fortunate" to miss the myriad of anticipated side effects. When they did not experience the expected vomiting, nausea, hair loss, etc., they became paranoid and suspected that they were receiving placebos instead of legitimate anticancer treatment. After all, was it not reasonable to expect severe side effects from chemicals that would kill cancer? Incompatible criteria for coping (treatment) outcomes clearly stimulated distress and a sense of isolation and persecution.

The nature of the patient's perspective also makes it difficult for him/her to appraise medical procedures. For example, a mother whose youngster had a sore throat rejected the physician's recommendation for treatment, nose drops, because the child's difficulty was in his/her throat and not in his/her nose. The practitioner had failed to explain that a postnasal drip was responsible for the throat irritation. Mothers have also been found to stop medication before the time recommended in the prescription; they watch for the disappearance of symptoms rather than treating for the disappearance of the underlying microbial agent (Elling, Whittemore, & Green, 1960). In summary, coping and appraisal based on the patient's perspective may be incompatible with coping and appraisal based on the technical criteria of the practitioner.

Engel (1977) points out that the biomedical or disease model has become a cultural dogma. As believed by the layman, the model suggests that illness can be cured by passive acquiescence to the practitioner's manipulations. One only needs to lie still, be operated on, take a pill, etc. to achieve a complete and permanent cure. This creates special problems for prevention and rehabilitation for chronic conditions, where complete adherence is unusual or nonexistent and complete prevention or reversal of an illness condition unrealistic. Adherence to diets, antismoking, or antidringing regimens is partial at best. Some adhere perfectly for a few days or weeks; most are back to their bad practice within 90 days of withdrawal. One serious problem in maintaining risk-reducing behaviors is the sense of hopelessness, entrapment (addiction), and lack of personal effectiveness that emerges from failures. Marlatt and Gordon (1980) point out that coping setbacks are the rule, not the exception, and that people interpret failures as a sign that they are unable to control their impulses and behaviors. They also point out that medically oriented models—acute-disease thinking—reinforce this belief; a single slip with a drink means one is again sick or diseased.

Failures to sustain coping seem especially likely when the individuals experience anger and frustration from severe environmental threat and feel that they lack the skills needed to cope, either with the threat or with the feelings of frustration generated by temptation. If the prohibited action (e.g., smoking or drinking) is seen as enhancing self-esteem and/or self-effectiveness, then the temptation itself becomes a means of conquering the distress aroused by the fear of succumbing (Leventhal & Cleary, 1980). In these circumstances, restraint is practically impossible.

We would like to highlight two important but little explored conditions that can generate frustration and conflict as a patient attempts to cope with illness, pain, and distress. First, culture or commonsense may lead to the selection of effective coping responses that increase both discomfort and risk, and when patients follow effective recommendations that are counter to such commonsense rules, they may be unable to accurately judge the benefits they have experienced. This is a common outcome in studies using sensory information and self-monitoring of specific body sensations as a way of reducing the emotional distress that is an integral part of pain. Individuals who monitor sensations report less distress than control subjects attempting to block out or ignore pain. Because the monitoring tactics are counterintuitive and because subjects do not try both blocking and monitoring in close sequence, they may believe monitoring to be ineffective when it has in fact reduced their distress (Reinhardt, 1979). This was graphically illustrated in a clinical study in which it proved extremely difficult to motivate pregnant mothers to monitor their contractions during labor, even though the mothers who did so were very much less distressed, anxious, depressed, etc. than control mothers during the second stage of labor. Having monitored their contractions, they were better able to regulate pushing contractions and felt less threatened when actively coping with labor and delivery (Leventhal, Shacham, Booth, & Leventhal, 1981).

The second problem arises when practitioners do not allow patients to regulate their treatment or refuse to treat when the patient requests it. For example, patients who are given detailed preparation for surgery or minor diagnostic procedures may be more active and more assertive in the postoperative and diagnostic setting. On some occasions, the active, self-regulating patient may be seen as disruptive, anxious, or even maladjusted (Richards & Schmale, 1974) and may even be given increased doses of tranquilizing medication to slow him or her down (Johnson, Dabbs, & Leventhal, 1970). This could happen if the practitioner confuses active self-regulation for anxiety or is threatened by the patient's active efforts to assert control.

The refusal of treatment, or the argument that treatment is not needed, is a complex issue. Patients often request unnecessary medication that the physician is wise to refuse. But patients may also request treatment for chronic conditions, such as hypertension, which their practitioner feels does not warrant treatment, despite randomized control trials showing the value of treatment, because it is mild or asymptomatic (Hypertension detection and follow-up program cooperative group, 1979a, b; Veterans Administration cooperative group study on antihypertensive agents, 1967). In either case, refusing treatment robs patients of a sense of control over their condition. If this is not dealt with, it can be the basis for a dehumanizing experience. The sense of wrong, neglect, and confusion may be exaggerated in the case of the patient seeking to control his or her hypertension after having made the effort to seek screening and advice on hypertension in accordance with information widely promulgated by a variety of mass media health promotional programs.

ENVIRONMENTAL FACTORS ENCOURAGING DEHUMANIZING BEHAVIORS

Certainly few, if any, medical practitioners wish to think of themselves as, or to act in ways that are, dehumanizing. Yet, their behavior often produces effects contrary to their benign intent. What conditions promote behaviors that contrast with stated intentions? And what is special about these factors that generates an imperviousness to the consequences of such actions? One can seek answers to these questions by first examining the biomedical model that dictates the current characteristics of medical environments, then by examining the nature of medical institutions fostered by that model.

The Biomedical Model and Dehumanizing Environments

The biomedical model has considerable impact on the thought of those formulating the policies and technology of medicine (Reiser, 1978). As Engel (1977) suggests, the model has become a dogma (i.e., it is no longer simply a paradigm underlying scientific inquiry and guiding treatment but an ideology that exerts a prescriptive and irrational hold on the design of medical systems, the teaching of medical students, and the justification of existent practices). In its pure, scientific form, the model argues for rational, empirical inquiry into the cause and treatment of the ills of man. A narrow version of the model argues that specific agents are necessary for the occurrence of specific diseases. It examines the vectors by which agents move from host to host, the physiological changes underlying their attack on the host system, how these physiological changes can be detected symptomatically and, more usually, instrumentally, and attempts to discover therapies to counter each specific agent (Broskowski & Baker, 1974). The level of detail can be inferential, as in Pasteur's demonstration of disease transmission, or detailed, as in the description of the biochemical, anatomical, and physiological changes underlying diabetes melitus. This narrow definition of biomedicine seems to promote a sense of ignorance and helplessness with respect to disease prevention, because the purist cannot see the value of general preventive activities; he or she requires exact cures and exact preventives, not half-way measures (Leventhal & Hirschman, in press; Thomas, 1977). Indeed, the biomedical advocate may resist the use of general interventions like hygienic practices or dietary changes to combat disease even though the major victories over infectious disease were won by hygiene, not wonder drugs (Dingle, 1973; Eckholm, 1977). And the true believer in the medical model finds it difficult to accept suggestions that many chronic illnesses can best be treated by life-style changes (e.g., dietary change, weight loss, and smoking cessation). We wish to single out two particular ways in which biomedical thinking appears to provide environments capable of generating dehumanization: one is technological, the other conceptual.

Technological Factors and Dehumanization.   Perhaps the most highly pub-
licized of the psychological changes that has had a marked impact on medical
care is the use of mechanization to sustain biological functions when human
functions are absent. Living bodies and dead brains, epitomized by the Karen
Quinlan case, captivate the public imagination and have led to a spate of writings
questioning the ethics of sustaining life functions by heroic technology
(Beauchamp & Childress, 1979). Although the issue of discriminating death
from life is of importance and has focused attention on the problem of ethics and
dehumanization, it is peripheral to the central issue of dehumanization as experienced by the patient.

Less dramatically, technology creates a great number of dehumanizing experiences by interposing itself between the practitioner and patient. The size and
strangeness of the machinery and the need to modify one's residence and patterns
of eating and sleeping to be looked at by a machine, stimulate a sense of self as
an object handled by other objects. The reliance on instruments can be so great as
to generate doubt and uncertainty about the validity of everyday experience: How
can one be sure of anything if what one sees, hears, and touches could be a
fallible guide to illness? Reiser (1978) suggests that reliance on instruments has
led doctors to doubt the value of all subjective experience, their own as well as
the patient's, when making diagnostic and treatment decisions. By ruling out the
patients' subjective experiences, as though the experience of an instrument were
not subjective, patients' reactions to their illness and treatment are automatically
denigrated as unimportant for treatment planning.

Finally, because it is there, technology may be used when its costs far out-
weigh its benefits. A high technology treatment that gains a few months and even
a year is of dubious value if the extra time is filled by pain and mutilation of self.
Worse yet are the heroic and painful measures that have virtually no chance of
gain (e.g., treatment failure of severely burned patients).

Our refined technologies can create a new set of dehumanizing and life-
destroying stresses if used for the early detection of disease threats for which we
have no known treatments (Sackett, 1975). For example, Robin (1978) questions
the use of axial tomography to detect pancreatic masses, many of which are
benign and if detected by tomography would require further invasive diagnostic
procedures. Is the gain in longevity from such early diagnosis sufficient to offset
the procedural stress? And if one does not act aggressively, what of the anxious
doubt and suffering while waiting for the positive signs of illness? We all live
with uncertainty, but there are limits to how much uncertainty one can or should
tolerate. Technology opens the gates for uncertainties as well as certainties and
experiences of self as an object that we might never have imagined.

Conceptual Factors and Dehumanization.   Biomedicine's and bioengineer-
ing's proliferation of technology is part of a proliferation of data and knowledge

that have led to the development of new medical specialties. Practitioners have been forced to narrow their focus: to be concerned with lungs, or liver, or intestines, or cardiovascular disease. Each specialist looks at a part of the patient: An organ or an organ system, not a person, is the focus of inquiry.

The fragmentation has also led to a realistic sense of the difficulty in communication. What and how does one tell patients about their condition? Can people think probabilistically or in terms of multiple causes? Technical complexity can create barriers to communication and sharing.

The medical model has also spawned the clinicopathologic conference, a forum that emphasizes and teaches diagnostic skills. Accurate labeling of agent and process is an important step, but as Robin (1978) points out, the end product of the diagnostic conference is not the same as that produced in "the clinical management conference" where the goal is: "the integration of data into proposals designed to provide the contented and more well-adjusted life for our patient [p. 2275]."

The medical model also seems to lead to a focus on the *process* of treatment and its *immediate outcomes* (Donabedian, 1978). Surgery is deemed successful if the procedure is completed and the patient survives the operation. Medical treatment is successful if the patient is discharged. It is only recently that medicine has examined longer-term outcomes: Does the patient live for weeks, months, or years? And is the quality of life poor or excellent? These questions, some of which are exemplified in the debate on surgical versus medical treatment of angina (Murphy et al., 1977), reflect a shift in focus that will require increased attention to the patient's experience of the illness and treatment and the way illness and treatment impact on the patient's life. But this focus has not been part of classic biomedicine that narrowly regulates a process of detecting agents and following tightly prescribed, technical treatment protocols with the goal of an immediate change in biological process.

In summary, the biomedical model has provided a rigorous way of looking at disease causation emphasizing the impact of single agents on narrowly but well-defined biological processes. It has fostered an enormous technology and encouraged a highly specialized form of training. It is suspicious of subjective experience both for data and for making medical decisions. Treatment has focused on the effective application of technology to amend errant biological processes. Evaluation of treatment effectiveness has focused on the performance of the technique (i.e., was it done correctly and what were its immediate effects?). Did the patient survive the operation and was he or she discharged to home? As a model of causation it has fostered a model of helping in which the patient is not responsible for illness: Illness is an unwelcome or chance event from a cruel world. Nor is the patient responsible for detection and treatment; the medical-care system screens and treats. Although this active expert to passive recipient definition of helping is not a necessary consequence of current biomedical thinking, such thinking has contributed to this view of helping and is used to justify and maintain it.

Institutional Structures

If the biomedical model has done nothing more than provide a justification for an expert-to-object model of helping, reducing dehumanization might not prove so formidable a task. However, the model and its knowledge base have also led to the proliferation of complex institutional and social structures, whose existence justify and are justified by the model. The already mentioned overspecialization of the physician leading to the treatment of organs and not people removes attention from the patient's subjective experience of illness and its impacts on his or her life.

Specialization has also led to a particular structure for medical care: The general practitioner and internist typically provide the only source of patient-oriented medical contact. Specialists, from radiologists to surgeons, are ensconced in hospital settings and may contact the patient (if they do at all) only before and after a specific procedure. Separation of specialists in space and time means that seeing the surgeon is a visit to another floor of the hospital at a time different from that when the internist is available. In addition to added problems in access, the patient must decide to whom to address specific questions, whose advice to weight most heavily for a given problem, and so forth.

Changing these structures is no simple matter given the vested interests of each specialty, the higher status of most specialties, and the economics of medical care. At an earlier time physicians looked down on the surgeon, their inferiors, who were mostly barbers. However, that is no longer the case. The surgeon has become the hero of the medical-care system: In the relatively concrete-minded commonsense representation of the patients, the removal of the lump or replacement of the coronary artery is removal of the disease. This form of concrete biomedical dogma, when carried to its extreme, fails to recognize the difference between tumor and clogged artery on the one hand and the underlying disease process on the other. The reverence for surgeons makes it difficult to modify their dehumanizing behaviors.

But even if surgeons were suddenly to become psychotherapeutic in orientation and active foes of poor communication, they would be ill-paid for their efforts. The fee-for-service concept is ingrained in our medical-care system; surgeons are paid for removing and repairing organs, not for preparing and communicating with patients. The fee-for-service system is entrenched in a large and complex third-party payment system initiated 60 years ago. Whereas insurance was started to protect patients against catastrophic loss, it was also clearly designed by a relatively narrow biomedical view of illness and treatment; the expansion of payment to cover time spent in procedures for patient education, psychological preparation, etc. is slow and reluctant (Klarman, 1977; Saward, 1977).

AN EXPANDED VIEW OF BIOMEDICINE AND ITS IMPLICATIONS FOR BEHAVIORAL RESEARCH

The vast achievements of biomedicine are sometimes presented as a necessary excuse or justification for the dehumanization experienced during treatment. But must we accept the uncaring, dehumanizing aspects of the medical system in order to reap the benefits of expert, biomedical technology? We think not. Indeed, we do not see any necessary connection between the use of biomedical theory and technology on the one hand and inhumane treatment on the other. Nevertheless, to remove dehumanization, we believe that it is necessary to provide a new biomedical model of disease causation. Adjustments in institutional arrangements (e.g., group practice, prepaid health-maintenance organizations, etc.) can help, but they do not necessarily alter the relationships among practitioners (doctors, nurses, social workers) and between practitioners and patients. The new model will provide the justification for attention to the patient's subjective states, symptoms and feelings, and perceptions of the impact of the illness on his or her life; will broaden the use of technologies; and will foster changes in education, institutional arrangements, and face-to-face communication.

Although this chapter is not the appropriate place to develop such a model, we believe that both medical, biological, and social scientists can contribute to its formulation, and, therefore, we discuss it briefly. It will, of necessity, be interdisciplinary as it will recognize the multivariate nature of disease causation, the multivarite nature of the individual's defenses against disease, and the multivariate nature of treatment. Moreover, it will recognize that these factors are hierarchically arranged from cellular through hormonal and neurological levels to the psychological social and cultural levels of functioning.

The traditional version of biomedicine described in our early sections focused on single agents, single vectors, and the alteration of relatively isolated, underlying physiological process that produced specific symptom patterns. This model is close to that developed for infectious disease. Contemporary textbooks of medicine state that many of man's chronic illnesses involve multiple agents operating through multiple vectors and interacting with a physiological system that is not only complex but capable of defensive reactions in depth (Beeson, McDermott, & Wyngaarden, 1979). Multiple causes may call for multiple therapies. General rather than specific changes in life style may be important in inoculating against a wide range of known and other yet unknown carcinogens.

Defense is also more complex and involved than simple administration of sulfanomide or penicillin. The concept of the complexities of the defense system is clearly emerging in biomedical thought. At the molecular level is the immune system with both its immunoglobulins (subcellular particles) and sensitive vigilant scavenger cells that identify and attack alien agents. At a more molar level are the various neuroendocrine functions (e.g., catecholamine activity important in maintaining internal homeostasis during intensive energy output to meet environmental demands). At yet a more integrative level are neural activities or problem-solving skills that avoid risks by directing the organism into safe settings and seeking social (and medical) assistance. At a still more molar level is the social system that cushions environmental demands and provides additional resources for dealing with such demands when they arise. Examples of the latter are seen in studies comparing the incidence of cardiovascular disease in socially integrated, traditional communities in contrast to more isolated, cosmopolitan communities. The settlers to both community types had been drawn from similar areas of the old world. The findings are fairly striking: Coronary disease rates are less in the traditional setting (Bruhn & Wolf, 1979). In a recent study comparing hormonal changes in air traffic controllers under stressful and nonstressful work conditions, Rose (1979) suggested that the social environment was the first level of defense against disease-inducing neuroendocrine changes. By rotating controllers through stations more rapidly during peak-load times, assigning less-demanding tasks to individuals who feel ill, etc., the social organization functions to minimize stress and smooth out fluctuations in psychophysiological states.

New Uses of Old Technologies

With few additional expansions, we have the makings of what Engel (1977) calls a biosocial medical model. One of its merits is that the focus on disease causation and disease management now includes the cultural, social, and psychological levels of description in addition to an expanded, multilevel, and multivariate view of the biology of illness. How patients feel and how they interpret their disease affects behaviors that affect their illness and recovery. These factors alter their selection and use of treatment (a better perspective than compliance). They change their emotional states and struggling that alter neuroendocrine balance and resistance to disease agents. Advanced technology (formerly only the domain of the specialist) can serve to facilitate the active, self-regulating role of the patient to reduce dehumanization and enhance recovery and quality of life.

An interesting example of this was seen in the last author's adaptation of a radiographic study not only as a diagnostic tool but also as a tool for promoting psychological change.

Mr. J. H. was a 39-year-old Mexican–American who had the onset of seizures as a child, although there had been no birth trauma, accidents, or head injuries, infections or family history of epilepsy. He used antiseizure drugs intermittently.

Because he had some acquaintances in a large northern city, he migrated there from Texas. He was hospitalized at a university-affiliated hospital after he had been brought to the emergency room by the police in *status epilepticus*. He then underwent his first thorough neurological examination. A large arteriovenous malformation was found on arteriography, deep in the left parietal lobe. Because of its position, it was considered inoperable at that time, and seizure control was attempted with anticonvulsants. J. H. subsequently had multiple admissions to the neurology service in *status epilepticus* precipitated by alcohol ingestion.

During his last admission, after the resolution of the postictal phase, I came to examine him and take an admission history. I found him in four-point leather restraints, side rails up, unkempt, and unshaven. He apologized for being so dirty and admitted that he had been drinking very heavily. He also said that he did not take his pills often. He stated that the seizures were becoming more frequent and he was unable to keep a job. He had a woman friend who was crippled and who participated in his drinking bouts. He also had a rent-free room that was payment for maintenance and meal preparation for his wheelchair-bound landlord. His social world revolved around his handicapped lady friend who depended on him for emotional as well as physical support, and the Hispanic Center, though he said he was treated with some suspicion there because of the fits.

I then examined him and found a minimally depressed sensorium with no localizing neurological signs. The remainder of his examination was unremarkable. During these examination, he expressed a few feelings of worthlessness, "nobody can do anything for me ... I'm not good enough to have an operation ... doctors don't care" I asked him to tell me about his family, friends. He recounted a long series of rejections: "you must be bad to have fits ... you can't stay home if you can't work" He said he had never hurt anybody or stolen anything, but if everyone said so, he must deserve so much trouble.

I tried to talk to him and explain about the increased irritability of the brain to alcohol but obviously had no impact and was dismissed as a gringo who could not understand that he only felt whole and free from ridicule when he was drunk (i.e., when he could not feel or care about the outside world).

Two themes ran throughout the interview and examination: (1) worthlessness, not worthy of being treated; and (2) hopelessness, isolation, and abandonment, first by his family, then by the physicians, and finally by himself. He was not worth the effort of taking care of himself, though he could take care of other dependent persons. He refused to assume control over drinking and taking medications.

I then asked him if he would like to see exactly what was wrong inside his head, what was causing the fits. He seemed surprised at my offer, was quiet for a few moments, and then said yes, he wanted to see the pictures of his head. I arranged to have the arteriograms brought to the ward the next day.

I set the film series up on the viewing box and compared the normal right side of his head with the left, pointing out the position of the large vascular lesion. I showed him frontal and lateral views, told him a little about the normal function of the left cortex, and then tried to make clear that there was no safe surgical approach and also commented that this was not a progressively expanding lesion but a developmental abnormality.

He was silent for several minutes after I had finished talking; he continued to look at the x-rays. He then said, "it would be even worse to be paralyzed, drag my leg . . . not use my right arm . . . maybe not talk so good." He then asked, "why did it happen to me?. . . . Can kids get it from their father?" I told him that what causes these developmental mistakes is not understood, but they are random events and don't appear to be inherited. He told me that he had fathered a son and had been terrified that the child would also have fits. He then thanked me and returned to his room.

On the day before his discharge, he asked if the hospital social worker and his closest friend, the counselor at the Hispanic Center, could see his x-rays. I said I would arrange to have them view the films and would discuss the findings with them.

A month later, J. H. called the hospital and had me paged. He asked me for a prescription renewal and told me he was working as an aide at the Hispanic Center. He told me he had been drunk only once since his discharge. Three months later, he called to say that he was going home to Texas to see his family. Six months later, the hospital received a letter from a physician in Galveston requesting a copy of his records. The letter noted that J. H. was medically stable, was being seen as an outpatient, and was working.

Thus, by using the complex technology of an angiographic study, which visualizes anatomy clearly and positions it in the head concretely, the patient was able to make the appropriate association between his symptoms and a discrete intracranial abnormality. The technique of the study also allowed him to compare a normal image with an abnormal condition and understand the surgeon's decision that the lesion was inoperable because the risks of functional loss were too great. By presenting a concrete image, the patient's concept of self could be changed because something was really wrong; the epilepsy was the result of a real abnormality, not the result of "bad" behavior, "bad" spirits. By making the etiology of his symptoms concrete, the barrier to the development of an effective coping strategy could be removed. Destructive behaviors such as alcohol injection and nonuse of antiseizure drugs could be rejected. J. H. could reassess his feelings of worthlessness. He clearly made a decision to assume responsibility for himself; he humanized himself.

A case does not a science make. But a case can vividly illustrate the vast range of possibilities for integrating biomedical concepts and technologies with a broader problem-solving framework that recognizes the multivariate and multilevel nature of human illness and functioning. By examining the process through which patients cope with their illness problems, we open up rich investigate opportunities that may increase comfort and caring and reduce the frequency of dehumanizing experiences.

REFERENCES

Abramson, L. *Induced mood and the illusion of control.* Presented at the annual meeting of American Psychological Association, Montreal, Canada, 1980.

Antonovsky, A. *Health, stress, and coping.* San Francisco: Jossey-Bass, 1979.

Bandura, A. Self-efficacy: Toward a unifying theory of behavioral change. *Psychological Review* 1977, *84*(2), 191-215.

Beauchamp, T. L., & Childress, J. F. *Principles of biomedical ethics.* New York: Oxford University Press, 1979.

Becker, M. H., & Maiman, L. A. Sociobehavioral determinants of compliance with health and medical care recommendation. *Med Care* 1975, *13*, 10-24.

Beecher, H. K. *Measurement of subjective responses.* New York: Oxford University Press, 1959.

Beeson, P. B., McDermott, W., & Wyngaarden, J. *Cecil textbook of medicine* (15th ed.). Philadelphia: Saunders, 1979.

Ben-Sira, Z. The structure and dynamics of the image of diseases. *Journal of Chronic Disease,* 1977, *30*, 831-842. (a)

Ben-Sira, Z. Involvement with a disease and health promoting behavior. *Social Science and Medicine,* 1977, *11*, 165-173. (b)

Bettelheim, B. Individual and mass behavior in extreme situations. *Journal of Abnormal Social Psychology,* 1943, *38*, 417-452.

Brickman, P., Karuza, J., Cohn, E., Rabinowitz, V. C., Coates, D., & Kidder, L. *Models of helping and coping.* Unpublished manuscript, University of Michigan, 1980.

Broskowski, A., & Baker, F. Professional, organizational, and social barriers to primary prevention. *American Journal of Orthopsychiatry,* 1974, *44*, 707-719.

Bruhn, J. G., & Wolf, S. *The Roseto story: Anatomy of health.* Norman: Oklahoma University Press, 1979.

Carver, C. S. A cybernetic model of self-attention processes. *Journal of Personality and Social Psychology,* 1979, *37*, 1251-1281.

Cohen, E. A. *Human behavior in the concentration camp.* New York: Norton, 1953.

Dingle, J. H. The ills of man. *Scientific American,* 1973, *229*, 77-84.

Donabedian, A. The quality of medical care: Methods for assessing and monitoring the quality of care for research and for quality assurance programs. *Science,* 1978, *200*, 856-864.

Eckholm, E. P. *The picture of health: Environmental sources of disease.* New York: Norton, 1977.

Elling, R., Whittemore, R., & Green, M. Patient participation in a pediatric program. *Journal of Health and Human Behavior,* Fall 1960, *1*, 183-191.

Engel, G. The need for a new medical model: A challenge for biomedicine. *Science,* 1977, *196*, 129-136.

Garfield, S. R. The delivery of medical care. *Scientific American,* April 1970, 15-23.

Garrity, T. F. Medical compliance and the clinician patient relationship: A review. In R. B. Haynes, M. E. Mattson, & T. O. Engebretson, Jr. (Eds.), *Patient compliance to prescribed antihypertensive medication regimens: A report to the National Heart, Lung, and Blood Institute.* Washington, D. C.: U. S. Department of Health and Human Services, NIH Publication No. 81-2102, 1980, 113-137.

Gibson, J. J. *The senses considered as perceptual systems.* Boston: Houghton Mifflin, 1966.

Gutmann, M. Personal correspondence, March 21, 1981.

Hayes-Bautista, D. E. Modifying the treatment: Patient compliance, patient control and medical care. *Social Science and Medicine,* 1976, *10*, 233-238.

Haynes, R. G., Taylor, D. W., & Sackett, D. L. (Eds.), *Compliance to health care*. Baltimore: Johns Hopkins University Press, 1979.

Herzlich, C. *Health and illness: A social psychological analysis*. New York: Academic Press, 1973.

Horowitz, M. J. *Image formation and cognition*. New York: Appleton–Century–Crofts, 1970.

Howard, J., & Strauss, A. (Eds.). *Humanizing health care*. Health, Medicine, and Society Series. New York: Wiley, 1975.

Hypertension detection and follow-up program cooperative group: I. Five-year findings of the hypertension detection and follow-up program. Reduction in mortality of persons with high blood pressure, including mild hypertension. *Journal of the American Medical Association*, 1979, *242*, 2562–2571. (a)

Hypertension detection and follow-up program cooperative group: II. Mortality by race, sex, and age. *Journal of the American Medical Association*, 1979, *242*, 2572–2577. (b)

Janis, I. L. *Air war and emotional stress*. New York: McGraw–Hill, 1951.

Janis, I. L. *Psychological stress: Psychoanalytic and behavioral studies of surgical patients*. New York: Wiley, 1958.

Jarvinen, K. A. J. Can ward rounds be a danger to patients with myocardial infraction? *British Medical Journal*, 1955, *1*, 318–320.

Johnson, J. E. Stress reduction through sensation information. In I. G. Sarason & C. D. Spielberger (Eds.), *Stress and anxiety* (Vol. 2). Washington, D. C.: Hemisphere, 1975.

Johnson, J., Dabbs, J., & Leventhal, H. Psychosocial factors in the welfare of surgical patients. *Nursing Research*, 1970, *19*, 18–29.

Kanfer, F. H. The many faces of self-control, or behavior modification changes its focus. In R. B. Stuart (Ed.), *Behavioral self-management: Strategies, techniques and outcome*. Brunner/Mazel, New York, 1977.

Klarman, H. E. The financing of health care. In J. H. Knowles (Ed.), *Doing better and feeling worse*. New York: Norton, 1977.

Lazarus, R. *Psychological stress and the coping process*. New York: McGraw–Hill, 1966.

Leventhal, H. Findings and theory in the study of fear communications. In L. Berkowitz (Ed.), *Advances in experimental social psychology* (Vol. 5). New York: Academic Press, 1970.

Leventhal, H. The consequences of depersonalization during illness and treatment. In J. Howard & A. Strauss (Eds.), *Humanizing health care*. New York: Wiley, 1975.

Leventhal, H. Toward a comprehensive theory of emotion. In L. Berkowitz (Ed.), *Advances in experimental social psychology* (Vol. 13). New York: Academic Press, 1980.

Leventhal, H., & Cleary, P. The smoking problem: A review of the research and theory in behavioral risk modification. *Psychological Bulletin*, 1980, *88*, 370–405.

Leventhal, H., & Everhart, D. Emotion, pain and physical illness. In C. Izard (Ed.), *Emotions and psychopathology*. New York: Plenum, 1979.

Leventhal, H., & Hirschman, R. S. Social psychology and prevention. In G. S. Sanders & J. Suls (Eds.), *Social psychology of illness and health*. Hillsdale, N. J.: Lawrence Erlbaum Associates, in press.

Leventhal, H., Meyer, D., & Nerenz, D. The commonsense representation of illness danger. In S. Rachman (Ed.), *Contributions to medical psychology* (Vol. 2). New York: Pergamon, 1980.

Leventhal, H., Safer, M., & Panagis, D. The process underlying individual responses to health communications: Some practical implications. *Health Education Monographs*, in press.

Leventhal, H., Shacham, S., Booth, C., & Leventhal, E. *Attention and coping in the control of distress from childbirth*. Unpublished manuscript, University of Wisconsin, Madison, 1981.

Ley, P. Psychological studies of doctor–patient communication. In S. Rachman (Ed.), *Contributions to medical psychology* (Vol. 1). New York: Pergamon Press, 1977.

Lifton, R. J. *Thought reform and the psychology of totalism: A study of 'brainwashing' in China*. New York: Norton, 1961.

Mandler, G. *Mind and emotion*. New York: Wiley, 1975.

Marlatt, G. A., & Gordon, J. R. Determinants of relapse: Implications for the maintenance of behavior change. In P. O. Davidson & S. M. Davidson (Eds.), *Behavioral medicine: Changing health life styles*. New York: Brunner/Mazel, 1980.

Mechanic, D. Social psychological factors affecting the presentation of bodily complaints. *New England Journal of Medicine*, 1972, *286*, 1132–1139.

Meyer, D. *The effects of patients' representation of high blood pressure on behavior in treatment.* Unpublished doctoral dissertation, University of Wisconsin-Madison, 1980.

Meyer, D., Leventhal, H., & Gutmann, M. Symptoms in hypertension: How patients evaluate and treat them. *New England Journal of Medicine*, in press.

Milgram, S. *Obedience to authority: An experimental view*. New York: Harper & Row, 1974.

Miller, G. A., Galanter, E. H., & Pribram, K. H. *Plans and the structure of behavior*. New York: Holt, 1960.

Mineka, S., & Kihlstrom, J. F. Unpredictable and uncontrollable events: A new perspective on experimental neurosis. *Journal of Abnormal Psychology*, 1978, *87*, 256–271.

Morris, W. (Ed.). *The American Heritage dictionary of the English language*. Boston: American Heritage & Houghton Mifflin, 1969.

Murphy, M. L., Hultgren, H. N., Detre, K., Thomson, J., Takaro, T., and participants of the Veterans Administration Cooperative Study. Treatment of chronic stable angina. *New England Journal of Medicine*, 1977, *297*, 621–627.

Nerenz, D. R. *Control of emotional distress in cancer chemotherapy*. Unpublished doctoral dissertation, University of Wisconsin-Madison, 1979.

Nisbett, R. E., & Schachter, S. Cognitive manipulation of pain. *Journal of Experimental Social Psychology*, 1966, *2*, 227–236.

Oden, G. C., & Massaro, D. W. Integration of featural information in speech perception. *Psychological Review*, 1978, *85*, 172–191.

Parsons, T. The sick role and the role of the physician reconsidered. *Milbank Memorial Fund Quaterly*, Health & Society, 1975, 257–277.

Pennebaker, J. W., & Skelton, J. A. Psychological parameters of physical symptoms. *Personality and Social Psychology Bulletin*, 1978, *4*, 524–530.

Pennebaker, J. W., & Skelton, J. A. *Selective monitoring of bodily sensations*. Unpublished manuscript, University of Virginia, 1980.

Platt, F. W., & McMath, J. C. Clinical hypocompetence: The interview. *Annals of Internal Medicine*, 1979, *91*, 898–902.

Powers, W. T. *Behavior: The control of perception*. Chicago: Aldine, 1973.

Reinhardt, L. C. *Attention and interpretation in control of cold pressor pain and distress*. Unpublished dissertation, University of Wisconsin, Madison, 1979.

Reiser, S. J. Humanism and fact-finding in medicine. *New England Journal of Medicine*, 1978, *299*, 950–953.

Richards, A. I., & Schmale, A. H. Psychosocial conferences in medical oncology: Role in a training program. *Annals of Internal Medicine*, 1974, *80*, 541–545.

Ringler, K. Dissertation in progress. University of Wisconsin-Madison, 1981.

Robin, E. D. Determinism and humanism in modern medicine. *Journal of the American Medical Association*, 1978, *240*, 2273–2275.

Robinson, D. *The process of becoming ill*. London: Routledge & Kegan Paul, 1971.

Rogers, R. W. A protection motivation theory of fear appeals and attitude change. *Journal of Psychology*, 1975, *91*, 93–114.

Rose, R. M. Psychophysiological and hormonal responses in air traffic controllers. *Proceedings of the 1979 meeting of the Academy of Behavioral Medicine Research*.

Rosen, T. J., Terry, N. S., & Leventhal, H. The role of esteem and coping in response to a threat communication. *Journal of Experimental Research in Personality*, in press.

Rosenstock, I. M. Historical origins of the health belief model. *Health Education Monograph*, 1974, *2*(4), 328–335.

Sackett, D. L. Screening for early detection of disease: To what purpose. *Bulletin of the New York Academy of Medicine*, 1975, *51*, 39-52.

Safer, M. A., Tharps, Q., Jackson, T., & Leventhal, H. Determinants of three stages of delay in seeking care at a medical clinic. *Medical Care*, 1979, *17*(1), 11-29.

Saward, E. W. Institutional organization, incentives, and change. In J. H. Knowles (Ed.), *Doing better and feeling worse*. New York: Norton, 1977.

Scheier, M. F., & Carver, C. S. Self-focused attention and the experience of emotion: Attraction, repulsion, elation, and depression. *Journal of Personality and Social Psychology*, 1977, *35*, 624-636.

Schein, E. H. The Chinese indoctrination program for prisoners of war—a study of attempted 'brainwashing.' *Psychiatry: Journal for the Study of Interpersonal Processes*, 1956, *19*, 149-172.

Seligman, M. E. P. *Helplessness*. San Francisco: W. H. Freeman, 1975.

Snow, C. P. Human care. *Journal of the American Medical Association*, 1973, *225*, 617-621.

Solzhenitsyn, Alexandr I. *The Gulag archipelago 1918-1956: An experiment in literary investigation*. Thomas P. Whitney, (trans. from Russian). New York: Harper & Row, 1974.

Sternbach, R. A. *Pain patients: Traits and treatment*. New York: Academic Press, 1974.

Svarstad, B. Physician-patient communication and patient conformity with medical advice. In D. Mechanic (Ed.), *The growth of bureaucratic medicine*. New York: Wiley, 1976.

Thomas, L. On the science and technology of medicine. In J. H. Knowles (Ed.), *Doing better and feeling worse: Health in the United States*. New York: Norton, 1977.

Urrutia, A. M. Anxiety and pain in surgical patients. *Journal of Consulting and Clinical Psychology*, 1975, *43*, 437-442.

Veterans Administration cooperative group study on antihypertensive agents. Results in patients with diastolic blood pressure averaging 115-129 mm/Hg. *Journal of the American Medical Association*, 1967, *202*, 1028-1034.

Weisman, A. D. *Coping with cancer*. New York: McGraw-Hill, 1976.

Weiss, J. M. Psychological factors in stress and disease. *Scientific American*, 1972, *226*, 104-113.

Zajonc, R. B. Feeling and thinking: Preferences need no inferences. *American Psychologist*, 1980, *35*, 151-175.

Zborowski, M. Cultural components in response to pain. *Journal of Social Issues*, 1952, *8*, 16-30.

Zola, I. Problems of communication diagnosis and patient care. *Journal of Medical Education*, 1963, *38*, 329-338.

5 Environmental and Sensory Cues Affecting the Perception of Physical Symptoms

James W. Pennebaker
Gregory L. Brittingham
University of Virginia

Our living and working environments vary in the amount of stimulation and potential information. At times, these settings may demand our full attention, whereas, at others, they can be devoid of information. The basic tenet of the present chapter is that individuals are constantly processing information from a variety of sources—both from within their bodies as well as from the external environment. Further, the probability that people will notice and report internal physical symptoms or sensations is highly dependent on available external information. Consequently, environments that require individuals to process a great deal of external information can often reduce the degree to which physical symptoms and other internal states are noticed and reported. All this implies, then, that internal and external information are in competition. Processing one type of information can preclude the processing of another.

The relationship between internal and external information in the symptom-reporting process has important implications for environmental psychology. Environments vary considerably in their information value as well as their potentials to elicit physiological change. For example, certain architectural structures that may not be physiologically arousing can be either interesting or boring. Similarly, settings that may be equally interesting can elicit different levels of arousal due to differing ambient noise levels. An understanding of environments in terms of their informational value to the individual can aid in assessing when settings will promote or discourage attentiveness to internal state.

As advertisors in the various media are fond of reminding us, we are constantly plagued with assorted physical symptoms ranging from indigestion to the heartbreak of psoriasis. The awareness of symptoms results in millions of dollars being spent to purchase prescription and nonprescription drugs, physician visits, and countless hours of lost job time, anxiety, and discomfort. National estimates indicate that the average American is restricted to his or her activity due to illness and physical symptoms 10 days per year (NCHS, 1979). Although researchers have recently begun to examine the psychological factors influencing illness and physiological change, proportionately less research effort has been devoted to the understanding of the psychological and perceptual variables that affect our awareness of the physical symptoms themselves.

In examining the symptom-reporting process, we first discuss the psychological elements that define a symptom. We then propose a model that describes the relationship between internal and external stimuli and awareness of physical symptoms. Next, we present a review of our own and others' research efforts that supports the model. Finally, the roles of specific environmental variables on the symptom reporting process are presented.

Elements of the Physical Symptom

Very simply, a physical symptom is the *awareness* of some aspect of *internal state*. Note that this definition does not mean that there necessarily is any physiological concomitant of the symptom. Rather, the symptom is a perception. As percepts, then, we must examine both the perceptual processes involved as well as the stimulus factors (e.g., physiological change) that may influence them. A core assumption of the present chapter is that the perceptual processes that have traditionally been implicated in our perceiving external information (e.g., sights, sounds) are the same processes involved in our perceiving bodily information. Consequently, by examining research in visual and auditory perception, we can begin to understand factors influencing our awareness of physical symptoms.

As researchers in perception have long known, our awareness of an object or event depends on several factors related to both the perceiver as well as the stimulus. Some of the assumptions that we must make include the following:

1. The organism is limited in the amount of information that can be processed in a given time. Although the capacity may vary from time to time (e.g., when on the verge of sleep versus when moderately aroused), the capacity is always finite (Navon & Gopher, 1979).

2. Potential information exists both within and outside of the organism. Consequently, the search for information can oscillate between external and internal stimuli. Such an assumption is consistent with research on self-focused attention (Wicklund, 1975).

3. The probability that a given stimulus will be encoded is dependent, in part, on the number of competing stimuli available at the same time. Consequently, an organism will be more likely to encode stimulus X if no competing stimuli are present than if stimuli A, B, and C are also present in conjunction with X.

4. Similarly, certain stimulus characteristics are more likely to be encoded than others. For example, stimuli that are unique, moderately complex, or display motion will be examined in greater detail than stimuli that are redundant, simple, or stationary (Berlyne, 1960).

5. The organism is an active and selective perceiver (Gibson, 1966; Neisser, 1976). Rather than passively encoding potential information, the organism selectively searches for information that may be relevant to its past experience, needs, and expectancies. The organization of past knowledge, needs, expectancies, etc. is defined as a *schema* (also set or tentative hypothesis). The schemata that the organism holds or adopts, then, often determine which information is most likely to be attended to and encoded. The role of schemata and selective search has been discussed at length elsewhere (Garner, 1974; Newtson, 1976; Snyder, 1979). Additional assumptions concerning schemata and selective search are discussed later.

6. An individual holding a given schema is more likely to encode schema-relevant information than schema-irrelevant (Taylor & Crocker, 1978). For example, if a person was in a situation where he expected to feel tense, he would be more likely to attend to sensations that were relevant to tension than to sensations that could indicate hunger.

7. Schemata or tentative hypotheses can be adopted and discarded in a number of ways. Enduring schemata may be the result of early learning, expectancies, or interaction with others who hold given schemata. For example, a person who has had a heart attack may chronically attend to sensations that are cardiovascular relevant. Similarly, if a person has read about a given illness, he or she may selectively search his/her body for symptoms that may be indicative of the illness (Woods, Natterson & Silverman, 1966).

8. The processing of information may occur at very low levels; that is, the individual need not be aware of the fact that he/she holds a given schema nor of the way in which the external or internal environment is searched (Pennebaker, 1980).

Each of these assumptions is congruent with views of perception that deal with the encoding of external information. In order to understand how individuals perceive internal state, then, we must consider both stimulus factors as well as the cognitive structures that the individuals have adopted in dealing with their worlds.

A PERCEPTUAL MODEL OF SYMPTOM REPORTING

These assumptions about perceptual processes point to the importance of both external and internal sources of information that can affect awareness of internal state in general. Although we are primarily interested in physical symptoms and sensations, these perceptual processes should also influence the perception of other internal states such as emotion.

The preceding factors indicate that the awareness of physical symptoms can be expressed as a function of the ratio of the quantity (or salience) of potential internal information to external information. Or,

$$\text{Symptom awareness} = f \left(\frac{\text{Internal Information}}{\text{External Information}} \right)$$

Such a relationship implies that when internal information is constant, the amount of potential information in the external environment will be inversely related to symptom reporting. Similarly, when external information is invariant, the degree of potential internal information will be positively correlated with symptom reporting. At this point, the previous equation is merely intended to express the general relationship among the variables involved. We are greatly restricted in applying the relationship, because quantifying the variables is extremely difficult at this time. In the remainder of this section, we discuss the stimulus variables related to internal and external information. In addition, we point to the interdependence of the two types of information.

Internal Information.   By internal information, we mean any potential physical sensations that can be encoded. The primary stimulus factors related to internal information result from physiological activity. Various receptors throughout the body can detect mechanical deformation or pressure, temperature, physical or chemical damage in the form of pain, and, in some cases, chemical level. Stimulation of these receptors produces neuronal transmission of the information along afferent fibers within either the dorsal column or spinothalamic systems to the central nervous system. Perception of internal sensations brought about by exercise, hunger, the body's reaction to damage or disease, emotion, etc. typically derive from stimulation of appropriate receptors, which are then organized and encoded in the brain.

Two physiological factors are important in assessing potential internal information. Firstly, receptors within the body are always firing in both random and systematic ways. For example, pressure receptors from the skin are constantly firing when in contact with clothing even though we may not always perceive the sensations (unless we "consciously" attend to such stimulation). In addition, during times of heightened autonomic activity, such as during periods of anxiety, a large number of sensations are potentially available for processing. This fact is especially important during times when we may have certain body-relevant schemata. These schemata may direct our search to specific parts of the body with the result being that the schema is verified. For example, if during a period of heightened autonomic activity we adopted the schema "I might be sick," we would have an increased probability of finding some internal sensations that would verify that schema.

A second important physiological consideration is that firing of internal receptors varies in intensity. Pain or pressure can be subtle or intense. As the number of firing receptors increases, the greater the probability that we will notice internal stimulation. Further, as has long been known by psychophysicists (Stevens, 1951), the perception of sensations is a power function of the intensity of stimulation. Note that this power relationship between perception of sensation and receptor stimulation assumes that all other sources of information are controlled.

In sum, when external information is held constant, perception of internal sensations is directly related to physiological change. In addition, the intact organism almost always has at least a minimal degree of potential internal information.

External Information.   We are defining potential external information as the perception of any stimuli outside the body. Sights, sounds, and other external stimuli serve as the bases of external information. In perceiving a complex array of stimulus events, the person must provide structure for them to have meaning (Garner, 1974; Gibson, 1966). External information, then, is the organized perception of stimuli emanating outside the body. External stimuli can vary in their potential information to the individual as a function of their inherent structure. Hence, when external stimuli are random, redundant, or repetitive, they may have very little information value.

Various researchers have noted that certain types of external stimuli will contain more potential information for the perceiver than others. For example, Berlyne (1960) notes that stimulus arrays that are unique, moderately complex, or display motion will be examined in greater detail than redundant, simple or stationary arrays. Extrapolating this reasoning to potential sources of information in the natural environment, work or living settings that are constantly repetitious, bland, boring, or even random, will discourage external focus of attention and, hence, will increase the probability of processing internal sensory information.

Interdependence of External and Internal Information.   Only in very few settings is information from either internal or external stimuli constant. On occasions, the perception of an external event (e.g., seeing a bear) will result in increased internal information (e.g., racing heart, sweating, etc). Consequently, there is often a corresponding change in both external and internal information. However, as noted earlier in the hypothesized model of symptom awareness, the perception of a physical symptom is dependent on the *relative* processing of internal versus external cues.

The remainder of the chapter presents research findings from a variety of sources that offer converging support for our model of symptom awareness based on the competition of internal and external cues. Many of the cited studies are merely suggestive. Several of the large surveys are correlational rather than experimental. Nevertheless, our model serves as a simple conceptual tool by which to organize several divergent literatures.

RESEARCH EVIDENCE

Evidence supporting the contention that symptom reporting is dependent on the relative processing of internal and external cues is based on several sources. Because our own research program has attempted to experimentally test this idea directly, it is presented first. Our research falls into two categories. The first series of studies manipulated the salience of potential external information, wherein physiological change was held constant. These studies indicate that lack of external information increases awareness of internal sensations. The second series of experiments manipulated both potential internal and external information in order to evaluate their interplay.

After presenting our experimental evidence, we review several lines of research that are consistent with the competition of cues model. The literatures to be discussed include surveys of residential status, living and working environments, crowding, and relevant dispositional measures related to the reporting of physical symptoms and other internal states.

Experimental Evidence

Manipulation of External Information.   As noted previously, the probability of processing internal cues is partially dependent on the potential information in the external environment. Consequently, when external information is lacking, individuals would have a higher probability of noticing (and perhaps dwelling on) internal sensations. In situations where there is a great deal of external information to process, however, internal sensations would not be as likely to be encoded. Over the past 2 years, we have conducted several experiments to test the competition of cues idea. Three are briefly presented. The first two dealt with self-reports of physical symptoms and fatigue in exercise settings (Pennebaker & Lightner, 1980). It was predicted that subjects would report more symptoms and greater fatigue in settings where external information was lacking. The third experiment examined coughing behavior in naturalistic classroom settings (Pennebaker, 1980). We reasoned that people would be more likely to notice tickling or itching sensations in their throats and, subsequently, emit a cough, when portions of a movie they were watching were boring as compared to periods of the movie judged to be interesting.

In the first experiment, male subjects walked for 11 minutes on a treadmill on 2 days separated a week apart. During the first week, all subjects wore headphones but heard no sounds over them. During the second week of the study, subjects were randomly assigned to one of three headphone conditions. In the Sounds condition, subjects heard a variety of moderately interesting street sounds while they walked on the treadmill. The street sounds were designed to simulate sounds a person might hear as they walked from building to building (e.g., portions of conversations, music, passing cars, etc.). In the Breathing condition, subjects heard their own breathing piped over the headphones. The Control-condition subjects heard nothing over the phones. On both days of the study, blood pressure and heart rate were measured before and after walking on the treadmill. In addition, self-reports of physical symptoms and fatigue were taken immediately after the treadmill task.

Despite the fact that there were no differences in heart rate or blood pressure between conditions, large and significant self-report differences were found. As can be seen below, a composite symptom index indicated that Sound subjects reported the least symptoms, Control the next, and Breathing subjects the highest degree of symptoms. Although there was a significant overall decline in symptom reporting from Day 1 to Day 2, it was most pronounced for the Sound subjects. Comparable results were found for self-reports of fatigue. These data indicate that, although potential physiological information was constant across conditions, subjects differed substantially in the degree to which this information was processed. In the Sounds condition, subjects monitored the street sounds that they were hearing over the headphones. They had proportionately less time and

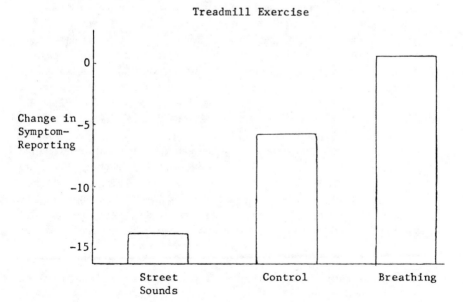

FIG. 5.1.   Change in symptom reporting from day 1 to day 2 following treadmill exercise.

capacity to encode any sensations that were related to the exercise. Breathing subjects, on the other hand, were forced to process internal sensations. Their labored breathing was apparent over the headphones and was not particularly interesting. Consequently, they devoted a great deal of time attending to all sensations related to exercise.

The second experiment was a field study in the truest sense of the word. Based on the findings of the first experiment as well as informal reports from others, we expected that the types of tracks that beginning joggers use varied considerably in the potential amount of external information. Two common types of jogging tracks are the cross-country track and the standard circular lap track. A cross-country track typically meanders through fields and woods. The jogger must be constantly alert to obstacles, turns, and bends. The standard lap track, however, simply requires the jogger to run in one lane around and around the course. There are no obstacles, no danger of collisions, and very few distractions in general. In short, a lap track is lacking in external information relative to a cross-country track.

For the second study, two jogging courses were constructed—a 200-meter circular lap track and an 1800-meter cross-country course. Both courses had an equivalent number of turns and bends. Thirteen beginning joggers ran on the two courses on alternating days for 2 weeks (excluding weekends). The joggers were required to run nine laps on the lap course and one lap on the cross-country course. Heart rate and blood pressure were measured before and after jogging each day by an experimenter. In addition, subjects completed a symptom and fatigue checklist after each day's run. One of two predictions were made. The first assumed that subjects would run at equivalent paces on the two courses but would report more symptoms and fatigue following jogging on the lap course. Alternatively, subjects could have set their jogging pace in line with their perceived fatigue levels. If so, we predicted that subjects would actually jog faster on the cross-country track but would report comparable levels of fatigue on the two courses. The results supported this second line of reasoning. Although there were no differences in self-reported fatigue and symptoms between the two courses, there were large differences in running time. When subjects ran on the cross-country course, their average time was 9.2 minutes, whereas the mean time for the lap course was 10.1 minutes. In other words, subjects ran the more interesting cross-country course almost 1 minute faster than the lap. In addition, there were no differences in heart rate or blood pressure between courses despite the large differences in running time. These two studies taken together offer support for the fact that when the external environment is lacking in information, the person is more likely to encode internal sensations related to fatigue.

One problem with using self-reported physical symptoms as dependent measures is that we have no way of knowing if the subjects are truly experiencing them. By definition, an internal sensation is a private event that cannot be monitored. The third study dealing with competition of cues used coughing as the dependent variable. A cough is typically a reaction to the perception of an itching or tickling throat (Beecher, 1959). Fortunately, for the experimenter, it is a public reaction to an internal sensation that can be monitored without the subjects' being aware of it. In one of several studies on coughing behavior (Pennebaker, 1980), we required 50 subjects to view a 17-minute movie on approach avoidance. Every 30 seconds during the movie, the subjects rated how interesting the movie had been during the previous 30 seconds, along a 7-point scale ranging from 1 = not interesting to 7 = interesting. The movie was then shown to three Introductory Psychology courses of 200, 90, and 40 students. Total number of coughs in each class was recorded every 30 seconds corresponding to the same intervals that the initial 50 subjects had rated for interest value.

The mean number of coughs per 30-second interval was then correlated with the mean interest ratings. It was predicted that during the interesting portions of the movie, subjects would process proportionately more information from the movie and less information about their irritated throats. Boring parts of the movie, on the other hand, offer less-potential external information for the viewer, which should increase the probability of each person's attending to his/her throat and subsequently emitting a cough. In fact, the data support this reasoning. The correlation between number of coughs and interest rating was a highly significant $-.57$; that is, the more interesting the movie, the fewer the number of coughs.

Each of the preceding three studies offers converging evidence for the fact that internal sensory cues are more likely to be processed when external information is lacking. Clearly, there are boundary conditions to these findings. The most obvious concerns the case where there are an overabundance of external cues that must be taken in. As various studies have shown, when persons are in a state of cognitive overload, autonomic activity increases. The increase in autonomic activity will heighten the salience of the internal information, which may then be reported as physical symptoms or sensations. This aspect of the symptom-reporting process is discussed later.

Manipulation of External and Internal Information.   Each of the preceding studies manipulated potential external information. No differences in potential internal information—as measured by heart rate and blood pressure—were found in the treadmill or jogging studies. Although no physiological indexes were monitored in the coughing study, we assume that none occurred between interesting and boring parts of the movie. The two experiments discussed here attempted to manipulate the ratio of internal versus external information (Pennebaker & Brittingham, 1979).

The studies were conducted in order to evaluate the perceptual and physiological processes that may underly recent research on person–environment (P–E) fit (French, 1973; Jaque, 1966). As is discussed in greater detail in the following section, one can express the relationship between persons' abilities and the demands of their jobs along a continuum ranging from settings where $P > E$ (i.e., the persons' abilities exceed job demands), to $P = E$ (where abilities and job demands are well-matched), to $P < E$ (abilities are below demands). In commonsense terms, when $P > E$, the job is seen as boring and represents an underload for the person. When $P < E$, the job is extremely taxing and is called an overload for the individual. The allure of the person–environment fit concept is its relationship to symptom reporting, absenteeism, and reported job dissatisfaction among workers in the "real world." Specifically, symptom reporting (Coburn, 1975) and job dissatisfaction (Caplan, Cobb, French, Harrison & Pinneau, 1975) are highest in both underload and overload settings relative to settings where there is a person–environment match. Of particular relevance to the symptom-awareness model is that although P-E fit researchers typically find a "U" relationship between degree of P-E fit for self-reports, physiological measures typically find increased autonomic activity only in overload settings (Caplan et al., 1975; Sales, 1970).

Our P-E fit analog experiments were conducted to suggest that in underload and overload settings there was a constant ratio of internal to external information resulting in comparable levels of symptom reports. However, when there was a match between task demands and the persons' abilities, external information would be encoded at the expense of internal, thus resulting in reduced symptom reporting.

Two similar laboratory experiments were conducted to learn it self-reported physical symptoms would exhibit a "U"-shaped function as a function of manipulated work-load demands. The studies differed in that the first experiment did not assess physiological change or a direct measure of attention to body, because any such measures may have artificially forced the subjects' attention to internal sensations.

In the first experiment, subjects worked simple arithmetic problems (e.g., 4 + 6 − 3) that were serially presented on a memory drum on two different occasions. On the first occasion, subjects selected their own preferred pace. The second time, pace was set by the experimenter to be either 50% faster (Fast condition), the same speed (Moderate), or 50% slower (Slow) than the original pace. Subjects completed symptom checklists after each arithmetic session.

Predictions for symptom reporting were based on the relative processing of internal and external cues. In the Moderate condition, subjects were expected to report the least number of symptoms, because they had to process on optimum amount of external information, whereas the task would not arouse them sufficiently to provide much internal information. In the Slow condition, there was expected to be very little internal as well as external information. Similarly, the Fast-condition subjects would have access to a great deal of both types of information. In both the Slow and Fast conditions, then, subjects would be more likely to report symptoms than subjects in the Moderate cell. As can be seen in Figure 5.2, change in symptom reporting from the first series of arithmetic problems to the second confirmed the prediction.

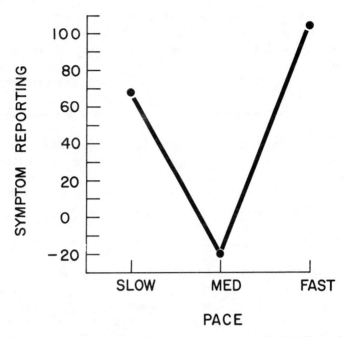

FIG. 5.2.   Change in symptom reporting from pretest to posttest for P-E fit experiment.

The second experiment was designed to tap the hypothesized perceptual and physiological processes that may have underlain the first study. In the experiment, subjects again worked on two sets of problems—the first set where they fixed the pace; the second set where the experimenter manipulated the pace to be either 50% faster, 50% slower, or the same pace as the subjects had chosen. The primary difference between the two studies was that the second experiment employed measures of autonomic activity (skin conductance) and of attention to body during the second series of working on the problems. The measure of attention to body was based on the subjects' abilities to recall six subtle bursts of air that were delivered to the subjects' forearm during the course of the study. We reasoned that if subjects were attentive to their bodies, they would be more likely to notice how many air blasts they received.

The results of the study showed that subjects again reported equivalently high levels of symptoms in the Slow and Fast conditions. Again, subjects in the Moderate cell reported a decrease in symptoms. In terms of skin conductance, Fast subjects evinced heightened autonomic activity throughout the study relative to the Slow and Moderate subjects. In terms of accuracy of recall about air blasts to the arm, only Slow subjects were consistently accurate. Both Fast and Moderate subjects were equally poor at recalling the number of air blasts that they received. These data, then, indicate that Moderate subjects were not autonomically aroused (relative to Fast subjects) and, hence, had very little potential internal information. Further, they were sufficiently preoccupied with the task that they did not notice the air blasts. Slow subjects were not greatly aroused but, unlike the Moderate subjects, had so little potential external information that they were extremely attentive to the blasts. Fast subjects had to process information from a variety of sources. They had a great deal of potential internal and external information. Even though the Fast subjects were poor at recalling the number of air blasts, the blasts represented only a portion of the potential internal information.

In sum, the second experiment points to the importance of the processing of both internal and external cues in the symptom-reporting process. Lack of external information as well as an overabundance of internal information can lead to far greater symptom reporting than situations characterized by high degrees of external and low volumes of internal information.

Environmental Research

The studies discussed previously were intended to demonstrate that the competition of cues model can account for differential symptom reporting in controlled experiments. In the present section, we present a number of studies—from Sociology, Psychology, and related disciplines—that have found evidence that is highly consistent with the competition of cues idea. All the studies discussed were examining other types of effects. Nevertheless, when considered in light of the preceding research, these studies add additional weight to the importance of considering unstimulating environments as causally related to self-reports of physical symptoms and poor health. Three environmental categories are discussed: residential status, occupation and work environment, and crowding. Additional supporting evidence from studies on personality is also presented.

Residential Status. Individuals who live alone or in social isolation could be considered to have less-external information than those living with others. The presence of others may indeed serve as one of the most powerful sources of all external information. All things being equal, one would expect the isolated individual to lack a great deal of external stimulation and information, thereby increasing the chances of attending to internal sensations. Consequently, it would be predicted that individuals who live alone would be aware of and report more physical symptoms than those who live with others. Survey data support such a claim.

One of the most common findings in the literature is that unmarried college students and adults report more physical symptoms and claim to be in worse health than their married peers (Comstock & Slome, 1973; Greenley & Mechanic, 1976; Pennebaker & Funkhouser, 1980; Wan, 1976). Similarly, the number of people living together in a household is highly related to health variables. For example, Wan (1976), in a national survey of the individuals between the ages of 58 and 63, found that people living alone reported being in worse health than if living with one or two others. In a study by Moos and Van Dort (1976), students living in social environments characterized low in unity and cohesion, student participation, and social activities complained of having far more physical symptoms than students living in more cohesive dormitories.

A related measure of attentiveness to physical symptoms is the use of aspirin and sleeping pills. In surveys conducted by the National Center for Health Statistics (NCHS, 1979), it was found that these over-the-counter-drugs were highly related to living arrangements. For example, the percentage of individuals over age 20 who use aspirin once a week or more was highest for those living alone (24.2%). Rates of weekly aspirin use among respondents living with spouse (23.4%), relatives (21.4%), or nonrelatives (16.8%) were lower. Comparable patterns of weekly use of sleeping pills were found as a function of living arrangements; living alone (8.2%), with spouse (5.2%), with relatives (6.2%), with nonrelatives (6.7%).

Another interesting line of research by Baum, Aiello, and Davis (1979) examined symptom reporting in two neighborhoods that differed in the number of daily social contacts. Although residents in the more crowded neighborhood visited physicians with slightly greater frequency, the subjects in the less-social area reported more physical symptoms. Further, as the authors point out, the residents in the less-social neighborhood spent proportionately more time indoors than outdoors and were characterized as more withdrawn in general. The various measures, then, indicated that the residents of the less-social neighborhood confronted fewer novel and/or social external information than those residing in the social neighborhood.

All the preceding studies are closely linked to research in social support and health (see Cobb, 1976, for review). There is abundant evidence indicating that individuals who have positive social networks are much less likely to have health problems in general. This appears to be due to several interdependent factors. Firstly, an adequate social support system helps to buffer individuals from the deleterious effects of major life stresses. When confronted with upheavals such as divorce, death of a loved one, etc., the person with an intact social support system can turn to others. Secondly, having access to close friends allows individuals to gain information about any physical symptoms that they may be experiencing. Such social comparison information can either alleviate anxiety about the symptoms (that would have the dual effect of reducing autonomic activity that could aggravate the problem and lessen the probability that the person would continue to focus on it), or result in the persons' receiving advice to seek medical attention concerning the symptoms. The third probable advantage of the social network is that it forces the individual to focus proportionately more time on others as opposed to one's own internal cues.

Obviously, all the previous survey findings are not strong tests of the competition of cues idea. It can easily be argued that individuals who are chronically sick or overly attentive to internal state are undesirable to live with. Hence, the physical symptoms determine the living arrangements instead of the obverse.

Occupation and Work Environment.   Whether or not a person is employed as well as the type of occupation he or she holds can also be related to the amount of external stimulation available. An employed person who enjoys his or her job should spend considerably less time focusing on and analyzing his or her internal sensations. Normative data from health surveys and recent research concerning person–environment fit support this reasoning.

Simply being employed is highly related to measures of self-reported health. For example, among Wan's (1976) sample of 58–63-year olds, the percentage of respondents who rated themselves as being in unsatisfactory health was much lower for employed subjects (11.9%) than those who were "keeping house" (32%), looking for work (15.4%), or retired (37.5%). Comparable statistics are available for aspirin and sleeping-pill use (NCHS, 1979). For example, the weekly use of aspirin was much higher for those unemployed or not in the labor force (27.8%) than among either white-collar (19.5%) or blue-collar (18.4%) workers. A similar pattern of results is found for regular sleeping-pill use: unemployed or not in labor force (9.1%) versus white-collar (3.3%) and blue-collar (2.9%) workers.

Although whether or not a person is employed is related to perceived health problems, a more interesting and direct test of the competition of cues idea in natural settings concerns the nature of the job itself. As many researchers have noted, jobs vary tremendously in their degree of complexity, interest, and stimulation. A work environment that would be seen as boring or repetitious would by definition discourage maximal processing of external cues (if, indeed, many novel external cues were present). In such situations, the employee should have a greater probability of processing internal sensations relative to workers who held more interesting occupations. Evidence for this assertion is abundant.

Moos (1975) examined people in military basic training companies to learn if recruits differed in their reported health problems as a function of the type of jobs they held. He found that his subjects were more likely to report to sick-call if they found their work boring and repetitious than if they found their job interesting. This finding is consistent with an intriguing study by Wright et al. (1977). Wright and her colleagues administered questionnaires assessing job satisfaction and symptom reports as well as physiological measures of respiratory dysfunction to 1100 smelter and mine workers of Kennecott Corporation. The researchers were interested in the relationship between self-reported lung symptoms and an objective measure of these symptoms. Overall, they found that those employees who were least satisfied with their jobs overreported respiratory symptoms (relative to the objective measure) compared to those employees who were relatively satisfied. If job satisfaction is an indicant of people's attending more to the various aspects of their job, then satisfied workers would devote less time dwelling on their internal sensations related to lung problems.

Perhaps one of the more convincing lines of research relevant to the differential processing of internal and external cues has evolved from work on person-environment fit. As discussed earlier, the degree of incongruence between workers' abilities and job demands is highly related to symptom reporting (Coburn, 1975), self-reported illness (Weiman, 1977), somatic depression (Harrison, 1976), and measures of job dissatisfaction (Caplan et al., 1975; Seybolt, 1976). The person–environment relationship can be conceptualized along several dimensions, including the congruence between the person's ideal versus actual job complexity (French, 1973), role or status (Kasl & Cobb, 1971), or work load (Caplan et al, 1975). Despite examining different continua between person and environment, researchers have consistently found the "U" function for self-reported health problems; that is, reports of illness, job dissatisfaction, etc. are higher when $P > E$ and $P < E$ than when there is a match between person and environment ($P = E$).

Although $P-E$ fit researchers typically find the "U" function for self-reports, actual physiological measures of stress (e.g., heart rate, blood pressure, catecholamine levels) are usually either nonsignificant or linear with overload workers evincing greatest autonomic activity (Caplan et al, 1975; French, 1973; Sales, 1970). The composite view of these self-report and physiological findings indicates that our previously discussed analog study may have mirrored the perceptual processes underlying the $P-E$ fit phenomena; that is, in underload settings external information is minimal, with the result being that any internal information has a higher probability of being encoded. In overload settings, both external and internal information is salient and encoded to some degree. In other words, the ratio between internal and external information is comparable in both underload and overload settings. Only in situations where there is a match between person and environment is the ratio between the two sources of information different; that is, when $P = E$, there is an optimal amount of external information to be processed relative to low levels of sensory information.

As with the studies on residential status, the present review of occupation and work settings is based on correlational survey research. Again, it is possible that individuals with chronic illness or who are predisposed to complain about their health have difficulties finding employment, and, when they do, they end up in objectively unsatisfying jobs. Although this alternative explanation may account for a portion of the variance, the converging findings continue to be consistent with the competition of cues explanation.

Crowding.   An environmental stimulus that has received much interest in the past few years is that of high population density and its effect on human performance, mood, and health. Beginning with the animal research by Calhoun (1962) and Christian (Christian & Davis, 1972; Christian, Flyger, & Davis, 1960), it was assumed by many researchers that the existence of high density always results in negative consequences for the individual—both mentally and physically (Sundstrom, 1978). As research has progressed, it has become clear that the experience of crowding is not a simple phenomenon but one that is mediated by situational, social, and even physiological factors. Most researchers now feel that crowding is characterized by an increase in autonomic activity. Interestingly, it has been posited that states of increased arousal due to crowding is not necessarily negative or aversive (Epstein & Karlin, 1975; Freedman, 1975; Worchel & Teddlie, 1976). These views, then, imply that the experience of crowding is related to the type and quantity of information that the individual encodes.

Recent explanations of crowding stress many of the same factors that have been advanced by person–environment fit researchers. For example, Altman (1975) argues that crowding is a problem of privacy regulation. According to this view, crowding is the result of excessive social stimulation—excessive in that it is greater than the desired level for the individual at that time. Similarly, Milgram (1970) proposes that the complexity of the environment is critical to crowding. The individual becomes overloaded by too much external stimulus information. The experience of crowding, then, should increase as environmental complexity increases. These approaches are in general accord with other research demonstrating that crowding occurs more often in large groups, even when density is relatively constant (Sundstrom, 1975).

It is important to note that although the previous approaches differ in their theoretical perspectives, they share one important assumption; that is, high density is neither necessary nor sufficient for the psychological state of crowding to occur. Because both demographic (Mitchell, 1971; Ward, 1975) and laboratory studies (Freedman, 1975; Freedman, Klevansky, & Ehrlich, 1971) have failed to find negative consequences on behavior solely as a result of density, a simple density = crowding model is not viable (Stokols, 1972, 1978). In order to understand crowding, then, it has become important to examine both perceptual and physiological variables.

In light of the framework presented on symptom reporting and competition of cues, it is possible to consider the perception of being crowded as a symptom in that it represents a perception of internal state. Clearly, crowding studies have found that the experience of crowding is related to potential internal information in the form of increased physiological activity (Aiello, Epstein, & Karlan, 1975; Bergman, 1971; Evans, 1975; McBride, King, & James, 1965; Middlemist, Knowles, & Matter, 1976; Saegert, 1974). Interestingly, increased autonomic activity does not always result in the perception of crowding; that is, the amount and type of external information that the person encodes is often highly related to self-reports of crowding.

An interesting example in the literature illustrates when subjects may be differentially processing internal versus external information, thus resulting in varying perceptions of crowding. Both Joy and Lehmann (1975) and Baum and Davis (1976) found that increased visual interest or variety may lead to a decrease in perceptions of crowding. Similarly, Worchel and Teddlie (1976) reported finding a reduction in crowding when pictures were added to a room. Although Desor (1972) found that one type of visual array (the number of doors in the setting) resulted in increased perceptions of crowding, this disparity may be due to the fact that, across studies, there are different degrees of potential internal and external information. Unfortunately, it is difficult to assess the degree of autonomic activity from study to study due to the fact that in many cases physiological measures were not used, or the indexes that were monitored differed. Nevertheless, it is becoming increasingly clear that subjects are differentially processing internal and external cues in making subjective estimates of perceived crowding. Future research in this field may benefit from trying to determine when and what types of information the crowded and uncrowded subjects are encoding.

Personality Measures. Just as individuals differentially process internal and external cues over time, individuals vary in the degree to which they chronically process information from their body versus the external environment. Some of the dispositional factors that have been found to be related to the differential processing of internal and external information and the reporting of symptoms include measures of inner attentiveness and the Type-A coronary-prone behavior pattern.

A person who chronically processes internal information should, by definition, report more physical symptoms. For example, Greenley and Mechanic (1976) note that students who report identifying with introspective others report more symptoms than students who do not. Similarly, measures of repression sensitization are correlated with the frequency and severity of reported illness and health-center utilization (Byrne, Steinberg, & Schwartz, 1968). Sensitizers process more internal sensory information and, according to the researchers, more readily perceive the onset of illness. Of particular relevance is recent correlational data concerning self-consciousness (Fenigstein, Scheier, & Buss, 1975). Individuals who score as high in private self-consciousness are attentive to their thoughts and moods. In several large-scale surveys, we have found that self-consciousness consistently correlates positively and significantly with symptom reporting (Pennebaker & Skelton, 1978; Skelton & Pennebaker, 1978). A particularly intriguing measure that appears to be related to the processing of internal sensory information is anxiety level. In fact, about 25% of the items on the Manifest Anxiety Scale (Taylor, 1953) are symptom items (e.g., "I often have butterflies in my stomach"). Not surprisingly, then, trait measures of anxiety correlate highly with other indexes of symptom reporting (Lipman, Rickels, Covi, Derogatis, & Uhlenhuth, 1969). In an interesting article on test anxiety, Wine (1971) suggests that high test-anxious individuals perform poorly on exams because they are processing a disproportionate amount of information from their bodies than from the tests or task at hand. If Wine's hypothesis is true, it serves as an excellent example of dysfunctional processing of internal cues.

Another individual difference measure, the Type-A coronary-prone behavior pattern, appears to tap differential processing of internal and external cues. The Type-A individual is characterized as hard driving, competitive, and time urgent (Glass, 1977). The Type-A's counterpart—Type B—lacks these traits. The importance of the A–B distinction is that the Type A is seven times more likely to succomb to heart failure than the B. Recent research indicates that A's and B's differ radically in the degree to which they process external information. At resting levels, Type A's actually report slightly more physical symptoms (Skelton & Pennebaker, 1978) and evince marginally greater autonomic activity (Glass, 1977). However, recent research by Weidner and Matthews (1978) indicates that while involved in a complex task, the A reports significantly fewer physical symptoms than the B; that is, when required to complete an important task, the Type A processes external information to the exclusion of internal sensory information relative to the Type B.

Although no systematic attempts have yet been made at devising a direct dispositional measure of the relative processing of internal sensory and external environmental information, the findings based on inner attentiveness and Type A suggest that systematic individual differences exist. Why they exist is not entirely clear. Early parental training, bouts with major illness or accident, and even heritability factors are prime candidates. To repeat an oft-made expression, further research is needed.

SUMMARY

In this chapter, we have sketched a model for symptom reporting based on how individuals differentially process internal and external cues. Laboratory and survey studies consistently find that when potential internal information is constant, the probability of reporting physical symptoms is inversely related to the amount of potential external information extant in the environment. When the environment is boring, redundant, insufficiently unique or complex, the individual is more likely to search his or her body for any sensory cues.

Our approach is based on current perspectives of perception and information processing. The ways in which we perceive private sensory events parallel the processes involved in the perception of external events. The body represents a source of information for the individual. Note that we have focused exclusively on the competition of internal and external cues. Perception is obviously far more complex and dynamic. A major aspect of the perceptual process that we have intentionally neglected is the role of schemata and selective search. Although this portion of the perceptual process as it relates to physical symptoms is discussed elsewhere (Pennebaker, 1981; Pennebaker & Skelton, 1978, 1981), it cannot be overlooked.

Individuals are active and selective perceivers. We do not passively wait for internal or external stimuli to bombard our senses. Rather, we constantly search for any type of information that may be self-relevant. Consequently, the schemata that we adopt may result in biased search and thus misperception of either internal or external stimuli. A symptom-relevant example can be seen in cases of "medical students' disease" (Woods et al., 1966). First year medical students are under constant stress (i.e., have a great deal of potential internal information). In addition, they read and hear about many types of exotic diseases characterized by specific constellations of symptoms. When reading about a given disease, they are likely to focus on highly specific sensations that they too may have (i.e., schema-guided search) and subsequently believe that they, too, have the disease. This example suggests that a variety of environmental settings may prompt selective search for sensations. Consequently, the awareness and reporting of physical symptoms can depend on the schemata that are held rather than solely on the potential ratio of internal and external stimuli present at the time.

Despite the importance of schemata and selective search, environmental psychologists and other researchers must weigh settings for their potential to provide optimal external and internal stimulation. Any work, living, or social setting that promotes heightened awareness of benign physical symptoms may result in needless medical expenses, discomfort, and anxiety. Future research must consider how such factors as architectural design, noise and light levels, and a host of related environmental stimuli can influence the perception of internal state.

REFERENCES

Aiello, J. R., Epstein, Y. M., & Karlin, R. A. Effects of crowding on electrodermal activity. *Sociological Symposium*, 1975, *14*, 43–57.

Altman, I. *The environment and social behavior: Privacy, personal space, territory and crowding*. Monterey, Calif.: Brooks/Cole, 1975.

Baum, A., Aiello, J., & Davis, G. *Urban stress, withdrawal and health*. Paper presented at American Psychological Association, New York, 1979.

Baum, A., & Davis, G. Spatial and social aspects of crowding perception. *Environment and Behavior*, 1976, *8*, 527–544.

Beecher, H. K. *Measurement of subjective responses: Quantitative effects of drugs*. New York: Oxford University Press, 1959.

Bergman, B. A. The effects of group size, personal space, and success-failure on physiological arousal, test performance, and questionnaire response. Unpublished Doctoral Dissertation, Temple University, Department of Psychology, Philadelphia, Pa., 1971 (*Abstract, Dissertation Abstracts International*, 1971, 2319–3420-A).

Berlyne, D. *Conflict, arousal, and curiousity*. New York: McGraw-Hill, 1960.

Byrne, D., Steinberg, M., & Schwartz, M. Relationship between repression sensitization and physical illness. *Journal of Abnormal Psychology*, 1968, *73*, 154–155.

Calhoun, J. B. Population density and social pathology. *Scientific American*, 1962, *206*(2), 139–148.

Caplan, R. D., Cobb, S., French, J. P. R., Harrison, R., & Pinneau, S. *Job demands and worker health*. Washington, D. C.: U. S. Government Printing Office, 1975.

Christian, J. J., & Davis, D. E. Endocrines, behavior, and population. In C. Toepfer, A Bicknell, L. Fox, W. Krik, & R. Sayre (Eds.), *Environmental Psychology: Selected Readings*. MSS Information Corporation, New York, 1972.

Christian, J. J., Flyger, V., & Davis, D. E. Factors in mass mortality of a herd sika deer (Cervus nippon). *Chesapeake Science*, 1960, *1*, 79-95.

Cobb, S. Social support as a moderator of life stress. *Psychosomatic Medicine*, 1976, *38*, 300-314.

Coburn, D. Job-worker incongruence: Consequences for health. *Journal of Health and Social Behavior*, 1975, *16*, 198-212.

Comstock, L., & Slome, C. A health survey of students, 1: Prevalence of problems. *Journal of American College of Health Associations*, 1973, *22*, 150-155.

Desor, J. A. Toward a psychological theory of crowding. *Journal of Personality and Social Psychology*, 1972, *21*, 79-83.

Epstein, Y. M., & Karlin, R. A. Effects of acute experimental crowding. *Journal of Applied Social Psychology*, 1975, *5*, 34-53.

Evans, G. W. *Behavioral and physiological consequences of crowding in humans*. Unpublished Doctoral Dissertation, University of Massachusetts, Department of Psychology, Amherst, 1975.

Fenigstein, A., Scheier, M., & Buss, A. Public and private self-consciousness: Assessment and theory. *Journal of Consulting and Clinical Psychology*, 1975, *43*, 522-527.

Freedman, J. L. *Crowding and Behavior*. San Francisco: W. H. Freeman, 1975.

Freedman, J. L., Klevansky, S., & Ehrlich, P. R. The effect of crowding on human task performance. *Journal of Applied Social Psychology*, 1971, *1*, 7-25.

French, J. Person role fit. *Occupational Mental Health*, 1973, *3*, 15-20.

Garner, W. *The processing of information and structure*. Potomac, Md.: Lawrence Erlbaum Associates, 1974.

Gibson, J. J. *The senses considered as perceptual systems*. Boston: Houghton Mufflin, 1966.

Glass, D. C. *Behavior patterns, stress, and coronary disease*. Hillsdale, N. J.: Lawrence Erlbaum Associates, 1977.

Greenley, J., & Mechanic, D. Social selection in seeking help for psychological problems. *Journal of Health and Social Behavior*, 1976, *17*, 249-262.

Harrison, R. *Job stress as person-environment fit*. American Psychological Association, Washington, 1976.

Jaques, E. Executive organization and individual adjustment. *Journal of Psychosomatic Research*, 1966, *10*, 77-82.

Joy, V. D., & Lehmann, N. *The cost of crowding: Responses and adaptations*. Unpublished manuscript, New York State Department of Mental Hygiene, 1975.

Kasl, S., & Cobb, S. Physical and mental health correlates of status incongruence. *Social Psychiatry*, 1971, *6*, 1-10.

Lipman, R., Rickels, K., Covi, L., Derogatis, L., & Uhlenhuth, E. Factors of symptom distress. *Archives of General Psychiatry*, 1969, *21*, 328-338.

McBride, G., King, M. G., & James, J. W. Social proximity effects on galvonic skin response in human adults. *Journal of Psychology*, 1965, *61*, 153-157.

Middlemist, R. D., Knowles, E. S., & Matter, C. F. Personal space invasions in the lavatory: Suggestive evidence for arousal. *Journal of Personality and Social Psychology*, 1976, *33*, 541-546.

Milgram, S. The experience of living in cities. *Science*, 1970, *167*, 1461-1468.

Mitchell, R. E. Some social implications of high density housing. *American Sociological Review*, 1971, 36, 18-29.

Moos, R. *Evaluating correctional and community settings*. New York: Wiley, 1975.

Moos, R., & Van Dort, B. *Student physical symptoms and the social climate of college living groups.* Unpublished manuscript, Stanford University, Social Ecology Laboratory, Department of Psychiatry and Behavioral Sciences, 1976.

National Center for Health Statistics. *Acute conditions: Incidence and associated disability, United States, July 1977–June 1978.* Public Health Service Series 10, Number 132. Washington, D. C.: Government Printing Office, 1979.

National Center for Health Statistics. *Use habits among adults of cigarettes, coffee, aspirin, and sleeping pills.* Public Health Series 10, Number 131. Washington, D. C.: Government Printing Office, 1979.

Navon, D., & Gopher, D. On the economy of the human-processing system. *Psychological Review,* 1979, *86,* 214-255.

Neisser, U. *Cognition and reality.* San Francisco: Freeman, 1976.

Newtson, D. Foundations of attribution: The perception of ongoing behavior. In J. Harvey, W. Ickes, & R. Kidd (Eds.), *New directions in attribution research* (Vol. 1). Hillsdale, N. J.: Lawrence Erlbaum Associates, 1976.

Pennebaker, J. W. Perceptual and environmental determinants of coughing. *Basic and Applied Social Psychology,* 1980, *1,* 83-91.

Pennebaker, J. W. Social and perceptual factors influencing symptom reporting and mass psychogenic illness. In M. Colligan, J. Pennebaker, & L. Murphy (Eds.), *Mass psychogenic illness: A social psychological analysis.* Hillsdale, N. J.: Lawrence Erlbaum Associates, 1982.

Pennebaker, J. W., & Brittingham, G. L. Situational and attentional factors influencing health: Person-Environment Fit. *American Psychological Association,* New York, 1979.

Pennebaker, J. W., & Funkhouser, J. E. *The influences of social support, activity, and life change on use of medication among an elderly population.* Unpublished manuscript (mimeo), University of Virginia, 1980.

Pennebaker, J. W., & Lightner, J. Competition of internal and external cues in an exercise setting. *Journal of Personality and Social Psychology,* 1980, *39,* 165-174.

Pennebaker, J., & Skelton, J. Psychological parameters of physical symptoms. *Personality and Social Psychology Bulletin,* 1978, *4,* 524-530.

Pennebaker, J. W., & Skelton, J. A. Selective monitoring of physical sensations. *Journal of Personality and Social Psychology,* 1981, *41,* 213-223.

Saegert, S. C. *Effects of spatial and social density on arousal, mood, and social orientation.* Unpublished Doctoral Dissertation, Department of Psychology, University of Michigan, Ann Arbor, 1974.

Sales, S. Some effects of role overload and role underload. *Organizational Behavior and Human Performance,* 1970, *5,* 592-608.

Seybolt, J. Work satisfaction as a function of person–environment interaction. *Organizational Behavior: Human Performance,* 1976, *17,* 66-75.

Skelton, J., & Pennebaker, J. Dispositional determinants of symptom reporting: Correlational evidence. *American Psychological Association,* Toronto, 1978.

Snyder, M. Self-monitoring processes. In L. Berkowitz (Ed.), *Advances in experimental social psychology* (Vol. 12). New York: Academic, 1979.

Stevens, S. S. *Handbook of experimental psychology.* New York: Wiley, 1951.

Stokols, D. On the distinction between density and crowding: Some implications for further research. *Psychological Review,* 1972, *79,* 275-277.

Stokols, D. A typology of crowding experiences. In A. Baum and Y. Epstein (Eds.), *Human Response to Crowding.* Hillsdale, N. J.: Lawrence Erlbaum Associates, 1978.

Sundstrom, E. An experimental study of crowding: Effects of room-size, intrusion, and goal-blocking on nonverbal behaviors, self-disclosure, and self-reported stress. *Journal of Personality and Social Psychology,* 1975, *32* (4), 645-654.

Sundstrom, E. Crowding as a sequential process: Review of research on the effects of population density on humans. In J. Baum and Y. Epstein (Eds.), *Human Response to Crowding*. Hillsdale, N. J.: Lawrence Erlbaum Associates, 1978.

Taylor, J. A personality scale of manifest anxiety. *Journal of Abnormal and Social Psychology*, 1953, *48*, 285-290.

Taylor, S. E., & Crocker, J. Schematic bases of social information processing. *Paper presented at First Ontario Symposium on Personality and Social Psychology: Cognitive structure and processes underlying person memory and social judgment*. August, 1978.

Wan, T. Predicting self-assessed health status: A multivariate approach. *Health Services Research*, 1976, *11*, 464-477.

Ward, L. Overcrowding and social pathology: A re-examination of the implications for the human population. *Human Ecology*, 1975.

Weidner, G., & Matthews, K. Reported physical symptoms elicited by unpredictable events and the type-A coronary-prone behavior pattern. *Journal of Personality and Social Psychology*, 1978, *36*, 1213-1220.

Weiman, C. A study of occupational stressor and the incidence of disease/risk. *Journal of Occupational Medicine*, 1977, *19*, 119-122.

Wicklund, R. A. Objective self-awareness. In L. Berkowitz (Ed.), *Advances in experimental social psychology* (Vol. 8). New York: Academic, 1975.

Wine, J. Test anxiety and direction of attention. *Psychology Bulletin*, 1971, *76*, 92-104.

Woods, S., Natterson, J., & Silverman, J. Medical students' disease: Hypochondriasis in medical education. *Journal of Medical Education*, 1966, *41*, 785-790.

Worchel, S., & Teddlie, C. The experience of crowding: A two-factor theory. *Journal of Personality and Social Psychology*, 1976, 34, 30-40.

Wright, D., Kane, R., Olsen, D., & Smith, T. The effects of selected psychosocial factors on the self-reporting of pulmonary symptoms. *Journal of Chronic Disease*, 1977, *30*, 195-206.

6

Hospital Design and Human Behavior: a Review of the Recent Literature

Janet E. Reizenstein
University of Michigan

INTRODUCTION

The effects of hospital environments on their human users have long been of interest. From the time of Florence Nightingale, the design of the hospital has been viewed as an important and integral part of the therapeutic milieu. As more hospital environments are studied, an increasing amount is learned about the various impacts of this environment on patients and staff. Yet, some of the same design concepts are used over and over in hospital design, regardless of their often negative effects on users. This leads one to ask if this existing literature on hospital design and behavior is utilized in design decision making.

The question of research utilization has been a major concern of many in the Environment-Behavior field. One major approach has been to focus on the architecture profession as the intended recipient of this research, often however, with unsuccessful and unsatisfying results. There has been much speculation as to why this "research translation" or "interdisciplinary collaboration" has not lived up to enthusiasts' expectations (Reizenstein, 1975).

The problem with this approach appears to lie in its assumption that architects are synonomous with all design decision makers. One reason for making this assumption is that many in the Environment-Behavior field are interested in looking at buildings as they are designed, rather than in observing how they are utilized and altered over their life cycle. Looking at design decision making as something that happens only in relation to the design of new buildings leads many to conclude, although falsely,[1] that architects should be the major beneficiaries of research findings.

---

[1]Because others are making decisions at this stage as well.

Taking a more long-term approach, it is clear that the architect's contractual responsibility ends when the building is first occupied and that many others are responsible for design decisions over time (allocation, furnishings, policies, renovation, etc.). However, we know very little either about those who make these ongoing spatial decisions or about what criteria they use (Reizenstein, 1977).

Thus, the problem of utilization of the literature on hospital design and human behavior seems to rest on the answers to three questions: (1) What research is available that could potentially be applied to hospital design decisions?; (2) what characterizes ongoing spatial decision-making processes in hospitals?; (3) how best might there be a match between the two? This chapter is a response to the first of these questions: What research is available that could potentially be applied to hospital design decision making? However, claims for the exhaustiveness of this review should be qualified. Firstly and most important, this is a review of literature that specifically focuses on hospital design and human behavior. None of the rest of the body of Environment–Behavior research literature is included, although much of it is applicable to this setting. The somewhat negative conclusions that are drawn about the scope and quality of this research do not mean that there is not a great deal that can be contributed by Environmental Psychologists and Sociologists to humanizing hospital design and ongoing hospital-design processes. Secondly, this literature review is not exhaustive because it does not cover every article or book ever written on this topic. Rather, it focuses on work that appeared during a 10-year period, roughly from 1969–1979. Thirdly, the review is not exhaustive because it omits a number of articles and/or books from those that appeared during this period. The most important reason for rejection was if a piece was purely descriptive, having no empirical basis.

The following bibliographic sources were searched:

1. Dissertation Abstracts (1974–1980).
2. Hospital Literature Index (1975–1979).
3. Abstracts of Hospital Management Studies (1974–1979).
4. Index Medicus (1975–1980).
5. Sociology Abstracts (1970–1980).
6. Architectural Index (1973–1978).
7. Council of Planning Librarians Bibliographies (All).
8. Proceedings of the Environmental Design Research Association Conferences (1969–1980).
9. Man–Environment References (1969–1974).

The next section on characteristics of the literature forms the main body of the chapter. Topics of discussion include: type of source in which the piece of literature is found, the country in which it was written, the type of hospital studied, the nature of the study, factors affected by hospital design, and design and planning issues discussed. This is followed by a brief discussion of utilization of this research in health facility planning and of areas in which further research is needed.

CHARACTERISTICS OF THE LITERATURE

Type of Source

Sources include both books (including chapters, monographs, dissertations, pamphlets) and journals. As described in Table 6.1, four types of journals contained articles on behavior and hospital design: hospital journals, architectural journals, medical journals, and one sociological journal. The largest number of relevant pieces was found in books (34), followed by hospital journals (21), architectural journals (17), and medical journals (14).

This breakdown demonstrates that there is a problem merely locating literature on hospital design and human behavior; a strike against its easy utilization by hospital design decision makers. It is clear from Table 6.1 that one cannot obtain all the relevant information from any single source. However, if professionals are likely to read only journals that are in their own field (and few are able to read even all of these), then a hospital administrator, hypothetically speaking, would be exposed to only one quarter of the information available on this topic, an architect slightly less, and a physician less yet. In addition, one could speculate that almost no one would be willing or able to regularly scan 30 different journals and keep track of new books and monographs, conference proceedings, and the like.

Country

Although a majority of the works reviewed here are American in origin (69), a sizable number (18) come from the United Kingdom, especially Great Britain. Taking into consideration such factors as size of the two powers, this might not seem surprising. However, a somewhat different picture emerges when the literature emanating from each country is divided into empirical and nonempirical work, as shown in Table 6.2. This table shows roughly[2] that the United Kingdom has a much larger percentage of empirical work, given its total output, than does the United States: 78% of the British work is empirically based, compared with 45% of the American work.

---

[2]A limitation of this and other tables in this chapter is that books and articles are given the same weight regardless of size.

TABLE 6.1
Type of Source

(Numbers Refer to Bibliography)
Books (monograph, dissertation, pamphlet or chapter)

13, 18, 19, 22, 25, 28, 29, 31, 34, 38, 42, 44, 45, 46, 47, 48, 49, 52, 54, 57, 58, 60, 61, 63, 67, 68, 70, 72, 76, 77, 81, 82, 84, 87

Hospital Journals

Archives of Internal Medicine	85
Dimensions in Health Service	37
Health Services Research	80
Hospital Administration in Canada	40
Hospital Progress	71
Hospital Topics	16, 32, 62
Hospitals	7, 8, 9, 15, 17, 59, 73
Modern Health Care	2, 33, 78
Nursing Research	56
Nursing Times	5
Topics in Health Care Financing	39

Architectural Journals

American Institute of Architects Journal	35
Architects Journal	21
Architectural Record	4, 53
Ekistics	75
Environment & Behavior	41, 79, 86
Human Factors	50, 69
Interior Design	6
J. of Architectural Education	10
J. of Architectural Research	12, 20, 65, 66
Progressive Architecture	14

Medical Journals

Am. J. Orthopsychiatry	27
Anasthesia	43
Hospital and Community Psychiatry	3, 11, 26, 55, 74, 83
J. Counselling Psychology	23
J. Hygiene	51
J. Psychosomatic Research	36
Medical Journal of Australia	1
Mental Hygiene	24
Practitioner	30

Sociological Journals

Sociological Review	64

TABLE 6.2
Type of Research by Country

		Country	
		United States	United Kingdom
Type of Research	Empirical	10, 13, 14, 23, 24, 35, 41, 42, 45, 46, 47, 50, 52, 54, 55, 56, 60, 61, 63, 66, 67, 68, 70, 73, 74, 76, 77, 79, 83, 84, 86	12, 20, 21, 22, 38, 43, 44, 51, 57, 58, 64, 65, 80, 85
	Non-Empirical	2, 3, 4, 5, 6, 7, 8, 9, 11, 15, 16, 17, 18, 19, 25, 26, 27, 28, 29, 30, 31, 32, 33, 34, 37, 39, 48, 49, 53, 59, 62, 69, 71, 72, 75, 78, 81, 82	1, 36, 40, 87

Summary of Table 6.2

		United States	United Kingdom
Empirical		31 studies	14 studies
		(45%)	(78%)
Non-Empirical		38 studies	4 studies
		(55%)	(22%)
		100%	100%

Type of Hospital

It would seem from these tables that the British, more than the Americans, see a need to base decisions related to hospital design on research. In fact, the British are responsible for one of the landmark studies in this field: a large, early series of empirical studies on the design and function of hospitals (Nuffield, 1955). There appears to be nothing comparable in the American literature, then or now.

Table 6.3 shows how the reviewed literature falls with regard to its relevance to acute-care hospitals versus nonacute-care facilities. Slightly over three quarters (78%) deal with acute-care facilities, such as small community general hospitals or large teaching hospitals. Just under one quarter (22%) apply to nonacute-care or specialized facilities. Of these, the kind of facility having the most literature associated with it is the psychiatric hospital. Some work has been done in children's hospitals (one of these was a children's psychiatric facility), and one study was done in an obstetrical hospital.

TABLE 6.3
Type of Hospital

(Numbers refer to Bibliography)

Acute Care

1, 2, 4, 5, 6, 7, 8, 9, 12, 13, 14, 15, 16, 17, 19, 20, 23, 25, 27, 28, 30, 31, 32, 33, 36, 37, 39, 40, 42, 43, 44, 45, 46, 47, 48, 50, 51, 52, 53, 54, 56, 57, 58, 59, 60, 61, 62, 63, 64, 65, 67, 69, 71, 72, 76, 77, 78, 79, 80, 81, 82, 84, 85, 87

Non-Acute or Specialized Care

Psychiatric
3, 10, 11, 22, 24, 26, 34, 35, 41, 55, 73, 74, 75, 83

Children's
21, 49, 86

Obstetric
70

Other
18, 29, 38, 66, 68

Again, as with the US/UK comparison, it would seem tempting to merely conclude that there is more work in the area of human behavior and hospital design done in acute-care rather than nonacute-care facilities. However, Table 6.4 shows how this picture is altered when the type of hospital is cross tabulated with type of study (empirical versus non-empirical). If empirical research is taken as a proxy for good quality research, then we can see that a much larger percentage of the literature on nonacute-care facilities such as psychiatric hospitals is empirical (67%), compared to the percentage of empirical literature relevant to acute-care hospitals (44%).

Why should this be the case? One reason might lie in perceived characteristics

TABLE 6.4
Type of Study by Type of Hospital

		Type of Hospital	
		Acute Care	Non-Acute or Specialized Care
Type of Study	Empirical	12, 13, 14, 23, 42, 43, 44, 45, 46, 47, 50, 51, 52, 54, 56, 57, 58, 60, 61, 63, 64, 65, 67, 77, 79, 80, 84, 85	10, 21, 22, 24, 35, 41, 55, 70, 73, 74, 83, 86
	Non-Empirical	1, 2, 4, 5, 6, 7, 8, 9, 15, 16, 17, 19, 20, 25, 27, 28, 30, 31 32, 33, 36, 37, 39, 40, 49, 53 59, 62, 69, 71, 72, 78, 81, 82 87	3, 11, 26, 34, 48, 75

Summary of Table 6.4

	Acute Care	Non-Acute or Specialized Care
Empirical	28 studies (44%)	12 studies (67%)
Non-Empirical	35 studies (56%)	6 studies (33%)
	100%	100%

of patients; that is, one characteristic common to both children (sick or not) and psychiatric patients is that they have little or no control over their lives. Especially in hospital settings, they have little power or say in what happens to them. Their tendency to participate in research without questioning it makes them seen by some as excellent potential research subjects. Another characteristic of psychiatric patients that makes them desirable subjects is their average length of stay, which tends to be longer than that for acute-care patients. Thus, studies on long-term effects of environment on behavior are much more feasible with this group.

Another reason for more empirical work being done in nonacute-care facilities such as psychiatric hospitals stems from philosophy of care. The term *therapeutic milieu* connotes the idea that the entire system that the patient experiences may contribute to his or her care. The physical environment has traditionally been seen as part of this therapy, at least in psychiatry. As described in Good, Siegel and Bay (1965), Dr. T. S. Kirkbride's (1880) book, entitled *On the Construction, Organization and General Arrangement of Hospitals for the Insane,* was based on his observations of the ways people used and behaved in buildings. He advocated a cheerful and comfortable appearance: "everything repulsive and prisonlike should be carefully avoided." He suggested an average of 15 patients to a ward and a design based on "a central hallway with parlors at the end and an alcove protruding." (p. 41)

Gordon (1976) hypothesizes another reason why more empirical work is done in psychiatric hospitals: "In the past fifteen years, psychiatrists have expressed increasing awareness of the effect of hospital and treatment environments, though published observations from surgical and medical colleagues remain sparse. Hospital staff soon develop defenses to protect themselves in their work environment and become less perceptive of its potential effects on others [p. 363]." This is an interesting hypothesis, probably worthy of testing.

Type of Study

Table 6.5 divides the reviewed literature into the empirically based and the nonempirical. About half the cited works fall into each category. The nonempirical work is further divided into the purely descriptive, guidelines based on some sort of research, guidelines not based on research, and two literature reviews.

TABLE 6.5
Type of Study

(Numbers refer to Bibliography)

Empirical

10, 12, 13, 14, 20, 21, 22, 23, 24, 35, 38, 41, 42, 43, 44, 45, 46, 47, 50, 51, 52, 54, 55, 56, 57, 58, 60, 61, 63, 64, 65, 66, 67, 68, 70, 73, 74, 76, 77, 79, 80, 84, 85, 86

Non-Empirical

Descriptive
2, 3, 4, 6, 7, 8, 9, 11, 27, 33, 36, 59, 71, 78, 87

Design Guidelines (Research Based)
15, 25, 26, 28, 31, 37, 39, 48, 49, 53, 62, 69, 72, 75, 81, 83

Design Guidelines (Not Research Based)
1, 5, 16, 17, 18, 19, 30, 32, 40

Literature Review
29, 82

Other
34

Empirical

Unfortunately, there is not a great deal of published empirical research in the area of hospital design and behavior. Most of these are described later in the section on factors affected by hospital design, but four studies are particularly worthy of note: those by Canter (1972), Kenny and Canter (1978), Noble and Dixon (1977), and Olsen (1978).

Olsen (1978) compared the effects of design and social-program differences seen on a traditional surgical floor and a "progressive patient care" floor in an acute-care hospital on behaviors and attitudes of patients. One notable aspect of Olsen's work is his focus on the patient as the key user and respondent. He (Olsen, 1978) describes the hospital setting as a "low choice" environment because: "Occupants live in settings with minimal amounts of space to use, finite and frequently small ranges of available activities to pursue and restricted opportunities for human contact. The choice of where to go, what to do and when and with whom to do it is curtailed in these total settings to a degree incomparable with the outside world [p. 3]."

He (Olsen, 1978) points out the symbolic function of the physical environment of the hospital, saying that it can transmit messages to patients that they are: "independent, competent individuals on the road back to health," or it may tell them that they are: "very sick and dependent and should behave in an accordingly passive manner, even though their physical condition no longer requires it [p. 7]."

Olsen found that patients on the progressive patient-care floor that had more "spatial options" and a less-institutional appearance rated their environment as more pleasant and cheerful than their counterparts on the more traditional surgical floor and also saw a more positive relationship between their setting and their mood (p. 126).

He also reports: "These patients were more mobile, more social, less passive, felt less confined and attributed specific positive affect to their unit and its options more frequently than did the comparable sample [p. 126]."

Canter (1972) evaluated a children's hospital in Scotland. His evaluation is divided into two parts: The first is an analysis of the concepts about the hospital held by the architect and a representative user, a senior nursing officer. The second part is an evaluation of satisfaction with the hospital, using nursing and medical staff, as well as mothers of the patients as respondents, because it was difficult to get useful information from the children themselves. He used both attitudinal measures (interviews and questionnaires) and behavioral measures (observation) and found a high level of satisfaction with most aspects of the hospital's design. Canter's study is notable for its careful consideration of the design process. It is an example of a fairly comprehensive empirical study of the effects of hospital design on behavior and is well-illustrated throughout. A drawback is that it is somewhat difficult to locate his major points, and implications of these findings for other projects are not made clear.

Using questionnaire data, Noble and Dixon (1977) evaluated three different types of ward design within a single hospital in London, England, from the viewpoints of both staff and patients. Their monograph is well-illustrated with floorplans and photographs and analyzes each ward in relation to doctors', nurses', and patients' requirements. A summary of findings and a discussion of which of these might be generalizable to other hospitals would have made this document more widely usable, but it is a good example of empirical work in the field.

As part of their "User Survey Evaluation Package (USEP)," Kenny and Canter (1978) surveyed 1921 nurses in 23 British hospitals concerning ward design. They present statistical and verbal descriptions of their findings as well as a series of design guidelines. This effort is laudable for its comprehensive instrument and large sample size. It seems unfortunate, however, that patients were not included.

NonEmpirical

Nonempirical: Descriptive.   Quality of the nonempirical articles reviewed is fairly uneven. Fifteen articles here are classified as purely descriptive. These are of a "show and tell" (Coutts, 1979) nature or what might be called a "fashion show" mode. They describe what was done, for example, in their own hospital and tell the reader (with no empirical basis whatever) how successful it was. Usually, the criteria described are aesthetic and behavioral. Two types of journals seemed to have a large number of these articles: hospital magazines, such as *Hospitals* and (nonresearch) architectural journals, such as *Architectural Record*. Many more of these show-and-tell-type articles were initially found in the literature search than are included in this review, because the same pattern seems to be repeated again and again, and often little can be learned that can be applied in other settings. The implication of the fashion-show article is, "If we could do this here, you can do this in your hospital," whereas the particular scheme may be totally inappropriate in another setting.

Consistent with the show-and-tell/fashion-show theme, imagery is often used and its appropriateness rarely questioned. It is interesting to note that many of these articles have no bylines. Thus, not only does the reader not know the opinion of the *users* of the facility, she or he does not even know in whose opinion it is pronounced an undeniable success. Pictures included with these articles rarely contain people in them. Thus, the reader is forced to judge the appropriateness of the environment only upon how it looks, empty, in glossy color pictures, and on what the journalist describes.

Some examples help illustrate this point. In an architectural journal ("The Goldberg Effect," 1976), one hospital is characterized as a: "quiet village" that engenders "an empathetic environment in which those taking cures feel closer to those giving them [p. 110]." A hospital journal ("Hospital's Design Details," 1977) positively evaluates a new hospital building: "The 176-bed $16 million building provides an environment that reflects the hospital's concern for individuality needs and comfort of its patients." (p. 38). This building may, in fact, do this, but the reader really has no way of knowing.

An example of a fashion-show article is provided by Schum (1975):

> The geometric design of lobby carpeting and the geometric precast concrete murals on the stairwells of the lobby as well as various other fabric patterns and art accents found throughout the hospital evoke an American Indian mood. Interestingly, these traditionally pagan elements reinforce rather than conflict with the religious symbols in the chapel and elsewhere [p. 35].

She goes on:

> Pattern and texture supply needed variety. The designers avoided matching patterns in favor of pattern interplay, adjusting the amount of interplay to the function of the respective areas i.e. the more public the area, the more unorthodox the pattern combinations [p. 36].

The notion of "pattern interplay" (others might call it "clashing" or "fighting" patterns) is an interesting one, as is the notion of different "interplay" in different areas of the hospital. The desirability, from the users' points of view, of correlating more public areas with greater "interplay" is one that does not appear to be mentioned anywhere else. Maybe this is only appropriate when an "American Indian mood" is evoked. In keeping with the uncritical stance often exhibited in articles of this kind, the author (Shum, 1975) is willing to make what are probably sincere, yet *totally unsubstantiated,* claims for this design: "Conducive to human relationship and endeavor, its atmosphere comforts patients and visitors, while providing efficiency among staff [p. 37]."

Depending on the esthetic and experience of the reader, examples presented in some of these descriptive articles may seem more desirable than others; however, it is important to remember that they are primarily individual opinions or anecdotes. One article of this kind described the use of color nature photography as a therapeutic agent in a radiation therapy department (Oberlander, 1979). The author's claims seem to make intuitive sense, but "harder" data are needed in order to really judge the effects of this design element on behavior: e.g. "Most radiation therapy departments with their cold grey walls and frightening machinery would strike terror in the bravest of hearts. When entering the linear accelerator room, however, patients feel as if they have entered a forest [p. 89]."

Another example of opinion based on experience is found in Brown (1961), who advocates more sensitivity to the patient's perspective than is usually found:

> Besides costs, appearance and utility seem to have been the primary considerations in the minds of architects, boards of trustees, hospitals administrators, medical chiefs of service, nurses in administrative positions and others who were responsible for the planning of new buildings. They brought to their task upper middle class perceptions of what were appropriate standards for a modern general hospital.... Probably they rarely had studies made of what patients would recommend in the construction and furnishing of a new building [p. 33].

Brown points out that there may be serious differences in perspective of medical staff and patients: "When staff members actually become patients, their perceptions of room limitations are quickly sharpened [p. 35]."

As reported in the *Medical Journal of Australia* (Anon., 1974) in a letter from a former patient, the environment in use by a sick person is often perceived very differently than when it is paraded in its initial fashion show:

> The hand basin has no vanity or mirror. To use it is to run the risk of collision with anyone entering the room. The drawers in the bedside cabinet roll awkwardly and it is positioned more for easy cleaning than for easy access by the patient. The emergency bell which is attached to the bed is out of order, but you do not discover that until late at night when you need pain relief and then the acute angle in the corridor outside the walls of your "sanctuary" muffles your cries [p. 302].

Sommer and Dewar (1963) explain this phenomenon:

> Aspects of the physical environment that are relatively unimportant to a well person may loom large upon the horizon of a person confined to a hospital bed . . . the well person can minimize the effects of unpleasant aspects of his environment either by changing or avoiding them [pp. 324–5].

Nonempirical, Research-Based Design Guidelines.   Fifteen of the nonempirical studies reviewed here were ones that gave design recommendations based on their own or other's research. These are some of the more exciting works to be found in the area of behavior and hospital design. Many of these take as their premise that the physical environment has certain effects on behavior, and, in a hospital setting where people are under stress more than in other environments, this relationship is a particularly important one to consider. Many of these give what are called "performance" criteria (specifying a desired end state and leaving the means up to the designer/decision maker) rather than "prescriptive" criteria (specifying exactly what is to be done, with regard to means and assuming that a desired end will result). Many of these pieces include both performance criteria and rationales for why each criterion makes sense.

Guidelines of this sort[3] vary in the levels of scale dealt with from whole hospitals to departments to particular environment–behavior issues. One of the few hospitals to carefully consider issues of behavior and design in their initial planning process was the Tufts New England Medical Center in Boston (Field, Hanson, Karalis, Kennedy, Lippert and Ronco, 1971). Knowing the enormous task they were setting for themselves, they decided to focus on the inpatient environment because: "It is the area with the greatest user dependency on the quality of the surrounding environment. It is at the same time in greatest need of humanizing [p. 14]."

A seemingly dedicated and forward-looking group of planners, architects, and social scientists worked very hard to get enough funding both for the kind of research they wanted to do regarding predesign programming and ongoing evaluation, once it was occupied. They were ultimately unsuccessful in obtaining this funding. However, the documentation of their process is almost 600 pages long, and it seems unfortunate that no other hospital has built on their legacy. In fact, design processes for new hospitals seem to have regressed since that time. For example, a description of the planning and design of the McMaster University Hospital in Hamilton, Ontario written by its architect (Zeidler, 1974) considers human behavior only in terms of the architect's perception of "emotions."

Another research-based planning document for a whole (children's) hospital was written by Lindheim, Glaser, and Coffin (1973), based on their observations

---

[3]These are works that place most emphasis on their guideline nature. A number of the works included in the "Empirical" section also suggest design guidelines. For example, see Petersen (1978).

in six children's hospitals over a period of several months. They also made use of existing literature on children in hospitals. They describe the design-related needs of each age group (infants, toddlers and preschoolers, grade schoolers, adolescents) and include separate chapters on family and staff. They give very general guidelines and then suggest a number of more specific approaches. An example of one of their general guidelines for toddlers and preschoolers is: Visual access is essential (kids need to see and be seen); exclude equipment apt to cause accidents; maintain links with home; accommodate both child and adult scale.

There are several examples of research-based design guidelines at the level of a single department. An excellent example of this type is the book by Clipson and Wehrer (1973) on Coronary Care Units. A meticulously researched, graphically well-presented and comprehensive document, it covers everything from needs of various user groups to sections on equipment and organization of the unit. The authors seem to have combed the literature on special coronary care and derived guidelines for design from these.

Another document, not nearly as extensive as the Clipson and Wehrer book, but good for a fairly quick, low-budget effort is that by Welch (1977) on Emergency Department design, based on existing literature and on her own observations. She organized the guidelines by activities rather than by room name, including: arrival, registration, triage, general waiting, examination and treatment, waiting during treatment, management, conferences, "backstage" staff activities, support services, and leaving. An example of one of her recommendations states:

> Accommodating people's physical and psychological needs helps them accept the inevitability of waiting because they realize it is an activity that has been planned for. This includes such items as convenient access to bathrooms, telephones, nourishment, diversions such as magazines, television, piped in music, furniture that is comfortable to sit in for long periods of time and that can be moved to adapt to a variety of social needs [p. 35].

It is interesting to compare the recommendations from this study with those of Petersen (1978), who did a more extensive study of one part of the Emergency Department, the waiting area. Two of his "general" criteria include: ease of self-orientation to the physical environment so that the available facilities are readily found and understood (p. 169) and availability of a number of self-selective activities which can be engaged in without inhibiting others' choices of activities (p. 169).

Two additional documents of design guidelines done for a single department both deal with radiology; one focusing on diagnostic radiology (Lindheim, 1971) and the other on therapeutic radiology (Conway, Zeisel, Welch, Clayton, & Heinig, 1977). In an early monograph that summarized her observations and

drew on the existing literature, Lindheim made some seemingly basic suggestions for improvements in the design of diagnostic radiology departments, yet
those that apparently had not been previously considered. Some of these included: providing special furniture for elderly patients; providing dressing rooms
large enough to use and that contain a place for storage of belongings; making
sure a toilet is in close proximity; and providing enough heat for the comfort of
undressed patients. Her major suggestions encompass a more flexible approach
to the organization of space and discuss the idea of "uncoupling"; that is,
understanding which components need to be spatially adjacent in order to function and which can be functionally linked but physically separated. The Conway
et al. study, done at the request of the National Institutes of Health, was based on
a combination of observation, interviewing, and use of existing literature. Their
document identified several significant differences:

> between the way radiation treatment centers are designed and the way their users
> use and perceive them. In some cases, modifications the staff made to the environ-
> ment made this conflict evident. In others, the conflict was suggested by the flagrant
> violation of "rules" which had been derived to make the space work the way its
> designers originally conceived it to be used [p. 4].

They organize their guidelines by user group and activity. The following are
an example of several of the guidelines related to patient gowning:

> Locating gowning area adjacent to but not directly off the waiting area means that
> patients going in and out of gowning cubicles do not feel like the focus of waiting
> patients' attention [p. 30].

> Organizing the gowning area clearly so that patients know where to find clean
> gowns, where to deposit used gowns, where to weigh themselves and how to find a
> lavatory, can add to patients' sense of control [p. 30].

> Identification on cubicles means that patients can identify in which one they left
> their clothes when returning from treatment [p. 30].

At the level of an environment–behavior issue, there is one good example of
design guidelines in the pieces reviewed here, that by Birren (1979) on light and
color. Building his argument on various empirical studies, he notes at the beginning:

> Current hospital decoration is often unduly pretentious. Choice of color is all too
> often based on personal feeling and personal whim [p. 94].

He makes a case against the use of the color white in hospitals:

> Akin to snow blindness, this combination of white walls and bright lights produces
> distressing glare, hampers vision, can cause headaches and nausea and may even
> damage the retina [p. 94].

Citing work by B. Brown (1974) who did research on human reaction to color, using the polygraph and EEG, he recommends:

Where there is high brightness (illumination) and warm colors (red, pink, orange, yellow), there is a tendency for human beings to be physically aroused and to direct their attention outward into the environment. Such a condition might be quite suitable for convalescent patients, maternity patients, or anyone on the way to recovery. Where there is less brightness and cooler colors, there is a tendency for human beings to be relaxed. This kind of environment would be good for chronic patients and for those who are likely to be institutionalized for long periods [p. 96].[4]

Nonempirical Design Guidelines, Not Research Based.   The last category of study types is that where recommendations for design are made without any apparent systematic basis. An example of one of these comes from the article by Edwards (1979) and provides contrast with research-based recommendations previously made by Birren: "It is therefore most important that colors in wards should not be overstimulating because patients find it impossible to 'let off steam' and the pent up emotion can become distressing or disturbing after a while, particularly for long stay patients [p. 746]."

In fact, Edwards is correct for *some* patients, but not for all. He goes on and discusses orientation/wayfinding as a potential problem in hospitals. He suggests that color can take care of the problem *without the need for signs*. For example, doors for different functions can be color coded: "These do not have to be different colors as variations *in tints or tones* are sufficient [my italics, p. 748]." One pictures the frustrated visitor madly searching for the men's room, while having to open numerous closets, supply room, and patient room doors, having unfortunately neglected to note variations in tone or tint.

To the person needing good information on which to base design decisions, this category is the most frustrating of all. It not only describes, it prescribes, and with no apparent basis for so doing. One has to question why administrators and other hospital-design decision makers are willing to accept this type of prescriptive fluff with regard to design when they are unwilling to do so for other decision-making areas, such as finance.

Factors Effected by Hospital Design

One way of examining some of the empirical works cited in this review is to describe what behavior the physical environment is seen as effecting. Table 6.6 lists these dependent variables alphabetically, with the numbers of the relevant studies.

---

[4]Reprinted with permission from Hospitals, J.A.H.A., published by the American Hospital Association, copyright July 16, 1979, Vol. 53, No. 14.

TABLE 6.6
Factors Effected by Hospital Design*

Confidentiality	20
Control over Social Interaction	14, 64, 67
Cross-Infection	51
Disclosure	23, 67
Image	14, 48, 59, 67, 70
Organizational Climate	13, 61
Perception	73, 74
Post-Operative Delirium	43, 85
Post-Operative Medication	56
Travel Time	33, 50, 76, 79

*Not all empirical studies are represented. Numbers refer to
Bibliography.

Confidentiality

Cammock (1975) looked at 32 health centers and five group practices in various parts of the UK, with regard to the issue of confidentiality of patient information and its relationship to design. She sees a threat to confidentiality because the move to health centers and group practices provides greater opportunities for "accidental leaks as confidential material passes between members of this larger team." She criticizes the existing British design guides because "they might have been designed to *maximize* risks to confidentiality [p. 6]." Cammock distinguishes between intentional and accidental breaches of confidentiality; the first being the responsibility of the organization through its policies and management, whereas the second depends more on design. She sees "architectural control of communications as a process of enclosure whereby people within are restricted in their communication with those who remain outside," (p. 7) and proceeds to discuss a hierarchy of possible enclosures from separate blocks, wings, or floors, to cupboards and drawers.

Control over Social Interaction

This dependent variable was looked at by several researchers. In a report on the design and evaluation of a 30-bed progressive patient-care wing, Beckman (1974) described the central purpose as: "a therapeutic corridor which would be structured with a variety of activity centers to encourage patients to venture out from the confinement of their rooms, to help each other, help themselves and to receive help and encouragement from families and professional attendants in realizing their cure" (p. 64). As part of this, the architectural details and furnishings were designed to provide as much control over their environment by patients and staff as possible. This included control over social interaction.

Pill (1967) observed the spatial ecology of two children's wards in England during the course of a year. One of his most striking findings relates to the difficulty of the nursing staff in controlling their social interaction with patients and visitors, due to the lack of space in which "to hide":

> The nurse while in the open ward, was under constant surveillance by her patients. Consequently, if she wished to relax, she would sometimes retire to the small linen cupboard. More often, however, the problem was solved by treating the whole ward temporarily as a back stage area. This was made easier by the fact that patients and even more so, child patients, are often treated in the normal functioning of the ward as if they were not there [p. 185].

Cross Infection

A study by McKendrick and Emond (1976) was conducted for 5 years in seven hospitals to assess the risk of cross infection with two highly infectious air-borne diseases in isolation wards of different design. A researcher recorded the distribution of susceptible contacts; their names, addresses, and ages; information from the ward sister (nurse) about any unusual behavior, and reason for discharge. This information was recorded 5 days a week for a 5-year period.

Causation between design and cross infection was not clear because "inadequate staff supervision could also be a factor." However, the researchers recommend that ward units be small with lateral rather than central corridors, that ventilation not take place into the corridor but outside the building, that rooms be entered through an airlock or anteroom with two sets of automatic doors, and that there be adequate numbers of trained staff (p. 31).

Disclosure

In a small study by Chaikin, Derlega and Miller (1976), the effects of a "hard" versus a "soft" environment on the intimacy of client self-disclosure (analogous to a counselling situation) were compared. Subjects were 52 college students, half males and half females. The experiment was conducted in a small, windowless room, 10 feet by 10 feet. The "hard" architecture condition was: brown asphalt tile floor, cement-block walls painted yellow; overhead fluorescent light; rectanglular table; straight-back chair for the subject. The "soft" architecture condition was: oriental rug covering most of the floor; indirect lighting; framed picture on the walls; an upholstered cushioned armchair for the subject and various small objects such as magazines and ashtrays. The researchers (Chaikin et al., 1976) found that: "subjects disclosed at a significantly more intimate level in the soft than in the hard room [p. 481]."

Reizenstein (1976) found a similar effect of the physical environment in her study of hospital social-work offices. Social workers were interviewed in conjunction with a predesign programming study for their offices and again after completion of the offices in a postoccupancy evaluation. They claimed that the improved physical facilities led to increased disclosure on the part of their clients.

Image

Quite a number of researchers have pointed up the importance of hospital image. For example, Lindheim et al. (1973) suggest that a monumental hospital building, although satisfying to donors and administrators, probably connotes a fortress to children, and the scary prospect of being "locked up" within. As mentioned earlier, Oberlander (1979) hypothesizes that the cold gray walls and frightening machinery in radiation therapy departments, "strike terror in the bravest hearts [p. 89]." Rosengren and Devault (1963) in their observation study of an obstetrical hospital argue that the father's importance in the delivery process is symbolized by his environment: "The father's room is adjacent to the recovery room—unattended and suggestive that the father is regarded as the least important in the process. By its sparseness of furnishing, its physical isolation and its small size, this room seemed to communicate symbolically the idea that fathers are unnecessary and functionally peripheral [p. 278]."

Organizational Climate

In a study of the effects of environmental modifications on the attitudes and behavior of different user groups in a small general hospital, Becker (1977) examined the "organizational climate." This included: mood/morale, quality of health care, perception of administration, and nursing and environmental awareness. He found that the physical renovations had a "positive effect" on these variables. Pendell and Coray (1976) also looked at organizational climate in their study of nursing-unit design in four hospitals. Their measures of organizational climate included: operational efficiency, workload balance, co-worker cooperation, visibility, and others.

Perception

In two articles, Spivack (1967, 1969) observed the design of two psychiatric facilities with regard to problems in perception. He discusses characteristics of corridors in detail, especially with regard to length and surfaces. These can lead to visibility problems such as glare and distortion, as well as to noise problems.

Post-operative Delirium

Keep (1977) reports Wilson's (1972) study of the effects of windows in intensive care units in Britain, with regard to surgical patient delirium. "In the windowless ICU, the incidence of post-operative delirium was twice as high as in the other unit. In patients with abnormal hemoglobin or blood urea levels, the incidence of delirium was three times as high [p. 599]."

Post-operative Medication

Minckley (1968), an operating-room supervisor, looked at the environmental issue of noise in her study of post-operative patients. She hypothesized that: "Post-operative patients already suffering from surgical pain are made more uncomfortable as the noise over which they have no control increases [p. 247]."

If this was true, she argued, then more pain medications will be requested and given per patient during periods of high noise level and less during periods of low noise level. Her procedure was to measure noise levels in a 10-bed recovery room (30 × 15 × 15) at half-hour intervals, using a portable sound meter. She found that: "The median noise level was found to be within 50–60 decibels. Periods of heightened activity, presence of large numbers of staff personnel, overcrowding of patients and certain sounds such as crying, laughing, groaning, snoring and the ringing of a telephone produced noise levels between 60–70 decibels [p. 250]." High noise levels were correlated with more pain medications being given, thus supporting her hypothesis.

Travel Time

One of the most frequently studied dependent variables relating to behavior and hospital design is nurse travel time on the ward. Thompson and Goldin (1975) and Trites, Galbraith, Sturdavant and Leckwart (1970) report empirical studies of this phenomenon, whereas Lippert (1971) reports on an approach (tour model) to studying this variable, and Girard (1978)[5] reports on a cluster design in his hospital that minimizes nurse travel time.

The Yale Traffic Index, done by Thompson (1959), is considered by some to be a classic study and is based on the notion that: "The way to determine the functional efficiency of units would seem to be to find a method of measuring the nursing steps each plan requires. . . . To trace nursing steps is to see how a whole unit functions [p. 282]." A 6-month study of traffic patterns was undertaken at Yale–New Haven Hospital in four nursing units: two medical and two surgical. Out of these data, they developed a single index by which design schemes for general medical and surgical nursing units could be compared for functional efficiency. The major variables are the distance between areas and the relative number of times this distance must be traversed.

A critic of this approach might suggest that travel is certainly one important factor to look at, but that perhaps it has been overemphasized due to its quantitative nature and to the difficulty of studying less-quantitative effects of hospital design on human behavior. In fact, this notion of measuring travel distance has literally appeared to cause some researchers to go overboard.

An example of this questionable obsession with studying nurse travel time is the research of Trites et al. (1970). Their mission was to look at radial, single corridor, and double corridor (racetrack) hospital floors to see which was most desirable. With the aid of a federal grant, the Rochester (Minn.) Methodist Hospital (570 beds) was constructed as a building that could be used as a labora-

---

[5]Interestingly, he participated in the Thompson study as a graduate student and is now a hospital administrator who has attempted to apply the findings of this study.

tory for such research.[6] Their study was extremely detailed and complex. Four units of each type of floor (12 in all) were observed and sampled over 82 days. Despite the veritable mountain of data (for example, they report, but do not publish, nine 71-variable intercorrelation matrices), their conclusions are almost meaningless: "It is obvious that much of the variance of the dependent variables remains unexplained by the independent variables included in this study [p. 322]."

In a somewhat desperate attempt to find something from this complex and extensive study, they employed a "single question direct approach" and *asked* the nurses which floor design they preferred. Radial design was the clear winner: "Expressed as time per 24 hours, the staff on the double corridor units spent 9.2 more hours in travel time and 9.7 hours on the single corridor than did the staff on radial units." (p. 331) It seems that if they had used the Yale Traffic Index to analyze the floorplans, they would neither have had to build a whole hospital to answer their questions nor have had to spend so much time, energy, and money studying it.

, What can be concluded from looking at some of the dependent variables that have been studied regarding hospital design and human behavior? Firstly, the range of possible behavioral effects of the physical environment has not been fully explored. Secondly, there have not been enough studies of any one dependent variable to give confidence in the replicability of findings. Thirdly, the quality of some of the research is lacking, and, fourthly, the most studied dependent variable, nurse travel time, has probably been overemphasized vis a vis other possible dependent variables.

Design and Planning Process Issues

Another way of analyzing this literature is to look at the ways in which various issues pertaining to the design and planning process are handled. Table 6.7 lists major process issues found in this review, with the associated bibliographic references. These issues include: cost containment, role of the external environment, user participation, planning for change, the role of research, social and physical systems working together, space allocation, and prioritization of needs.

Cost Containment

Clearly, one of the single biggest issues in the organization of medical care today is concern for wildly spirling costs. In addition to the benefits of user-sensitive design as measured in qualitative, humanistic terms, several authors

---

[6]It is difficult to understand why taxpayer dollars were used to build an entire hospital that was to be used for experimental purposes such as this. Two questions are immediately apparent: Why couldn't mock-up units of some kind be used for the purposes of experimentation, and what about all the patients and staff who have to live with the "undesirable" designs for the remainder of the building's life?

TABLE 6.7
Design and Planning Process Issues*

Cost Containment	14, 39, 62, 63
External Environment	62
User Participation	13, 22, 24, 48, 67
Planning for Change	17, 26, 35, 37, 49, 52, 53, 54, 80, 81
Role of Research	6, 22, 29, 42, 55, 63
Social & Physical Systems Working Together	14, 22
Space Allocation	2, 65
Prioritization of Needs	29, 69

*Not all empirical studies are represented. Numbers refer to Bibliography.

point out potential and actual benefits as measured in dollars. Petersen (1978) notes a growing interest by the field of hospital management in long-term planning of facilities as a means of cost containment (p. 18). Heckler and Sweetland (1977) note that operating costs rather than capital costs, as usually emphasized, may ultimately be a more important consideration: "Clearly, any sustainable savings in annual operating expenses will have a far greater effect than an equivalent reduction in capital expenditure [p. 66]."

Careful planning, they suggest, may reduce such ongoing operating costs as staffing, energy conservation, and maintenance (p. 56). Penkhus (1976) concurs, using the example of the private room: "review of costs by surveys has pointed toward higher internal capital investment, but lower operating expenses which may offset the former [p. 12]."

In a study of a specially designed wing for "progressive patient care," Beckman (1974) gives an example of user-sensitive design leading to cost savings: "Three years of operating experience has shown that the unit provides an economic advantage. Average costs of patient stay dropped 12% and it encourages rapid recovery when compared to more conventionally organized hospitals [p. 68]." In addition, he reports that average length of stay dropped by .8 days, and, thus, less staffing was required as well.

External Environment

In addition to considerations of costs, there are other factors stemming from outside the individual hospital that influence how spatial decisions are made. As Penkhus (1976) discusses, federal legislation is one major external factor. He mentions the Social Security Amendments of 1972 (PL 92–603) and the National Health Planning and Resource Development Act of 1974 (PL 92–641) as important examples that emphasize improved utilization of inpatient beds, more development of outpatient clinics, outpatient surgery, long-term care, and rehabilitation facilities. He also sees changing patterns of illness and new methods of treatment as other external variables influencing hospital design and function.

In addition to these, other external factors affect design, such as accreditation criteria (Joint Commission on the Accreditation of Hospitals), building codes, and other regulations such as those of OSHA (Occupational Safety and Health Act).

User Participation

A major theme in a number of the pieces reviewed here is that the *process* of including user needs in design and planning may be as important or even more important than the *products* of design. Specifically, the type of process that has been shown to be quite beneficial to both administrators and users is a participatory one. Several cases have shown that including staff in the design process has been so positively received by them that their satisfaction with the results seemed to be greater than it would have been if they were not included. For example, in Reizenstein's (1976) study of hospital social workers, most of the staff were interviewed concerning their satisfaction with existing office space and their desires for new space. These expressed desires, along with spatial and cost constraints, fed into a design that was constructed and occupied. After approximately 6 months of use, the social workers were interviewed concerning their satisfaction with the new offices. Most of them volunteered comments to the effect that they were very pleased to have had their opinions consulted regarding the design. Some of those whose new offices were actually smaller than their old ones responded to a questionnaire saying that they thought they now had more space. This was interpreted as being part of a halo effect stemming from the participatory process.

This effect is also borne out by Lindheim et al. (1973), who used a participatory programming process in a hospital for children: "Members of the staff who were involved in the planning and design process and thus had a commitment to the result have been more satisfied with the building than have those who started to work in the hospital after the design was complete [p. VIII]."

Cheek, Maxwell and Weisman (1971) came to a similar conclusion, although in a more indirect way. They report on social processes involved in the introduction and reception of carpeting in two different wards of a psychiatric hospital. On one ward, the staff had not been consulted about the carpeting issue, and they expressed great dissatisfaction with it due, ostensibly, to cleaning difficulties but probably due to their resentment at not having had a say.

On the other ward, even though specific staff people had not been around when the carpeting decision was made, an early informal survey of staff and patients showed that the idea of carpet was approved of. Despite the fact that they had to keep an eye on patient smoking, incontinence and spillage, they liked the carpeting. Cheek et al. (1971) explain this "success" as due to the administration's knowledge of the staff's "environmental definitions" and the administration's sensitivity to staff feedback on this issue.

Becker (1977) sees four factors as determining the perceived importance of participation in the design process by a setting's users: (1) normative expectations; (2) time in the setting; (3) perceived instrumentality of the setting; and (4) belief that participation will make a difference. He concedes that: "the administration will lose some 'power' by shifting responsibility for some decision-making to the nursing unit level, but there are types of decisions that can never be made very effectively by centralized administrators in any case [p. 153]."

Design participation has at least two additional advantages, as Becker sees it: It can legitimize staff's input (power) in decisions affecting their own work environment and can help to raise the "environmental consciousness" of staff, so that they will take the initiative in the future to use the physical environment as a resource.

Another advantage of user participation in design is pointed out by Canter and Canter (1979), who cite Holohan in saying that: "change in the physical environment is only likely to generate change in the behavioral and social system if the users of the setting are involved in the design [p. 24]."

Planning for Change

If there could be said to be one main theme running through the literature on hospital design and behavior reviewed here, it would be that of the necessity and difficulty of planning for change. McLaughlin (1976a.) states that the hospital is the: "most changing of building types and that its physical life is uniquely characterized by modification," and continues: "The demand for regular and small scale expansion of virtually every department is necessary and incessant. It frequently doesn't occur however, because the design of most buildings makes such an incremental, uneven process almost impossible [p. 118]." Boyar (1978) echoes this sentiment: "In a sense, the health care field is its own worst enemy for not demanding sound design concepts to provide for future unforseen yet inevitable changes in its rush to meet immediately targeted needs [p. 80]."

Lindheim (1971) warns that habits of spatial organization become "etched into the minds of both architect and client," yet these habits lag behind new technology unless the "tyranny of habit is overcome." She warns that designs will become functionally obsolete even as they are being built (p. 71).

Good and Hurtig (1978) would like to see buildings designed so that changes can be made without major alteration. Eisdorfer wants to take the responsibility for planning for change from the architect and put it on the client (Cochran, 1978): "Treatment modalities and the kinds of patients being hospitalized are changing rapidly and the architect should be told to build in as much flexibility as possible. The architect shouldn't be blamed if he's been told to design for only one kind of use [e.g. inpatient beds] and the use changes to offices for staff. And the client should expect to pay more for a flexible design [p. 534]."

An example of the widespread nature of this "inevitable" change in hospital design is reported by Welch (1977), who found in visits to a number of different Emergency Departments that: "none of these facilities were being used as they had been designed." She continues: "In some cases, organizational and administrative changes had necessitated change in the use of rooms or modification of the facilities: usually addition of counters, cabinet racks or partitions. In other cases, changes had occured as the staff discovered the misfit between their needs and what was provided. For example, in several hospitals, there was no provision for storing personal belongings of staff [p. 10]."

McLaughlin, Kibre and Raphail (1972b.) studied design changes in six existing hospitals between 1950 and 1970 on Radiology, Laboratory, Surgery, Emergency, Transportation, and Nursing Units. Nursing units accounted for almost half the total number of changes. Most of these (approximately 75%) were remodelings. About one third of these were minor changes to just one room to accommodate new uses or to improve the efficiency of use. Most other changes were made to improve operating efficiency and accommodate new or expanding programs.

At least two suggestions have been made for coping with changing hospital design. Weeks, Best, Cheyne and Leopold (1976) replicated Cowan's 1962-63 study of hospital room size. Cowan concluded that: (1) the majority of a hospital's activities can be successfully accommodated in a relatively small number of different-sized rooms, most being between 50 and 250 square feet. Weeks et al.'s findings tended to support Cowan's. Implications for hospital design are that a relatively small range of room sizes is capable of accommodating the activities that go on in hospitals.[7]

Another suggestion for coping with change is made by Lindheim (1971), who advocates "uncoupling." This means asking which components need to be spatially adjacent in order to function and which can be functionally linked but physically separated. She feels that: "many functional problems in hospital design could be solved with a more flexible approach to the organization of space [p. 76]."

Role of Research in Design Decision Making

Another theme of the literature reviewed here is that although the inclusion of research-based data in the design decision-making processes would be desirable, it is rarely if ever done.[8] For example, Canter and Canter (1979) note that: "there are many government publications which describe the physical layout and design to be achieved. However, it is rare for these documents to provide substantive evidence for the recommendations they are making [p. 7]."

Jaco (1972) explains this by observing that there is little systematic research available "concerning the effects of physical design on the care of patients by nursing and medical staffs, on patient and staff satisfaction, or on the organization, structure, and function of the hospital itself. He reviews some of the older work in this area, such as Sommer and Dewar (1963) and Rosengren and De-Vault (1963), but says these are more derived from "selected observations and

---

[7]However, there was no evaluation made of how well these work, only that they exist, and there was no discussion of causation (e.g., why these sizes were chosen in the first place).

[8]The next section also looks at this question.

impressions'' than from systematic statistical findings. However, he leaves the impression that more of the systematic type of studies are desirable:

> There are, however, other hospital researchers who either tacitly assume or overtly assert that the physical design of a unit conditions the activities of people in such settings. They are interested in testing hypotheses about the potential relations between various aspects of the physical setting and organizational and related behavior of individuals interacting in such surroundings. Studies of this kind are extremely rare to date, despite the potentially enormous contributions to hospital organization behavior and patient care research [p. 231].

Petersen (1978) echoes this sentiment and introduces his own empirical study of Emergency Department waiting areas as a way to: ''help behavioral scientists participate in the design process by adding to the existing body of knowledge and translating this information into a form usable by the designer [p. 13].''

However, not all writers in this field agree that research is desirable. Evidence of this was given in the section on the ''fashion-show'' type of article. These are writers who imply by their reporting style that personal impression is preferable to systematic evaluation. One interior designer who is quite vocal about this was quoted in an article entitled ''Psychology of Hospital Design (1977).'' The (unidentified) author calls this designer ''an authority on health care design'' who, unlike many other specialists who tend to be ''doctrinaire about their field of expertise, subscribes to individualistic evaluation and pragmatism geared entirely to the problem at hand. According to this interior designer: ''You can't go by sets of theories, for each case is conditional. For example, color alone cannot do the job because interior design of a hospital is never a surface thing . . . Nor can you go by the results of completed studies since many contradict themselves. That's why I don't start with preconceptions and don't know in advance just what I will do [p. 103].'' Others, such as architect Herbert McLaughlin (1976b), disagree: ''Useful breakthroughs in design generally result from a clear understanding of the problem and evaluation is probably the best tool available for developing useful design information [p. 571].''

In his review of some of the literature on hospital design, Coutts (1979) sees a change in the role of research: ''A trend in the literature away from hand wringing and toward the development of a factual data base appears to be taking place here and abroad. It seems logical that progress will take place not from a sudden breakthrough but from a broad-based effort by multidisciplinary researchers, each contributing in-depth reports with a limited scope [p. 8].''

Social and Physical Systems Working Together

Another theme running through the reviewed literature is that physical design cannot be examined in isolation from the social system in which it operates. This is implied in most of the articles on hospital design and behavior, but a couple of these specifically address this issue. For example, Beckman (1974) notes that:

"the administrators of this hospital use the facilities as a therapeutic tool . . . it takes an enlightened administration to creatively apply the opportunities provided by this experimental space [p. 68]."

Another example is provided by Rivlin and Wolfe (Canter & Canter, 1979) in their 6-year study of a children's psychiatric facility. They discuss something they call the "inadequacy of illusion equals reality," as a basis for design and planning. By this they mean that the design may convey a certain image (such as separation of units), but if the social program does not operate this way, the design becomes a sham.

Space Allocation

Very few articles reviewed looked at the process of space allocation in hospitals. One exception was Rawlinson's (1978) report on an ongoing study of this type. She finds that this process is different in hospitals than in other public-sector buildings due to their complexity, the rapid pace of change and development, and the interconnectedness of departments. She concentrates on quantitative aspects of space utilization and regards buildings: "as resources with a wide range of potential uses rather than as a collection of spaces each with a specific named use [p. 4]." She advocates a: "more flexible and less deterministic attitude toward space provision and use" (p. 4) and suggests three ways of achieving this: "more intensive use (for the same activity by the same users), shared use (by different user groups for the same activity) and alternative uses (by the same or different groups of users for different activities at different times.)" (p. 5)

Another article ("Computerized Space Planning," 1975) discusses computerized space allocation. Medical Planning Associates of Malibu, California has developed a program designed to assist short-term acute-care general hospitals: "Just tell the computer how many patients or tests . . . you want to accommodate and out will come specs and drawings showing exactly how much space is needed and how it should be arranged [p. 45]."

Neither of these articles looks at the spatial-allocation process as a political one or looks at *qualitative* aspects of space allocation.

Prioritization of Needs

One tendency of articles in this field is to concentrate on a single behavioral issue, for example, confidentiality, which the author argues should be the major consideration in hospital design. Few if any of the authors cited here paid attention to the problem of conflicting behavioral needs. One of the most important of these conflicts concerns which user-group's needs are to be given precedence (Coutts, 1979). Several authors, including Ronco (1972), argue that of all the possible user groups in a hospital (administrators, physicians, nurses, patients, staff, visitors) patients' needs should rank the highest.

Ronco feels that, from a psychological viewpoint, the patient has, on the whole, "been ignored if not forgotten in the (hospital) design process." Reasons for this include:

1. Lack of funds to permit designing what some might consider luxuries into function-oriented plans.
2. Minor involvement of the behavioral sciences in hospital and health-care fields (excepting mental health) until recently.
3. Insufficient data relating physical environments to behavior (p. 462).

UTILIZATION OF RESEARCH IN HEALTH-FACILITY PLANNING

Given the strengths and weaknesses of the available information that directly pertains to hospital design, the question remains, is this information used in design decision making? A study by Heath and Green (1976), done in Australia, gives some preliminary answers. They held structured interviews with 50 public and private health facility planners in Sydney, Australia in 1975, their aim being to: "discover how people went about obtaining information as a basis for decision-making and what they felt about the need for improvements in making information more readily available, applicable and understandable [p. 9]." The eight main topics covered by their study were: (1) availability of information within the respondent's own organization; (2) use of information sources outside the respondent's own organization; (3) mistakes caused by insufficient information; (4) who should provide information?; (5) information types found most valuable; (6) attitudes toward information sharing between organizations; (7) education of planners, designers, and users; and (8) roles for potential information brokers.

Heath and Green (1976) found that there is generally a "resistant attitude" regarding the use of information in decision making and problem solving, as well as limited awareness of the information available: "the various kinds of information services that are available do not appear to be used as effectively as they might be. This is partly due to problems of accessibility, but also to lack of awareness by information providers of the needs of practicing information users [p. 9]."

The most used information sources were "personal contacts" and state government departments, "although the reported success rate was low": "Many respondents tended to think of information as represented by the printed word only, but questioning revealed that in practice they made more use of colleagues' knowledge and experience and of information gleaned from seminars and visits than they did of publications [p. 33]."

Heath and Green also describe the kinds of mistakes made due to lack of information in design decision making. These include: (1) design inappropriate for function; (2) maintenance problems; (3) duplication of work already done; (4) inadequate services provided; (5) regulations ignored; (6) over-lavish provision of facilities; and (7) lack of appreciation of environmental effects. Results of these mistakes included: incurring additional costs, patient discomfort or distress, and staff discomfort or inconvenience. They conclude with a series of suggestions for making research information more easily utilized by health-facility design and planning decision makers.

A study of this sort makes it clear that it is not enough to simply call for more quantity or better quality research in order that it be applied in spatial decision making in hospitals. Thus, it seems that a better understanding of how that process *actually takes place* will lead to insights about how information could be more effectively "plugged in" than now seems to be the case in Australia or in the United States.[9]

SUMMARY

In this review of the recent literature on human behavior and hospital design, several patterns have emerged. Firstly, the literature is very widely scattered and can be found in books and journals in the hospital, architectural, and medical fields. It seems as if there is a problem merely coming into contact with much of it. Secondly, Great Britain seems to account for more empirical work (as a percentage of their total work) than does the United States. Perception of the importance of the physical environment may be one reason for this. Thirdly, more empirical work has been done in nonacute-care hospitals, especially psychiatric ones, than in acute-care hospitals. Several reasons for this were hypothesized, including the fact that psychiatric patients have less say in what goes on during their hospital stay than do acute-care patients and, for this reason, may be considered as more desirable subjects. Fourthly, about half the articles were empirical and half nonempirical. Some of both of these were of high quality and some not. There appears to be a great deal of the "show-and-tell" or "fashion-show" type of descriptive articles appearing in hospital and architectural journals, but which usually have no empirical basis for their claims. Fifthly, a number of dependent variables have been looked at in the empirical studies that have been done, but these do not appear to cover all the potentially important ones. Sixthly, a number of design and planning-process issues have been discussed, but none of the literature systematically looked at ongoing spatial decision-making processes. Finally, those who make design decisions in health facilities tend not to use the research that exists.

NEED FOR FURTHER RESEARCH

In order to provide a base of information on which design decision makers can rely, clearly more high-quality research is needed. One approach is to study more

---

[9]My own study of utilization of Environment–Behavior Research by architects and planners in the U. S. came to the same conclusions as this Australian study (see Reizenstein, 1975).

dependent variables. In addition, there need to be more studies made with regard to each variable. To take the patient-user group as an example, environmental needs might be categorized in the following way: wayfinding, physical comfort, symbolic meaning, social contact, security, convenience, special needs. For example, a series of case studies concerning how patients find their way through the often complex and confusing hospital environment would improve the state of the art in research and hopefully lead eventually to more easily negotiable hospitals.

Research on a range of settings within the hospital is also needed. From the building as a whole, to the design of public spaces such as lobbies and waiting areas, to the layout of certain rooms and choice of furnishings and surfaces, more information is needed on the effects of the physical environmental features on attitudes and behaviors of users. In addition, more research is needed on the environmental needs of patients with various types of diseases. For example, do hematology patients have different environmental needs than neurology patients? In addition, we need to know more about how various demographic variables such as gender, age, socioeconomic status, and the like effect the environmental needs of hospital patients, if at all.

Another type of study useful for pointing out effects of the physical environment on behaviors and attitudes in hospitals are "before and after" case studies of physical changes. In addition, further investigation of differences in needs among various user groups (doctors, nurses, patients, visitors, administration, housekeeping, etc.) would be enlightening and help address the issue of conflicting user needs. Some user groups have been understudied to date, especially patients, visitors, and nonmedical, non-nursing hospital staff.

CONCLUSION

In conclusion, two types of changes are called for to improve the quality and quantity of available information related to human behavior and hospital design and to help increase the utilization of this research. Available information can be improved with: (1) more recognition by hospitals that the physical environment is a valuable resource that can and does impact everyone in the hospital and effort on their part to find out more about environment–behavior relationships; (2) more funding of this type of research by both government and private sources; (3) more systematic research covering a wider variety of settings and variables; and (4) more research-based design guides using performance criteria. One potentially fruitful approach to increasing research utilization in hospital-design decision making is to study those processes as they actually occur, and to then see what ways are most appropriate for the introduction of behaviorally focused, research-based information.

ACKNOWLEDGMENT

This chapter was written while under a traineeship from the National Institute on Mental Health (2T32-MH14598-04).

BIBLIOGRAPHY

1. "A Slightly Serious Look at a Serious Problem: Hospital Design and Policy Versus Patient Comfort." *Medical Journal of Australia* 2 (4 Aug. 1974): 301–2.
2. "Computerized Space Planning." *Modern Health Care* 4 (Oct. 1975): 45–8.
3. "The Kirkbride Plan: Architecture for a Treatment System that Changed." *Hospital and Community Psychiatry* 27 (July 1976): 473–7.
4. "The Goldberg Effect: The Architect of Marina City Casts a Spell on Concrete to Enclose Health Care Concepts." *Architectural Record,* July 1976, p. 110.
5. "Architectural Straitjacket." *Nursing Times* 72 (20 May 1976): 755.
6. "Psychology of Hospital Design." *Interior Design* 48 (Jan. 1977): 102–7.
7. "Patient Room Takes Shapes that Ensure Comfort and Efficiency." *Hospitals* 57 (16 Nov. 1977): 14.
8. "Hospital's Design Details Provide Efficient, Pleasant Environment for Patients." *Hospitals* 51 (16 Sept. 1977): 38.
9. "Simple, Efficient Departmental Design Suits Functions, Growth of Nuclear Medicine." *Hospitals* 51 (16 May 1977): 30.
10. ARC (Architecture, Research, Construction). "Behavior Change on Ward 8: Physical Elements and Social Interaction." *J. of Architectural Education* 29 (April 1976): 26.
11. Barton, R. "The Patient's Personal Territory." *Hospital and Community Psychiatry* 17 (Nov. 1966): 336.
12. Beattie, A. and Curtis, J. "Hospital Corridors as a Case Study in Architectural Psychology." *J. of Architectural Research* 3 (May 1974): 44–50.
13. Becker, F. D. "The Effect of Physical Design Changes on Organizational Climate and Behavior Patterns in a Hospital Nursing Unit." In *User Participation, Personalization and Environmental Meaning: Three Field Studies,* edited by F. D. Becker, Ithaca, N.Y.: Cornell University, 1977.
14. Beckman, R. "Getting up and Getting out: Progressive Patient Care." *Progressive Architecture,* Nov. 1974, p. 64.
15. Birren, F. "Human Response to Color and Light." *Hospitals* 53 (16 July 1979): 93.
16. Bowling, J. S. "Expansion: The Importance of Involving Department Managers in the Planning Process and How to Achieve It." *Hospital Topics* 55 (Mar.–Apr. 1977): 60–6.
17. Boyar, R. L. "Flexibility Planning Keys Cost-Effective Construction." *Hospitals* 52 (1 May 1978): 79.
18. Brown, B. *New Mind, New Body: Bio-Feedback: New Directions for the Mind.* N.Y.: Harper & Row, 1974.
19. Brown, E. L. *Newer Dimensions of Patient Care.* New York: Russell Sage, 1961.
20. Cammock, R. "Confidentiality in Health Centers and Group Practices: The Implications for Design." *J. of Architectural Research* 4 (Feb. 1975): 6.
21. Canter, D. "Royal Hospital for Sick Children: A Psychological Analysis." *Architects Journal,* Sept. 6, 1972, 525–64.
22. Canter, D., and Canter, S., eds. *Designing for Therapeutic Environments: A Review of Research.* New York: John Wiley, 1979.
23. Chaikin, A. L.; Derlega, V. J.; and Miller, S. J. "Effects of Room Environment on Self-Disclosure in a Counselling Analogue." *J. of Counselling Psychology* 23 (1976): 479–81.

24. Cheek, F. E.; Maxwell, R.; and Weisman, R. "Carpeting the Ward: An Exploratory Study in Environmental Psychiatry." *Mental Hygiene* 55 (Jan. 1971): 109-18.
25. Clipson, C., and Wehrer, J. *Planning for Cardiac Care.* Ann Arbor: Health Administration Press, 1973.
26. Cochran, B. "Design and Planning of Psychiatric Facilities." *Hospital and Community Psychiatry* 29 (Aug. 1978): 533-37.
27. Colman, A. D. "Territoriality in Man; A Comparison of Behavior in Home and Hospital." *American J. of Orthopsychiatry* 38 (1968): 464.
28. Conway, D.; Zeisel, J.; Welch, P.; Clayton, P.; and Heinig, P. *Radiation Therapy Centers: Social and Behavioral Issues for Design.* Bethesda, Md.: National Institutes of Health, 1977.
29. Coutts, A. *The Physical Environment of the Health Care Facility: A Literature Review and Annotated Bibliography.* Washington, D.C.: Veterans Administration, 1979.
30. Edwards, K. "The Environment Inside the Hospital." *Practitioner* 222 (June 1979): 746-51.
31. Field, H.: Hanson, J.; Karalis, C.; Kennedy, D.; Lippert, S.; and Ronco, P. *Evaluation of Hospital Design: A Holistic Approach.* Boston: Tufts New England Medical Center, 1971.
32. Gerberich, B. "Key Factors to Consider in Deciding on Location Space for Departments." *Hospital Topics 50* (March 1972): 24-6.
33. Girard, N. E. "Room Clusters Facilitate Nursing Care." *Modern Health Care* 8 (June 1978): 46-7.
34. Good, L. R.; Siegel, S. M.; and Bay, A. P., eds. *Therapy by Design: Implications of Architecture for Human Behavior.* Springfield, Ill: Charles C. Thomas, 1965.
35. Good, L. R., and Hurtig, W. E. "Evaluation: A Mental Health Facility, its Users and Context." *American Institute of Architects Journal* 67 (Fib. 1978): 38-41.
36. Gordon, A. M. "The Effect of Treatment Environments." *J. of Psychosomatic Research* 20 (1976): 363-66.
37. Hardy, O. "Flexible Planning Allows Hospital Expansion." *Dimensions in Health Service* 52 (Nov. 1975): 15-17.
38. Heath, M. & Green, J. *Information Usage in Health Facilities Planning and Design: The State of the Art,* Kensington, New South Wales (Australia), University of New South Wales School of Health, 1976.
39. Heckler, T. and Sweetland, J. "Minimizing Costs Through Facilities Planning." *Topics in Health Care Financing* 3 (Summer 1977): 55-77.
40. Hogg, W. "Solving Space Problems in New Areas" *Hospital Administration in Canada* (14 July 1972): 8-9.
41. Ittelson, W.; Proshansky, H.; and Rivlin, L. "Bedroom Size and Social Interaction of the Psychiatric Ward." *Environment and Behavior* 2 (Dec. 1970): 255.
42. Jaco, E. G. "Ecological Aspects of Patient Care and Hospital Organization." In *Organization Research on Health Insittutions,* edited by B. Georgopoulous. Ann Arbor: Institute for Social Research, 1972.
43. Keep, P. J. "Stimulus Deprivation in Windowless Rooms." *Anesthesia* 32 (1977): 598-601.
44. Kenny, C., and Canter, D. *Findings from the Development of U.S.E.P.* Guilford, Eng.: Hospital Evaluation Research Unit, Department of Psychology, University of Surrey, 1978.
45. Kerr, J. "Space Use By Medical and Surgical Hospital Ward Staff." Ph.D. dissertation, UCLA, 1979.
46. Kim, J. "Functional Obsolescence in Community Hospitals." Ph.D. dissertation, University of Michigan, 1977.
47. Kornfield, D. "The Hospital Environment: Its Impact on the Patient." in *Advances in Psychosomatic Medicine: Psychosocial Aspects of Physical Illness,* edited by E. J. Lipowski, Vol. 8. Basel, Switz: Karger, 1972.
48. Lindheim, R., Glazer, H., & Coffin, C. *Changing Hospital Environments for Children.* Cambridge: Harvard Univ. Press, 1973.

49. Lindheim, R. *Uncoupling the Radiology System*. Chicago: Hospital and Educational Trust, 1971.
50. Lippert, S. "Travel in Nursing Units." *Human Factors* 13 (1971): 269-82.
51. McKendrick, G., and Emond, R., "Investigation of Cross-Infection in Isolation Wards of Different Design." *J. of Hygiene* 76 (Feb. 1976): 23-31.
52. McLaughlin. H.; Kibre, J.; and Raphail, M. *Obsolescence and Hospital Design*, Kaplan and McLaughlin Architects, San Francisco, Ca., 1972(a).
53. McLaughlin, H. "The Monumental Headache: Overtly Monumental and Systematic Hospitals are Usually Functional Disasters." *Architectural Record*, July 1976(a), p. 118.
54. McLaughlin, H.; Kibre, J.; and Raphail, M. "Patterns of Physical Change in Six Existing Hospitals" in *Environmental Design: Research and Practice*, edited by W. J. Mitchell. Los Angeles: UCLA, 1972(b).
55. McLaughlin, H. "Evaluating the Effectiveness of Innovative Design for a Community Mental Health Center." *Hospital and Community Psychiatry* 27 (1976b): 27.
56. Minckley, B. "A Study of Noise and Its Relationship to Patient Discomfort in the Recovery Room." *Nursing Research* 17 (May-June 1968): 247-50.
57. Noble, A., and Dixon, R. *Ward Evaluation: St. Thomas Hospital*. London: Medical Architecture Research Unit, The Polytechnic of North London, 1977.
58. Nuffield Provincial Hospitals Trust. *Studies in the Functions and Design of Hospitals*. London: Oxford Univ. Press, 1955.
59. Oberlander, R. "Beauty in a Hospital Aids the Cure." *Hospitals* 53 (16 Mar. 1979): 89.
60. Olsen, R. *"The Effect of the Hospital Environment."* Ph.D. dissertation, City University of New York, 1978.
61. Pendell, S., & Coray, K. An Evaluation of Nursing Unit Design. In P. Suedfeld & J. Russell (Eds.), *The Behavioral Basis of Design, Book I*. Stroudsburg, P.A.: Dowden, Hutchinson, and Ross, 1976.
62. Penkhus, M. "External Forces are Changing Patterns of Inpatient Care" *Hospital Topics* 54 (Mar.-Apr. 1976): 12.
63. Petersen, R. "Behavioral Design Criteria for a Hospital Emergency Department Waiting Room. Ph.D. dissertation, Univ. of Utah, 1978.
64. Pill, R. "Space and Social Structure in Two Children's Wards." *Sociological Review* 15 (July 1967): 179-92.
65. Rawlinson, C. "Space Utilization in Hospitals." *J. of Architectural Research* 6 (July 1978): 4-12.
66. Reizenstein, J. "Linking Social Research and Design." *Journal of Architectural Research* (Vol. 4), No. 3, December, 1975.
67. Reizenstein, J. *Social Research and Design: Cambridge Hospital Social Service Offices*. Springfield, Va.: National Technical Information Service, 1976.
68. Reizenstein, J. "Spatial Decision-Making in a Complex Organization." Unpublished paper, Department of Sociology, University of Michigan, 1977.
69. Ronco, P. "Human Factors Applied to Hospital Patient Care" *Human Factors* 14 (1972): 461-70.
70. Rosengren, W., & DeVault, S. The Sociology of Time and Space in an Obstetrical Hospital. In E. Friedson (Ed.), *The Hospital in Modern Society*, New York: Free Press, 1963.
71. Schum, M. "Humanizing a Hospital Interior." *Hospital Progress* 56 (Jan. 1975): 34-7.
72. Sommer, R., and Dewar, R. "The Physical Environment of the Ward" in *The Hospital in Modern Society*, E. Friedson (Ed.), New York: Free Press, 1963.
73. Spivack, M. "Psychological Implications of Mental Health Center Architecture." *Hospitals* 43 (Jan. 1969): 39-44.
74. Spivack, M. "Sensory Distortions in Tunnels and Corridors." *Hospital and Community Psychiatry* (Jan. 1967): 24-30.

75. Spivack, M. "Hospitalization—Time Without Purpose." *Ekistics* 245 (April 1976): 200.
76. Thompson, J. D. "Yale Studies of Hospital Function and Design," Washington, D.C.: U.S. Public Health Service, 1959.
77. Thompson, J. D., and Goldin, G. *The Hospital: A Social and Architectural History*. New Haven: Yale Univ. Press, 1975.
78. Traska, M. "Private Rooms Prove Highly Adaptable." *Modern Health Care* 7 (Apr. 1977): 54-5.
79. Trites, D.; Galbraith, F.; Sturdavant, M.; and Leckwart, J. "Influence of Nursing Unit Design on the Activities and Subjective Feelings of Nursing Personnel." *Environment & Behavior* 2 (Dec. 1970): 303-34.
80. Weeks, J.; Best, G.; Cheyne, J.; and Leopold, E. "Distribution of Room Size in Hospitals." *Health Services Research* 11 (Fall 1976): 227-40.
81. Welch, P. *Hospital Emergency Facilities: Translating Behavioral Issues into Design*. Cambridge: Harvard University Graduate School of Design, 1977.
82. Wehrli, R., and Kapsch, R. *Hospital Bedrooms and Nursing Units: A Systems Approach*. Gaithersburg, Md.: National Bureau of Standards, 1972.
83. Whitehead, C.; Ellison, G.; Kerpen, S.; and Marshall, D. et al. "The Aging Psychiatric Hospital: An Approach to Humanistic Redesign." *Hospital and Community Psychiatry* 27 (Nov. 1976): 781-8.
84. Willems, E. "Behavioral Ecology, Health Status and Health Care." in *Human Behavior and Environment: Advances in Theory and Research*, edited by I. Altman and J. Wohlwill, Vol. I. New York: Plenum, 1976.
85. Wilson, S. "Intensive Care Delirium." *Archives of Internal Medicine*, 130: 225, 1972.
86. Wolfe, M. "Room Size, Group Size and Density: Behavior Patterns in a Children's Psychiatric Facility." *Environment & Behavior* 7 (June, 1975): 199.
87. Zeidler, E. *Healing the Hospital*. Toronto: The Zeidler Partnership, 1974.

7

Opportunity for Control and the Designed Environment: The Case of an Institution for the Developmentally Disabled

Craig Zimring
College of Architecture
Georgia Institute of Technology

William Weitzer
Department of Psychology
University of Massachusetts at Amherst

R. Christopher Knight
Amherst, Massachusetts

Despite ambitious renovations and building programs, little information is available for the planning and design of living environments for developmentally disabled people. It is unclear how physical settings affect people with poor cognitive and functional skills—and indeed whether such people are affected at all by the physical design of their living environment. The ELEMR Project (Effects of the Living Environment on the Mentally Retarded) was funded by the Developmental Disabilities Office of the Department of HEW in order to address these issues.

ELEMR was a 4-year longitudinal research program studying the effects of interior design changes at a large state institution for the developmentally disabled. Large open wards were divided to provide three interior design schemes that provided increased privacy in more pleasant settings. A move by residents and staff into these renovated facilities allowed the relative influences of the different settings to be monitored. The outcomes of the research program include both theoretical conclusions about the relationships of behavior to the designed environment and pragmatic conclusions about the planning, design, and management of living facilities for the developmentally disabled.

Over a 30-month period, the project monitored 141 randomly chosen residents labeled "severely and profoundly retarded" and 50 direct-care staff. A multiple method data-gathering strategy was used to record the move from traditional ward-type institutions to the different renovated environments. Interviews, direct observation, participant and nonparticipant observation, analysis of records, and other methods were employed to focus on three classes of activities: residents' use of their own spaces, residents' social and solitary activities, and resident–staff interaction.

It is useful to consider an overview of the sections that follow. The *Research Context* discusses: (1) the project origins; (2) the normalization principle, which was the treatment philosophy informally guiding the renovations; (3) the research setting before and after the renovations; and (4) the larger system of influences that were identified using an informal system approach. The *Research Methods* sections addresses: (1) the observation methods; and (2) other complementary method. The *Results* section presents an overview of the data analyses as they relate to changes in three categories of behavior: (1) resident and staff recognition and respect of the residents' personal and private spaces; (2) staff–resident interaction; (3) resident social and solitary behaviors. The *Discussion* section focuses on: (1) the concept of control as it relates to the designed environment; (2) a theoretical heuristic "opportunity for control,"as it helps explain the ELEMR data; and (3) the implications of the research findings.

RESEARCH CONTEXT

In the early 1970s, attention by the press and increasing activism by parents of residents prompted dramatic physical and programmatic changes at Belchertown State School. A class-action suit brought on behalf of the residents by the Friends of Belchertown resulted in a major settlement for the school from the Commonwealth of Massachusetts, with $2.6 million designated for physical renovations. Old open wards and large barren dayrooms were to be renovated and divided into private and semiprivate spaces. In addition, a dedicated, capable administration was assembled to oversee this transition in treatment models.

The ELEMR Project originated when the research team, which included the present authors, with Arnold Friedmann and Harold Raush as Co-Principal Investigators[1], was approached by a top administrator from the institution. Although the court-ordered renovations were already being planned, the administrators and architects were finding little information to guide them in their design decisions. A single building had been renovated earlier on private funds, and these renova-

---

[1] In addition, the ELEMR Project is indebted to many people. The observers spent many hours of tireless labor; the Steering Committee provided invaluable assistance at many points during the research; the Developmental Disabilities Office, and especially Doris Haar, was supportive over 4 difficult years; many, many other people enriched the project—they are too numerous to name but deserve acknowledgment.

tions were believed to provide significant benefits for the residents. Staff members working in this building reported more frequent and positive conversations by the residents and less stereotyped behavior. However, observations of these benefits were informal and more systematic observation was required. The court-ordered renovations, which involved most of the buildings on the grounds, provided an opportunity for measuring these behavioral changes and generating data about the effect of less institutional, more "home-like" environments.

The Normalization Principle

The designs of the renovations at the state school were guided to a large extent by the "normalization principle." This principle has gained increased acceptance as an organizing concept for both physical design and service-delivery systems (Wolfensberger, 1972). Wolfensberger has described the normalization principle as: "the utilization of means which are as culturally normative as possible, in order to establish and/or maintain personal behaviors and characteristics which are as culturally normative as possible [p. 28]."

In Wolfensberger's view, the normalization principle addresses the broad issues of social deviancy. "Deviancy" is a creation of society that is manifest in the differential and stigmatizing treatment of individuals with variant lifestyles, physical handicaps, minority racial origins, or other distinguishing characteristics. In its most general sense, the normalization principle is viewed as an ideology for altering the culturally held concepts of deviancy that label the mentally retarded as odd, subhuman, and menacing and relegate them to a separate and debilitating existence.

In our view, the normalization principle has been justified principally as an ethical civil-rights issue. It calls for an end to the societal practice of labeling retarded people as "deviant," a practice that has led to their isolation behind the walls of bleak, over-crowded, and dehumanizing asylums. The crux of the argument is that the developmentally disabled deserve the same rights and privileges as other citizens to pursue normal, rich, and meaningful lives.

Within the normalization principle there remains another important issue, a *behavioral hypothesis*. The behavioral hypothesis suggests that much of the bizarre behavior associated with the mentally retarded in large institutions (and perhaps their developmental dificit itself) actually stems from their relegation to a deviant position in society. Institutional environments and social stigmatization rather than organic problems account for much of the apparently deviant behavior. It is argued that when integrated within communities and given supportive social and physical climates, the developmentally disabled will act in a more normal manner. Stated very simply, not only do the developmentally disabled deserve to be fully integrated into our society, but these are the only circumstances in which they may fully develop important personal and social skills.

One important element of normalization for the developmentally disabled concerns their physical living environment. Although physically normalized environments are not the only issues addressed by the normalization principle, they constitute an important element that has not been well-investigated in the past; they serve as the focus of the ELEMR Project. Within the concept of normalization, more homelike living designs are thought to encourage resident behaviors that are less deviant and more culturally normative. Many questions remain, however, concerning the dimensions of "normalized physical design," "homelike" interior designs, and the meaning and effects of these environments for the developmentally disabled.

Before continuing we should note that normalization, normal environments, and normal behavior are all terms that may be criticized for their vagueness and implicit value content. They may imply typical, average, positive, or ideal. Moreover, the meanings of these terms are highly dependent on personal values, social class, and culture. In this sense the terms present some vexing conceptual problems. Throughout this chapter *normal behavior* refers to behaviors that are positively valued, adaptive, and socially acceptable in the wider culture (e.g., high personal and social competence, independence). *Normalization* of built environments is taken to suggest positive and healthy settings, facilitating adaptive behaviors within this same value context.

An additional caveat should be noted: This report is not to be taken as support for institutions as viable living facilities. The case has been made convincingly elsewhere for moving most or all institutionalized clients into the community (Wolfensberger, 1972). The present study permitted research on only selected elements of normalization: the transition from a very desolate living facility to a somewhat more homelike one. Within this domain, the research begins to elucidate some of the underlying relationships between environments and behavior that affect the normalization process. More importantly, however, this study may help to avoid the recreation of mini institutions in the community. Many of the same dynamics among residents, staff, and the built environment found in large institutions can be unwittingly transported to community settings. A better understanding of these institutional dynamics may help us to avoid similar problems when designing community settings.

The Research Setting Prior to Renovations

Belchertown State School (BSS) is a large rural institution for the developmentally disabled located in Western Massachusetts. Primarily constructed in the 1920s and 30s, BSS has an architectural design that reflects an institutional treatment model accepted at that time. At the origin of the project, most of the residents were housed in moderate-size buildings (40 to 50 residents) on a campus of rolling hills. Each building contained six 30-by-40-foot rooms, three of which slept 15 to 20 residents in an open-ward arrangement. These are illustrated in the accompanying photographs and floorplans (Fig. 7.1-3). The remaining rooms served as dayrooms, dining halls, or multipurpose rooms. These rooms were designed in a familiar institutional scheme, using linoleum tile floors, plaster or ceramic tile walls, and plaster ceilings. Plaster walls were usually painted in pastel colors, with glossy paint low on the walls and flat paint above. Furnishings were sparse, institutional in design, and were often in poor condition.

The population of *residents* at BSS changed dramatically in the period from 1970 to 1977. In that period, the population dropped from about 1500 to 700 residents, with the most functionally capable leaving the institution for community residences and other community facilities. Consequently, those observed in the study were predominantly those who have been labeled "severely and profoundly retarded." The residents participating in this study were ambulatory, physically healthy adult men and women, most of whom had spent the bulk of their lives in large institutions. The residents ranged in day-to-day functional skills from those who required considerable assistance in dressing and toileting to others who showed modest independence. In comparison to institutions that had not gone through a similar depopulation, these residents would represent the least functionally developed and least socially skilled, those for whom there had been least hope of improvement or development. This is important to note in relationship to the magnitude of behavioral change that can be expected to result from renovations.

The *direct-care staff* in this study had the greatest day-to-day contact with residents—far more than the professional staff. Despite the centrality of their role in the residents' lives, direct-care staff tended to have low status on the grounds of the school. They were poorly paid and often poorly educated, although the average level of education increased somewhat in the 1970s at this particular state school. A custodial-maintenance attitude toward residents was reinforced by high ratios between residents and direct-care staff (effectively 15 to 30 residents to each direct-care staff member on duty), by training that emphasized physical care of residents, and by a lack of material and educational support. It should be recognized, however, that these negative conditions were a product of the entire social context of service-delivery for the developmentally disabled. The administration at BSS was active and progressive and made significant strides despite poor funding and inadequate support.

Renovations

The early 1970s witnessed increasing activism by parents and by the general public. This activism resulted in a class-action suit on behalf of the residents of Belchertown State School (BSS). The court found that the constitutional right to treatment of the residents had been violated and awarded $2.6 million to BSS for physical renovations. The buildings included in the ELEMR research were

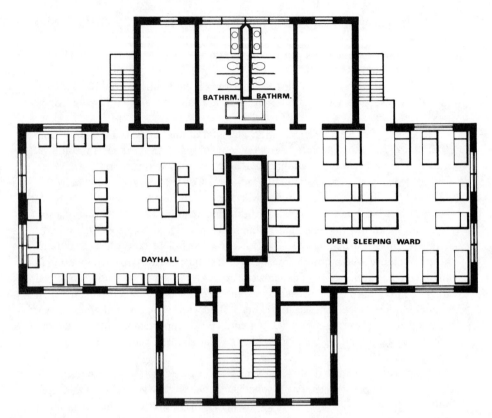

FIG. 7.1.   Open sleeping ward before renovations.

among those remodeled as a result of this court settlement. The court's consent decree established the time schedule and general physical characteristics of the renovations, with the actual form of the renovations determined by the court, the Friends of Belchertown, the administration, and the architects.

A very brief time period and low budget were allotted for design development. No formal document was provided to the designers that explicated spatial needs, room arrangements, and other architectural issues. Rather, the design was established more informally through interactions between the principal actors. Also, although the renovations were composed entirely of modifications of building interiors, no interior designer was involved. The designs that resulted were influenced by the perceptions of the various participants, and the quality of the designs clearly suffered from the fiscal and time pressures placed on the architects, Bradley Associates of Pittsfield, Massachusetts.

The ELEMR Project focused on three design schemes that were part of the normalization of the physical environment at BSS. These designs are illustrated

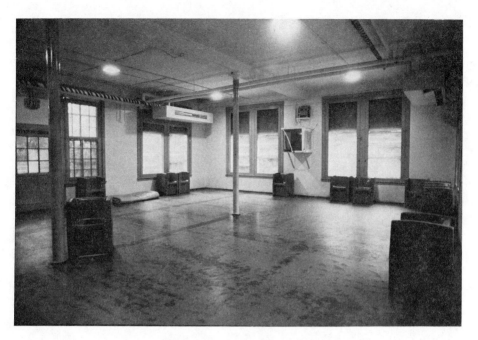

FIG. 7.2. Day hall before renovations.

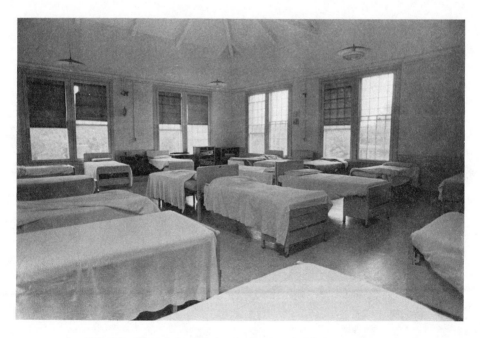

FIG. 7.3. Plan of open sleeping ward and day hall before renovations.

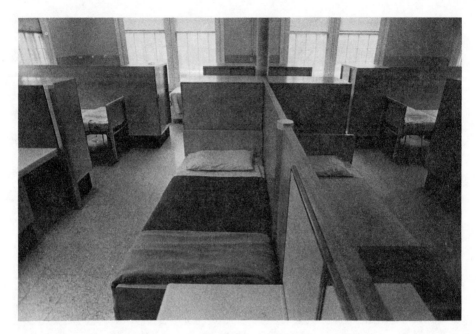

FIG. 7.4. Module bedroom.

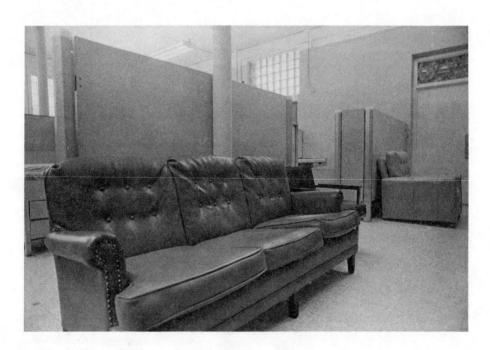

FIG. 7.5. Module lounge area.

in the accompanying plans and photographs. The first design was a renovation of the old institutional buildings inspired by the concept of landscaped offices: the *module design*. Shoulder-height partitions (4½ feet high) divided the large wards and day halls into 12 semiprivate modular units and a small lounge area. A plan of this renovation is shown in Fig. 7.4 (the dark vertical and horizontal lines represent partitions). Several views are presented in the photographs (Fig. 7.5, 6). Each modular unit had a bed, dresser/closet, desk, and mirror with corkboard. The low height of the walls created partial visual privacy that was only offered when seated or prone. Also, the placement of the walls and dressers provided less privacy for some modules than for others. The beds in the two modules in the center of each room were actually on pathways to the rear modules and were easily visible from the lounges as well. The corner modules provided a bit more privacy. Lighting was controlled by a central switch for each large room (wiring and lighting could not be altered as part of the renovations), and sound travelled easily from lounges to modules.

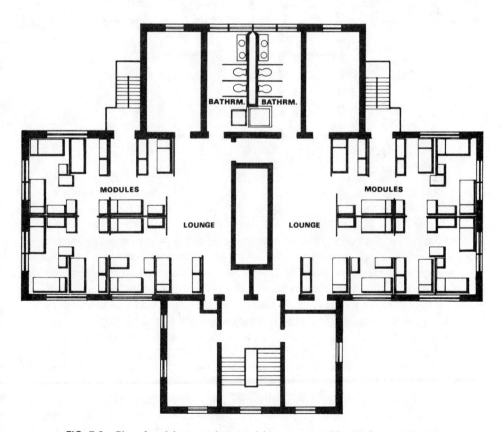

FIG. 7.6. Plan of module renovations (modules are separated by 4½ foot partitions).

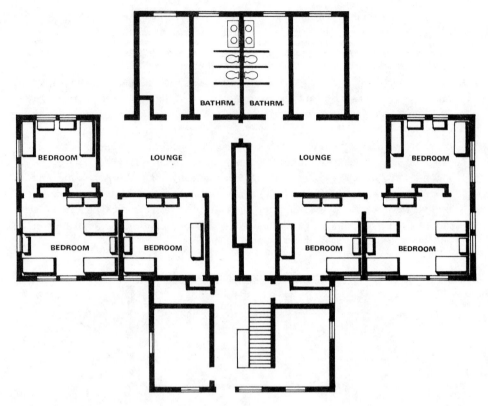

FIG. 7.7. Suite design bedroom.

The second renovation was a *suite design*. Eight-foot-tall partitions were introduced into the old ward rooms and day halls to provide four-room suites. However, because of the requirements of the heating system, there were gaps at the top of the partitions. Three of the rooms were 2-to-4-person bedrooms; the fourth served as a lounge. The bedrooms were attractively furnished with area rugs, drapery, dressers, chairs, and beds. However, as in the other designs, the furniture was vinyl covered and heavy. The bedrooms were individually lit by wall-mounted light fixtures in each room and were controlled by switches accessible to room occupants. The lounges were completely furnished. Each room had heavy vinyl-covered sofas and chairs, a television, and a coffee table, and some had lamps.

The third renovation was a *corridor design* resembling a college dormitory. The building that was renovated was constructed more recently (1968) and permitted a different design scheme as illustrated by the floor plans and photographs (Fig. 7.10–12). A central activity core included an entrance foyer, two large lounges, two smaller lounges, and staff and resident bathrooms. The large

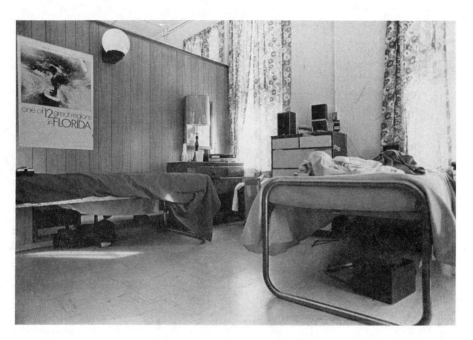

FIG. 7.8.   Suite design lounge.

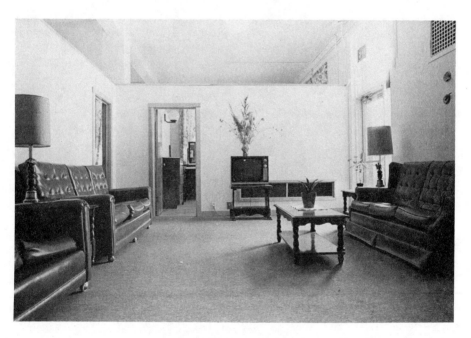

FIG. 7.9.   Plan of suite renovations.

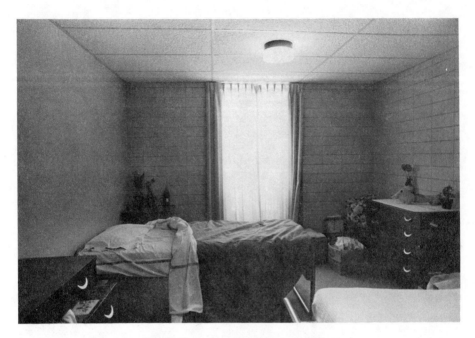

FIG. 7.10.   Corridor double bedroom.

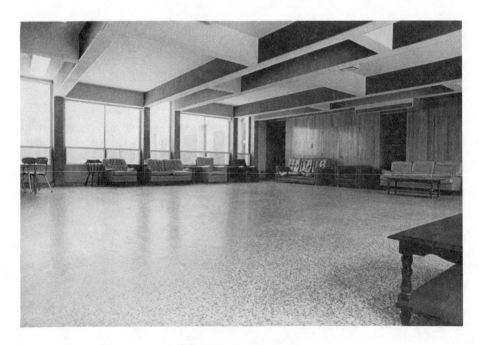

FIG. 7.11.   Corridor lounge.

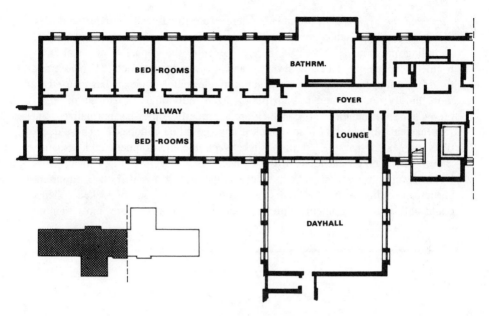

FIG. 7.12.   Corridor plan.

lounges had terrazzo floors, and wood and sheetrock walls. They were furnished with comfortable but very heavy vinyl-covered furniture. An attempt was made at acoustical treatment by adding carpet panels to ceiling beams and walls. The foyer, which was furnished with several sofas, had terrazzo floors and ceramic tile walls. The central activity core was flanked by two double-loaded bedroom corridors, one for men, the other for women. These hallways were carpeted and were separated from the central area by fire doors. Bedrooms were double or single rooms with dressers, mirrors, chairs, and closets. Bedroom doors were lockable, although they were usually left unlocked. Lights were individually controlled by occupants of each room.

The Larger System and Focal Problem

The renovated environments cannot be viewed in isolation from the institution in which they are situated. We sought to identify influential aspects of the renovations. For example, involvement by parents can alter treatment of residents by direct-care staff; administrative policies can encourage (or discourage) training; professional staff can potentially train residents to appropriately use the designed environment. These other agents within the BSS system were coined the *larger system*; they were not the focus of evaluation, yet, were important influences.

The *focal problem* was defined by the relationships within the larger system that were of greatest concern to the evaluation: *the relationship of residents, staff, and the designed environment.* There is a critical need to understand how developmentally disabled residents relate to the physical living environment, including questions such as: "Is there evidence of the impact of physical environments on people labeled 'severely and profoundly retarded'?." (Most optimism about social intervention and supportive research evidence has focused on more mildly retarded and less-institutionalized individuals.) "Do the different renovated environments, all of which are apparently somewhat normalized, affect residents differently? If so, which if any should be endorsed?" These questions suggested that the relationship between the environment and residents should be the empirical focus of this project.

However, observation and experience in the setting revealed other important participants: direct-care staff. Because doors were frequently locked, clients could only use environments with staff permission. Furthermore, most training

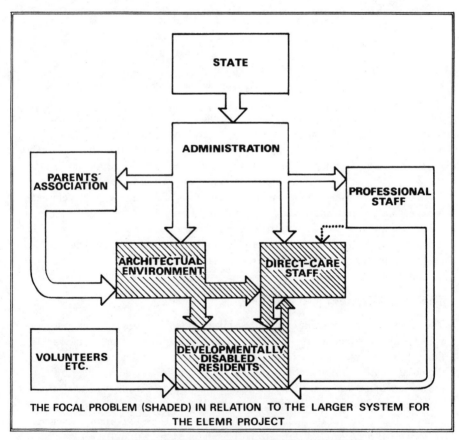

THE FOCAL PROBLEM (SHADED) IN RELATION TO THE LARGER SYSTEM FOR THE ELEMR PROJECT

(SIZE OF ARROW REFLECTS APPROXIMATE STRENGTH OF INFLUENCE

FIG. 7.13.   The focal problem in the context of the larger system.

of clients was performed by direct-care staff. If new environments were to be used appropriately, specific action by staff was required. For example, direct-care staff serve as examples by modeling appropriate (or inappropriate) behavior; they can also teach socially acceptable norms of privacy and modesty. Given the powerful role of the staff, a three-way focal problem was considered: residents, staff, and the built environment (Fig. 7.13).

Because the focal problem dictated an emphasis on the *living environment,* most attention was given to this area, and there were no direct observations of work or behavior-programming settings, administrative areas, or so on. Still, the larger system was monitored by formal and informal interviews, participant and nonparticipant observation, and frequent site visits.

RESEARCH METHODS

The ELEMR Project research methods were designed to examine the various ramifications of this attempt to create less institutional, more homelike settings. Reliable quantitative and qualitative techniques were used in a converging manner, allowing the strengths of some methods to compensate for weakness in others. The methods included direct observation of residents, direct observation of staff, structured and unstructured interviews, participant and nonparticipant observation, physical measurements of sound and acoustics, an experimental simulation of the impact of sound and acoustics on speech discrimination, and analysis of background and archival (Title XIX) data. These methods resulted in some 300,000 observations, 500 interviews, and thousands of pages of coded observations.

The ELEMR Project did not control changes in the research setting. It was anticipated that populations of residents and staff would shift unexpectedly because of renovation and building schedules or administrative decisions, and this in fact happened. For example, an infirmary ward was studied before renovations only to find the contractor's schedule delayed renovations until after all data collection was completed; at one point residents were partially reassigned to buildings according to their county of birth; some residents observed before renovations left for community placement, and so on. From the original number of environmental settings (buildings), residents, and staff in the research sample, we were able to use a reduced number of settings, selected because they allowed for clear comparisons and informative analyses.

Overview of Methods

An overview of the research strategy is presented in Fig. 7.14. The methodological approach of the project dictated that separate highly reliable schemes be used for direct observation of randomly selected residents and of staff. These, in turn, were supplemented by a broad range of qualitative techniques. This multiple-

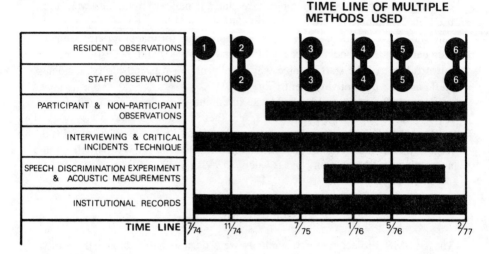

FIG. 7.14. Research strategy.

method approach permitted the relative strengths of some methods to compensate for weaknesses in others.

Resident observations included a behavior checklist with trained observers coding resident behaviors into discrete categories. Staff observations were also based on a behavior checklist but focused more specifically on interactions with residents and other staff. The observational measures were organized into 6-week observations. During each of these periods, each selected staff member and each selected resident was observed 550 times, with observations randomly distributed over afternoon and evening periods. Other methods included virtually continuous nonparticipant and participant observations, interviews, acoustic and noise measurements, a speech discrimination experiment, and utilization of institutional records. The use of various complementary measures facilitated an understanding of the complex social and physical changes represented by the renovations.

Observational Methods

Due to different needs, responsibilities, and behavior patterns of the residents and the staff, two different observation methods were developed.

Resident Observation Procedure.[2]   At observation period one, 17 to 20 residents were randomly selected from those living in each building being observed (building populations were 40 to 55 residents). At each subsequent observation

---

[2]The resident observation scheme was partially adapted from Viet, Simon, and Billings, 1974.

period, previously observed residents were included and additional residents from the remaining population were randomly selected to replace those who had moved from the building. The total sample for each building was maintained at 17 to 20.

The resident observation procedure was a *time-sampling* direct-observation scheme in which observations were randomly chosen at fixed time intervals. "Behavioral snapshots" were recorded every 15 seconds for periods of 10 observations, with 550 total intervals being recorded for each resident. The intervals were randomly sampled throughout a building during the afternoon and evening hours, when the residents were relatively free to use their building as they chose (2:00 p.m. to 9:00 p.m.). Each "behavioral snapshot" required coding the observed behavior of a specific resident into one of 41 mutually exclusive and exhaustive categories of interactive and solitary behaviors, such as "resident-staff verbal interaction" or "stationary intent." In addition, observers made judgments about the location of residents on a 4-by-4-foot gridded floor plan and coded the object nearest to the resident at the time of observation.

The analyses of resident behaviors included in this report were constructed by combining several specific observation codes into indices describing more general activities. A list of these larger behavioral classifications is presented in Table 7.1.

TABLE 7.1
Combined Resident Behavior Categories

1. *Resident Use of their Own Personal/Private Spaces*; included residents' presence in their own bed-area in the institutional design, or in the renovated designs, presence in their own module, private or semi-private rooms.

2. *Resident Intrusions into Others' Personal/Private Space*; included time spent in others' bed-area, module or room.

3. *Resident-Staff Interactions;* included all resident-staff interactive behaviors such as talking, touching, playing and aggression (although aggression was rare).

4. *Resident-Resident Interactions*; included all resident-resident interactive behaviors such as talking, hugging, cooperatively using an object, and aggression (which was again rare).

5. *Resident-Resident Positive Social Interactions*; included all interactions between residents but excluded aggression.

6. *Resident Verbal Interactions*; included all articulate interactions with other people such as utterances and physical gestures.

7. *Resident-Resident Verbal Interactions*; as in (6) included all articulate interactions, but was limited to interactions with other residents.

8. *Alert*; included solitary, noninteractive behavior that shows awareness of ongoing activities, such as watching passersby, watching television or walking purposefully.

9. *Withdrawn*; included solitary, noninteractive behaviors where the resident is not aware of ongoing activity such as stereotyped rocking or aimless pacing.

TABLE 7.2
Staff Behaviors Included in Final Analysis

1. *Staff Intrusions into Residents' Personal/Private Spaces*; included all behaviors in the residents' assigned bed-area, module or room.

2. *Staff Unjustified Intrusions into Residents' Personal/Private Spaces*; refers to time spent by staff in residents' assigned area without the residents being present.

3. *Staff-Initiated Interactions with Residents*; included all staff-resident interactions initiated by residents.

4. *Resident-Initiated Interactions with Staff*; included all staff-resident interactions initiated by staff.

5. *Interaction Context*; all interactions were coded into four contexts:

   (a) *Personal care*; included interactions where a member is caring for the physical needs of a resident;

   (b) *Ward activity*; included all staff-resident interactions where staff member is organizing residents;

   (c) *Formal training*; included all formal instruction of residents by staff;

   (d) *Social*; included all interactions not included in the above categories.

Staff (Attendant) Observation Procedure.[3]   All direct-care staff were observed in each building setting in the research design. The number of staff in each building varied from two to five (only one member refused to allow observation during the 2½-year period when observations took place). Due to frequent transfers and a high staff turnover rate, very few attendants were observed for more than one observation period. Supervisory and nursing staff were not included in the sample due to the incomparability of their work responsibilities to those of the direct-care staff.

The staff observation method was an *incident-sampling* recording scheme focusing on interactions of staff members with residents and other staff. Sampling of interactions was not based on time but rather on events, with events randomly selected and with both the frequency and characteristics of interactions noted. The data were collected by an observer focusing on one attendant and scoring his/her interactions (or noninteractions) during randomly selected 15-second intervals. During each 6-week observation period, about 550 intervals were recorded for each attendant in the sample. These observations took place in the building settings during the afternoon and evening hours (2:00 p.m. to 9:00 p.m.). As with the resident-observation method, each observer coded the 4-by-4-foot "grid-square" and the "object location" at which the behavior occurred. Table 7.2 lists the categories of staff behaviors derived from this procedure and used in the data analyses.

---

[3]The attendant observation scheme was partially adapted from Viet, Allen, Chinskey, Dailey, Harris, and Corcoran, 1974.

Validity and Reliability.   The reliability of coding for each variable for residents and staff was high. Each observation period spanned 6 to 8 weeks, and observations were randomly selected across time and situations. Prior to observing residents and staff, each observer was trained for 10 to 14 days. All observers achieved an interrater agreement rate of at least .85 for each behavioral category in the observation scheme before actual data gathering commenced. Most behavioral categories were reliably coded at a level between .95 and .99. Interrater agreement was rechecked at the midpoint of each observation period to insure continued reliability of coding.

Complementary Methods

Every data collection technique is limited in what it can detect, biased in the form of data it generates, and inherently incapable of achieving a fully satisfactory description of human phenomena. In the interest of addressing these problematic qualities of a single data-collection procedure, a variety of complementary techniques was used. These methods were used to corroborate and elaborate findings and to investigate ambiguities.

Participant and Nonparticipant Observation.   Participant and nonparticipant observations in the ELEMR Project included nearly 2 years observing staff routines, interactions with residents, and interactions among staff members, as well as 2 weeks of observation with the observer working as a full-time attendant in one residential building.

These qualitative techniques were employed to help grasp the underlying practices, values, and interactive networks that operated in the setting. Rather than attempting to develop specific categories and measure the frequency of behaviors, the participant observers attempted to synthesize their observations with information provided through discussions with informants and with consideration of the general interactive and language styles used by individuals in a setting. This technique was especially useful in that its flexibility allowed us to identify changing social concepts.

Interviews.   Throughout the 4 years of the ELEMR Project, both formal and informal interviews were conducted with staff members and administrators at BSS. At the most informal level, every site visit by the research team included conversations, questions, answers, and comments by attendants and administrators. This information became a part of the data for our analyses. More formally, several attendants and some lower-level administrators agreed to in-depth interviews concerning work routines, relationships between staff and residents, interstaff relationships, perceptions of the building renovation program, and other major issues of interest to them and to the research project.

Speech Discrimination Experiment and Acoustic Assessments. Acoustic measurements were conducted in both unrenovated buildings and in modular-unit designs in order to assess the reverberation qualities of rooms. In addition, noise-level readings were taken in a variety of buildings when dayrooms and wards were occupied by residents and staff. Using this information, an experiment using simulated conditions was conducted to determine the impact of typical reverberation qualities and noise levels on resident and staff abilities to discriminate spoken words.

Resident Institutional Records. As do most institutions, BSS keeps voluminous records on all residents. In the ELEMR Project, medical records and Medicaid Title XIX evaluations were used to assess individual difference characteristics of residents that might affect their responses to built environments. The records judged most meaningful and valid were used in data analyses, based on interviews with those supervising their collection. Among those evaluative characteristics analyzed were IQ, age, sex, and measures of abilities such as feeding, dressing, and bathing. A variety of analyses were conducted to understand the relationship of these variables to the behavioral observation data.

Research Design and Analysis of Data

As noted previously, the researchers had no control over the design of the renovations nor over the movement of residents between buildings. Renovations schedules and administrative decisions caused the residents and staff to change buildings with little warning and made a strictly controlled research design impossible. Despite this inconvenience, comparisons among buildings had to be made if the effects of the renovations were to be ascertained.

During the 30-month data collection period, nine different buildings were studied, with each building observed during one to five observation periods, totalling 17 building observations. From these observed settings, groups of residents were chosen who had moved together from a prerenovation setting to one or more renovated buildings. In most cases, residents moving as a group were observed, and randomly selected residents were added to the sample. Examination of the resident records and informal observations were used to confirm that groups used for comparison were similar on a large number of background variables and Title XIX evaluations.

Three resident/environment sequences were identified that allowed for renovation comparisons: (1) residents who moved from the institutional design to the corridor design to the suite design; (2) a different group of residents who moved from the institutional design to the corridor design only; and (3) groups of residents who moved from the institutional design to the module units. These comparisons allowed within-group analyses of residents moving from unrenovated to renovated buildings, and between-group comparisons of randomly chosen residents living in the different renovated settings.

Whenever possible in conducting the data analyses, standard statistical techniques were used. For example, in the case of the resident characteristic data, significance in correlation and regression analyses was determined by the proportion of variance accounted for, as is the standard procedure. However, some problems were presented in the analysis of trends for the observational data. A decision was made to focus on individual patterns of change and only secondarily on changes in group means (as would be a more standard method). The rationale for this view was that the residents were placed in BSS for very diverse reasons (e.g., epilepsy, brain damage, family problems, emotional difficulties), and to label the residents as a single group would have been highly misleading.

The problem in determining significance in the observational data was addressed in the following manner. Behavioral patterns were considered to be statistically reliable if the pattern of behavior changes of individuals in the within-group sample (those experiencing all building settings within a given comparison) met a predetermined criteria of consistency. These criteria, based on probability distributions, depended on the number of persons and settings involved.[4]

RESULTS

Having spent over 2½ years gathering information through a number of formal and informal methods, the task of integrating the sources of data was formidable. The quantitative nature of the resident and staff observation strategies and the large amount of information gathered through these strategies resulted in a heavy focus on these methods. However, without the additional qualitative and quantitative data derived from other measures, the full extent of the changes that took place at BSS would not have been revealed. At many stages during the data analyses, one method or another either suggested a direction for future analyses or shed light on results in hand.

In the following summary of the results, the intention is to provide an overview of the conclusions drawn from the data analyses and to highlight the sources of the information that directed these findings. The data from the resident

---

[4]For example, a group of five residents were observed in three settings. The probability of any resident's score, on a given variable, increasing or decreasing from one setting to the next is simply .5. Therefore, the probability of any one pattern occurring over two setting changes is $.5^2$ or .25 for any one individual. According to a binominal distribution, the probability of four out of five of these individuals showing the same pattern of change is less than .0156. Therefore, our criterion for accepting a pattern as significant was based on achieving similar patterns for four out of five residents.

and staff observations serve as the cornerstone of this summary, and, where appropriate, complementary methods are introduced.

Overview of the Results

The data collected from the observation of residents and staff and augmented by other methods were analyzed in terms of three specific questions:

1. Did staff and residents use, recognize, and respect personal/private space? It was taken as a necessary prerequisite that staff and residents use the new environments in some way before they experienced more profound personal and social changes.

2. Did staff–resident interactions change? Most teaching of residents occurred through direct interactions with direct-care staff members. Institutionalized residents needed training in order to learn to use more normalized environments most effectively.

3. Did resident social and solitary behaviors change? If the normalization of environments was to be valuable, it should have affected such behaviors as: amount of resident interactions with other residents, quality of resident interaction, and resident alertness.

The overall trend of the results indicated that even poorly functioning developmentally disabled residents exhibited improved social and solitary behavior in the more homelike renovated environments. However, the effects of the built environment were mediated by the staff responses to the environment and by the extent to which the residents were allowed to realize control over their environmental experiences. Although the very lowest functioning residents were more alert in some renovated buildings, improvements in their social behavior were limited by their poor cognitive abilities, paucity of existing social skills, and the absence of meaningful training by staff.

Comparison of the results in the different settings revealed that the corridor design was clearly more positive than the unrenovated buildings, the suite, or the module. The summary of these data, provided in Fig. 7.15, illustrates that little change from the unrenovated setting was evidenced in the module design, some appropriate changes were seen in the suite, and stronger appropriate changes occurred in the corridor design.

Earlier, we described the criteria that were utilized in determining whether these changes were significant. However, it is also relevant to note that significant changes in percentages of behaviors can be misinterpreted if not viewed in the context of the frequency of their occurrence. All the social behaviors listed in the table occurred on a relatively infrequent basis (for the most part, they comprised less than 20% of the observations) and the two nonsocial behaviors (alert and withdrawn) were exhibited quite frequently (often over 50% of the time). It is important to note the low frequency of these behaviors but also to note that, when compared to the frequency of social and nonsocial behaviors occurring in a

OVERVIEW OF MAJOR
QUANTITATIVE RESULTS
CHANGES FROM THE INSTITUTIONAL
DESIGN

○	=	NO CHANGE
▽	=	DECREASE
△	=	INCREASE
▼	=	SIGNIFICANT DECREASE
▲	=	SIGNIFICANT INCREASE

BEHAVIORS OBSERVED	MODULE	SUITE	CORRIDOR HIGHER FUNCT. RES.
STAFF INTRUSIONS INTO RESIDENT PERSONAL-PRIVATE SPACES *	○ *	▽ *	▼ *
RESIDENT INTRUSIONS INTO OTHER RESIDENTS' PERSONAL-PRIVATE SPACES *	○ *	▽ *	▽ *
RESIDENTS' USE OF THEIR OWN PERSONAL-PRIVATE SPACES	○	△	▲
OVERALL STAFF-RESIDENT INTERACTION	○	▽	▽
STAFF INITIATIONS TO RESIDENTS	○	▼	▽
RESIDENT INITIATIONS TO STAFF	HIGHER FUNCT. ○ RES.	▼	▽
OVERALL RESIDENT-RESIDENT INTERACTIONS	○	△	▲
RESIDENT RESIDENT VERBAL	○	△	▲
ALERT BEHAVIORS	○	△	▲
WITHDRAWN BEHAVIORS *	○ *	▽ *	▼ *

*THESE BEHAVIORS ARE NEGATIVELY VALUED, HENCE A DECREASE CAN BE CONSIDERED THERAPEUTIC CHANGE

FIG. 7.15.   Overview of findings.

typical American home, these proportions are not necessarily out of the ordinary. Comparisons of the renovation designs are discussed in three parts, each section addressing one of the questions identified earlier.

Resident and Staff Recognition and Use of Personal/Private Space.   Resident and staff recognition and use of personal/private space was an important prerequisite for more complex behavioral change. The measurement of recognition and use was seen as an initial check to see if there were any behavioral effects at all of renovations; if personal/private spaces were not used and recognized, it seemed logical that they would not have more subtle behavioral effects. Non-recognition of personal/private space was operationally defined as "intrusion"— the time spent by residents and staff in others' personal/private spaces. "Un-justified intrusion" was defined as the time spent in others' spaces without the "owner" present. The obverse of nonrecognition was "use of own personal/private space." "Use" was operationally defined as the time that residents spent in the area assigned to them (i.e., depending on the design, the resident's own bed, module, or bedroom).

The staff's and the residents' recognition and use of personal/private space increased significantly more in the corridor design than in the other renovation designs. The staff intruded less often into the residents' spaces, and fewer of those intrusions were unjustified (e.g., were without the presence of residents). Moreover, two groups differing in functional abilities were observed in this same setting, and this finding held true for both the higher- and lower-functioning resident groups.

However, the finding that staff intruded less often into resident spaces was not necessarily the result of a change in staff attitudes. Participant observation and informal interviews revealed that the staff found supervision to be more difficult in the more variegated renovated environments. Hence, the renovations in some cases reduced intrusions into residents' private spaces due to the increased diffi-culty in supervising these areas.

In the suite design, the frequency of staff intrusion was less than in the unrenovated institution, yet more than the corridor design. In the module design, however, the staff actually showed a slight increase in intrusions. Several months after the renovations, informal observations revealed that dictates by the adminis-tration to increase supervision of the spaces were causing the staff to spend more time with residents in the module areas. As a result, the level of staff intrusion increased dramatically in the last observation period. The participant observer, Hollis Wheeler, recorded the following observations:

> Prior to this (new administrative dictate), if a resident didn't want to clean their room, that was their privilege . . . Now we (the attendants) have to do all the clean-ing, and instead of being the resident's privilege, they can't leave the building until it's done . . . Doing this dusting and stuff in the resident's room is really a Catch 22 situation: We are not suppsoed to go into the rooms without knocking and being invited in . . . However, now we are under order to clean their rooms and make sure everything is picked up, so the attendants naturally think the whole deal is absurd and it frustrates them and they resent it.

The level of intrusions by residents was affected similarly to the level of staff intrusions. In the suite and corridor designs, intrusions by residents into others' personal/private space were reduced in comparison to the unrenovated institution. However, unlike the case of staff intrusions, where the corridor design was superior, both the corridor and suite designs had similarly low levels of resident intrusions. Further, in the corridor design even the lower-functioning group of residents did not intrude frequently into other residents' private rooms. And for both higher- and lower-functioning residents, a large proportion of the time in others' private rooms was not alone; much of the "intrusion" in the corridor design appeared to involve some form of socializing. Pecularities in the physical designs did not allow this to be measured in the other designs without actual intrusion by the observers. However, the qualitative measures showed socializing to be much less common in private spaces in other designs.

In the modular design, the level of resident intrusion was higher after renovations. However, the administrative change that increased supervision between the two postrenovation observations served to decrease resident intrusion during the last observation period (i.e., the constant presence of attendants helped keep residents in their own spaces).

Residents' use of their own personal/private spaces showed a similar pattern to the intrusion data. The suite design showed a moderate increase in use of the resident's own space in comparison to the unrenovated institution. However, the module design also showed an increase in use with the renovations. Once again, an administrative order caused residents to be kept in their own modules, which resulted in increased use of their own space. This increase was apparently due to the supervisory pressures by staff rather than residents spontaneously using their own spaces.

Regarding the resident characteristics, initial analyses indicated that conventional demographic characteristics (age, sex, age at admission, years in the institution) did not predict spatial behavior. This finding allowed all further analyses to be conducted ignoring these demographic distinctions. In addition, ratings of individual functional levels were found to be unrelated to the residents' use of private spaces and their respect of others' private spaces. In the next section, the role of resident characteristics in predicting social behavior is discussed.

Staff-Resident Interactions.   The second issue of the focal problem concerned the interactions among staff, residents, and environment. The residents had long institutional histories, and if they were to learn to use new environments properly they had to be trained to do so. At BSS most resident training was conducted by the direct-care staff. Obviously, if such training was to occur, residents and staff had to communicate; one rough index of staff-resident communication was simply the total level of interaction. The resident data allowed analysis of the overall proportion of resident time spent interacting with staff. The staff data allowed more fine-grained analysis, permitting the discrimination between staff-initiated and resident-initiated interactions.

Levels of staff-resident interactions changed in a manner apparently antithetical to effects on spatial usage. Indeed, the findings were somewhat paradoxical:

There was less staff-resident interaction in both the corridor design and the suites than in the unrenovated institution. This finding was corroborated by both the resident data and staff data and was generally true for both higher- and lower-functioning groups of residents. For the higher-functioning group, both resident and staff initiations decreased in the renovated environment; for the lower-functioning group, staff decreased their initiations to residents, but residents maintained a roughly constant level of initiations to staff.

A somewhat different pattern emerged from resident-staff interactions in the module renovations. Even before renovations there was a slight trend for interactions to increase, and this trend was somewhat accelerated with renovations. Detailed analysis revealed the sources of this trend. The staff data showed that staff initiations to residents increased, but resident initiations to staff did not. Thus, staff was responsible for starting more interactions with residents. Moreover, when residents were divided into high-IQ and low-IQ groups, with means of 30 and 17, respectively, the results were further clarified. The high-IQ group increased its interactions with staff after renovations; the low-IQ group did not. This effect was perhaps due to the staff being locked into the modular areas with residents. When they had no choice but to interact, they chose higher-functioning, more responsive residents.

The speech discrimination data were informative in this regard. In a controlled experiment, it was found that speech discrimination was affected by noise, reverberation time, and whether the subject was a resident or staff member. All participants could better discriminate words in low noise and in short reverberation time. And, although all participants were previously screened for perfect hearing, staff could discriminate words better than residents. There was a noise-by-group interaction: Residents' speech discrimination was more degraded by high noise than was the staff's. In addition, the residents were more affected than were staff by the overall prerenovation conditions, including long reverberation time and high noise (Gentry & Zimring, 1979).

These effects suggest that changes in levels of social interaction due to renovation can be explained in part by speech discrimination problems that may have been prevalent in the acoustically deficient prerenovation environment. For example, some of the perceptions of the staff that the residents were subnormal may have resulted from inappropriate responses by residents due to difficulties in speech discrimination.

Resident-Resident Social and Solitary Behaviors. The third aspect of the focal problem centered on the residents themselves. If residents are to make strides toward autonomous functioning either in institutions or in the community, they must show significant changes in several key interactive and solitary dimensions. Interactions were divided into resident-staff and resident-resident interactions. Whereas resident-staff interactions were described previously, resident-resident interactions are of equal importance, as much learning can potentially occur through peer contact.

The observational measures showed that residents in the corridor-style building spent more time interacting with each other than those living in the suite arrangement, and residents in both renovated styles interacted more with other residents than did those living in the institutional arrangement. Moreover, a greater proportion of this social interaction was positive and a greater proportion was verbal. In the module-style building there was no effect; resident–resident interaction remained virtually constant (and very infrequent) across the renovations.

When examining the residents on a continuum from lower to higher functioning, the analysis of the resident characteristic data revealed no relationship between measures of resident functional level and use of space by residents. However, these data do shed light on the observed social behavior. The analyses from the prerenovation environments revealed a positive relationship between resident functional level and social behavior. No such relationship was found in the new environments. This finding suggests that even lower-functioning residents were responding to the renovations with increased amounts of social behavior, and thus there was a marked weakening in the relationship between functional level and social behaviors.

Solitary behaviors by residents are important, too. Only a portion of day-to-day life is spent interacting with others. Solitary behaviors were operationalized using two large categories. ''Withdrawn'' was coded when a resident was out of contact with the surrounding environment, when he/she was performing stereotyped actions or was wandering aimlessly. ''Alert'' was the converse of ''withdrawn'' and was coded when a resident was not interacting but was following surrounding activities, or he/she was moving to a location in a purposeful manner.

Measures of solitary behavior once again demonstrated that the corridor design was the most beneficial. Residents were more alert and less withdrawn in the corridor design than in the suite or institutional design. This finding was consistent for both the higher- and lower-functioning groups. The modular design showed equivocal results. Though not significant, there was an apparent trend for decreased ''withdrawal'' and increased ''alertness'' immediately after the renovations to the modular design. This trend reversed by the last observation period, by which time these levels had returned to their prerenovation levels. It was not possible to discern whether this reversal was due to the increased supervision of staff, or to residents habituating to the new environment, or to some combination of these factors.

DISCUSSION

The corridor design had many beneficial impacts: Residents and staff recognized and used personal/private spaces; residents interacted more with each other; more of those interactions were verbal and positive; residents were more alert and less withdrawn. The suite design had similar, though weaker, effects. The modular design had no measurable effects on these behaviors.

These results suggest some vexing problems for interpretation. The homelikeness and visual appeal of the suite-style design did not facilitate the most dramatic changes in resident behavior. Rather, the most positive environment was the corridor design where, despite its institutional appearance, there were several socially appropriate changes in resident behavior such as: less resident intrusion into others' private spaces, increased use of the residents' own spaces, increased resident–resident interaction, increased alertness, decreased withdrawal, and other positive changes. A possible explanation for these broadly based behavioral impacts is that the corridor design better enabled the residents to control their environmental situation to fit their individual needs.

In the following section, the discussion begins with a look at environmental control as a mediator between human behavior and the built environment (Barnes, 1980; Baum & Valins, 1977) and examines several ways control operates in designed environments. Then, the usefulness of control as an explanatory heuristic for viewing the specific ELEMR Project findings is explored. Finally, environmental design and theoretical implications of the research are considered, and directions for future research are addressed.

Control in the Designed Environment

The Concept of Control.   The process of effecting a comfortable relationship between individual needs and environmental attributes—of increasing person-environment fit—requires the exercise of personal *control*. This issue has recently undergone intense scrutiny in psychology. Although the complexity of this issue is too great to untangle in the present chapter, research findings are generally consistent: Increased actual and perceived control generally provides positive effects for the individual. With control over their lives people feel more satisfied, less stressed, and perform tasks more effectively (Averill, 1973; Barnes, 1980; Barron & Rodin, 1978).

This section addresses issues directly related to control as it operates in *designed* environments. Firstly, we consider a useful conceptualization of needs that must be satisfied by the designed environment. Secondly, costs of lack of control are considered. Finally, mechanisms for exercising control are discussed.

Steele (1973) proposed that several individual needs are directly affected by the designed environment. Steele's conceptualization helps identify critical areas where the environment must fit the individual. To paraphrase Steele, these needs may be labeled: (1) *safety and security,* including physical comfort and safety from crime; (2) *social interaction,* including raucous activity, quiet conversation, visual privacy, auditory privacy, and so on; (3) *task support,* including all the various personal and professional tasks that must be accomplished; (4) *environmental knowing,* including the knowledge necessary to find one's way and to generally predict events in the environment; (5) *environmental messages,* including the various symbolic statements environments make to users; (6) *pleasure;* (7) *growth.* The ELEMR Project focused on the second issue, social interaction among residents, staff, and others, However, it is important to recognize the interrelatedness of these various needs. For example, because residents had little direct power to fill safety and security needs, they had to rely on social interactions with staff to achieve many of their basic needs; because the environment clearly communicated to all participants that the residents were to be maintained in a custodial manner, little growth was encouraged.

Secondly, there are at least two sets of costs attached to control. The costs most commonly associated with lack of control directly result from specific misfits or unfulfilled needs in a given situatio- and are independent of any more general feeling of lack of control or impotence. These specific stressors involve costs independent of any more general self-judgments. For example, if a resident needs to sleep but noise in the crowded dormitory prevents him or her from doing so, the resident directly suffers from tiredness. Similarly, if a staff member is trying to accomplish an assigned duty, and the lack of a conducive environment does not allow him or her to do a good job, the staff member may directly suffer from a low job evaluation. In these situations the individual may also feel generally helpless or out of control, but the point here is that he or she suffers directly from tiredness or poor job evaluation.

There are also potential costs attached to the processes used in resolving person–environment misfits (these have been more thoroughly studied in psychology than have been direct costs, Barnes, 1980; Baron & Rodin, 1978). These process–costs arise in at least two ways. Firstly, when there is a particularly serious misfit between person and situation, and when no graceful or socially valued methods are available for altering the misfit, the individual may choose adjustment processes that are themselves costly. For example, when residents are locked in a large barren dayroom and have no access to private space, they may limit interaction by fiercely protecting territories in the dayroom by using verbal or even physical aggression. These control strategies can be costly, in that they lead to physical harm or disciplinary action or may lead to long-term costs of fewer friendships and lower satisfaction.

A second type of process–cost results from the self-attributions individuals make based on their own behavior. If a person is ineffective in fulfilling important needs, he/she may feel impotent, powerless, out of control. These feelings then may become linked to listlessness, passiveness, and depression (Baum, Singer, & Baum, 1981; Seligman, 1975). For example, if a resident tries time and time again to change the channel on a television or to reduce the volume and is constantly thwarted, the resident soon gives up—learns that his or her efforts make no difference, anyway. Assessing these types of costs requires that the individual's experience be understood. These costs may only arise if the individual perceives his/her power or powerlessness.

It is important to realize, also, that the costs of coping strategies are highly dependent on one's perspective. To some direct-care staff members, a resident's assertive actions to fulfill his/her own needs may be seen as costly if they arouse others to similar actions. To other direct-care staff, this consequence may be viewed as a benefit rather than a cost, because it moves the residents toward independent behavior.

It is necessary to consider how person–environment fit is regulated. As a first step, it is necessary to acknowledge the complexity of the fit between person and environment. The environment is both a social entity and a physical entity. As a social entity, the environment includes both the expectations and past experiences an individual brings to an environment, as well as the existing social structure of the setting, including power relationships, rules, and other issues. As a physical entity, an environment can be seen as an increasingly large set of spaces, each having its own control mechanisms. These spaces include: clothing, rooms, buildings, cities, regions, etc.

Moreover, the person is also complex. He or she may have widely divergent skills, needs, desires. The diversity of environments and persons tends to make the regulation of person–environment fit an individual matter. Yet, environmental mechanisms can be identified that work for a broad range of persons.

Two sets of mechanisms are available to individuals to improve person–environment fit: changing personal needs and changing the environment. For example, if a resident comes to realize that his bedroom is not as attractive as desired, that it communicates an unfavorable environmental message about the resident's work and status, there are several alternatives. The resident may directly change the situation by beautifying or renovating the room, or he/she may exercise choice and move to another setting. These are probably the strategies that affluent people with power over their lives would choose. However, institutional residents frequently lack this power. Often, residents have little money and have little voice in any environmental changes. Moreover, the physical setting may provide the resident little choice of rooms (e.g., the unrenovated dorms at BSS had six large rooms for up to 55 residents), and the social system may not allow the resident to choose another setting. As a result, the resident is forced to change his/her own needs, to decide that the poor environment makes no difference, and to accommodate to the existing setting.

A similar scenario of the regulation of person–environment fit can be seen with the manipulation of social interaction. If an owner of a suburban house is bothered by the noisy play of her two sons, she can manipulate the situation by quieting them, or she may exercise choice by moving to another room. However, a resident in an institution may not have these options. If the resident is locked in a crowded, noisy day dayroom and wants peace, he/she may lack the power to quiet the other residents or to move to other rooms. Moreover, the building simply may not provide adequate choice. There may only be large public dayrooms, bathrooms, and sleeping wards, with no space for quiet reflection.

The physical environment allows the regulation of personal-environment fit by providing the *opportunity for control* of personal experience (Knight, Zimring, & Kent, 1977). The physical environment may offer both choice and direct manipulation of the physical environment. However, for a choice in settings to be possible, the environment must provide a variegated set of rooms; for direct manipulation of heat, light, and noise to be possible, the environment must provide physical control over those ambient qualities. However, the physical environment can only provide the *opportunity* for control. The social context will dictate whether this control is realized. Four walls and a door may define a resident's private room, for example, but this room is only private if it is respected by other people.

A related research program has examined similar designs in college dormitories and serves to exemplify this theoretical analysis. Baum and Valins (1977) examined several freshman dormitories at the State University of New York at Stony Brook and at Trinity College. At Stony Brook, freshmen were randomly assigned by the housing office to one of two different room arrangements: (1) rooms located on double-loaded corridors with 36 residents sharing a common lounge and bathroom; or (2) suites where six students shared a lounge and bathroom. Baum and Valins observed and interviewed the students living in the two dorm types and had them participate in several experimental studies. Despite having comparable floor area per person, residents felt more crowded and behaved differently in the long corridor settings than did the residents in suites.

Baum and Valins attributed the difference between the designs to the amount of control each offered. The suite and short-corridor arrangements provided semiprivate spaces (lounges and hallways) that served only a small number of people. In these designs, residents could more easily control social interactions, light, heat, and noise.

Opportunity for Control and the ELEMR Data.   The normalization principle as it relates to physical designs was only partially useful for understanding the impacts of renovated environments. The minimally normalized modular renovations did have little impact, as would be expected. Yet, some findings were not as would have been suggested by the normalization principle: The most aesthetic and homelike suites were *less* effective than the more institutional corridor design in encouraging socially appropriate behavior. However, if we view these results in terms of the opportunity for control each allowed, the findings become more comprehensible.

The prerenovation environment offered almost no opportunity for control. The sleeping wards were vast seas of beds that often provided little walking space, much less visual or auditory privacy. Day halls were large cacophonous rooms with blaring televisions and furniture lining the walls; control of social interaction was difficult or impossible. In addition, lights, television, radiators, and so on were controlled by the staff; residents had little control of their ambient environment. Residents were locked into the sleeping wards or day halls for hours at a time. They had no option to move to a more sympathetic setting.

The modules failed almost totally in normalizing behavior because they offered little opportunity for control. The 4½-foot-high partitions offered only a small amount of visual privacy and offered no control over heat, light, and noise. Moreover, the openness of the design presented no real choice among activities. A blaring television in the lounge area was just as loud in the private modules. And the lack of choice was exacerbated by the attitudes of staff, who were compelled to oversee the safety of the residents and to ensure the cleanliness of the building.

This supervisory attitude mandated that doors between the module areas be locked, preventing residents from exercising what little choice the design might have offered. Finally, the modules offered few symbols to aid in social control. The modules had as little as one wall defining the space; most "private" closets were in the corridor; there was no secure place to store possessions. These symbols simply did not communicate to residents or staff that private spaces were to be respected, nor did they allow teaching of appropriate activities such as knocking before entering.

The suites offered greater opportunity for personal control. Residents in each 2-4-person bedroom could control their own lights, and close and lock their doors. The 8-foot partitions offered good visual privacy from people other than roommates. The bedrooms and lounges were at least visually separated and hence quite different activities could occur in them. Also, the bedrooms were well-defined spaces and contained closets, lightswitches, and so on.

Yet, the suites were still limited in their opportunity for control. Because of heating problems, the top of the partitions ended short of the ceiling, and sound traveled over them. Noises from the lounge easily overflowed into the bedrooms. Moreover, there were no transition spaces to separate public and private areas. Open doors exposed private spaces to curious individuals in the lounge. Although the suite design offered a more homelike environment than the unrenovated dorm or modular units, it offered only limited personal control.

The corridor-style renovation had the greatest positive impacts; these impacts are comprehensible if it is understood that this design offered the greatest opportunity for control. Single-person bedrooms and double bedrooms offered considerable control over physical stimulation. Each person or pair could manipulate the lightswitch; they could close the door to limit the noise or discourage interaction. Moreover, the corridors provided a "hierarchy of spaces," with clearly indicated public and private spaces, and a buffer zone between them. Also, there were a wide variety of spaces in the building; small television rooms, large lounges, entrance foyers, corridors, bedrooms. The varied nature of these, and the full-wall construction, allowed many different activities to occur simultaneously.

The corridor design was clearly the most effective in aiding behavior change for these clients. However, it is critically important not to misconstrue the reasons for its relative success. The corridor design *was not an ideal setting* and, in fact, retained many institutional features. Nonetheless, it did offer a *meaningful level of control* for the users. The corridor design offered considerable physical control: If a person wanted to be quiet and sleep, he/she could close the door and quiet was provided. On the other hand, in the suites, if someone wanted to sleep while activity was going on in the lounge, he/she had to challenge the noisemakers or try to resort to symbolic control. Socially adept people might cope with this situation by yawning and commenting on their tiring day; if the people in the lounge were equally adept, they would understand these symbols and reduce noise levels. However, severely and profoundly retarded individuals with long institutional histories rarely have such sophisticated social skills; more explicit, physical control was needed, the kind of physical control that was more adequately provided in the corridor design.

Opportunity for Control and the Paradox of Staff-Resident Interactions. Staff involvement in the normalization process is critical, yet the data indicated a paradox. In the buildings where the residents showed greatest improvement, there was less staff–resident interaction. Does this mean that reducing staff involvement is somehow desirable?; that reducing the staff's role is necessary to the normalization process? The thrust of quantitative results, as well as participant observation and other qualitative data, suggests that residents improve, not *because* of the decrease in interaction, but *in spite* of it. Even in the corridor-style renovation, changes in resident behavior were fairly modest. Although important and statistically significant, changes were limited to relatively small shifts in social and solitary behaviors. Observations, analysis of institutional records and other evidence, suggest that residents were still operating below capacity. The only way that severely and profoundly retarded residents can fulfill their capacities is through comprehensive training, in which direct-care staff have a central role (as discussed earlier in the section on normalization; the impoverished and artificial institutional environment also places limits on the residents' growth).

So why did the staff interact less in the "better" buildings? The concept of opportunity for control sheds some light on this phenomenon; *renovated buildings also allowed the staff some measures of personal control.* However, the way staff used this control must be seen in the context of evidence from interviews, participant observation, and other data. Direct-care staff were generally very capable but were poorly paid, poorly trained, and, often, highly alienated from their work. They faced pressures to train residents, yet, had little support in these efforts. Staff were bored and harried. When provided the opportunity, they exercised personal control by withdrawing from residents.

The participant observation notes confirm this impression of the staff's attitudes. After participating in staff orientation, Hollis Wheeler wrote:

> My general impression of orientation was corroborated by an attendant who commented: "You know, that orientation was interesting but you know what it showed? It showed you're just beating your head if you want to change anything around here."

> Both Cher and Gloria, plus the charge, have given me the advice, "Just do what you can," i.e., "it is impossible to do everything so just do what is possible and don't worry about the rest."

In fact, in the corridor renovation, which offered the most varied spaces, there was least staff intrusion into personal/private spaces. This lack of intrusion was probably due, in part, to the symbolic meaning of the corridor rooms—such rooms were viewed by staff as relatively more "private" and, thus, were entered less often. However, the lack of intrusion was also in part caused by the fact that such "private rooms" provided the staff with a valid excuse to withdraw from residents and to maintain their own privacy. Thus, low staff intrusions in the corridor rooms were supported by both the symbolic meaning of the rooms, and by staff needs for privacy.

At the other extreme, the modular units offered little opportunity for the staff to withdraw. Locked with residents into a day hall, or into a modular area, the staff had little choice but to interact with residents. Nonetheless, although withdrawal was still difficult, the staff did exercise some choice. They initiated interactions with the most attractive and responsive residents: the higher-functioning individuals.

In summary, *an effective living environment is one that offers the appropriate level of choice and physical opportunity for residents to control their experience.* In a case such as the corridor design in this study, residents respond by respecting the privacy of others, being more social with each other, more verbal, less withdrawn, and more alert. At the same time, staff who are faced with institutionalized, frustrating working situations exercise control, when possible, by withdrawing from residents. Residents then seem to behave more positively on their own in these settings, although the residents' social development is less than it might be. If the entire setting were less institutionally defined, if staff efforts were reinforced by community and social attitudes, staff could be motivated to attempt more meaningful interactions. Opportunities for control would constitute opportunity for more effective staff work. Only then could staff participate with residents to assist in the achievement of their full developmental potentials.

Opportunity for Control and a Full Range of Living Environments for the Developmentally Disabled

The principal value of the concept of "opportunity for control" is that it allows us to understand a broad continuum of settings for developmentally disabled people as well as other groups. Had the findings been constructed as an atheoretical evaluation of environments, a clear and misleading conclusion would have resulted: Build more corridor-style renovations. Yet, these environments are not appropriate for community settings. More flexibility is gained if we view the results within a framework in which "opportunity for control" is a central organizing concept.

For example, this heuristic may help in choosing among many possible designs for community residences. A modern residence may be an open-plan design, with bedrooms opening directly onto a living area without corridors of any kind. The living area itself may be a large free-flowing space that combines living, dining, and cooking. In contrast, a residence may be a traditional home, with bedrooms clearly set off on hallways and providing a separate kitchen, living room, and dining area. Both are good designs. In fact, if anything, the modern design with its flexibility and liveliness is currently more popular among architects and builders. However, if we view these residences from the perspective of "opportunity for control," they take on a different cast. The traditional design offers better *direct control* and *choice* with its hierarchy of spaces (e.g., bedroom, hallway, living area), and with its variegated public spaces. We have seen that people lacking in social skills are best served by the availability of physical control; for developmentally disabled people, the traditional design may be a better choice.

In addition, we must consider control by staff. Staff in institutions are themselves victims of institutionalization and, hence, sometimes are not able to behave in the residents' best interests. When the staff in the present study were given control in the corridor and suite designs, their general job dissatisfaction led them to withdraw from residents. This withdrawal allowed some residents—the most capable—to draw on their own resources and improve. The lower-functioning residents showed some improvement: They increased their alertness in the corridor-style design. The higher-functioning residents showed more change: They improved in alertness and in a variety of social skills. Nonetheless, the development of everyone was clearly limited. Training by staff could have facilitated greater change and learning by all groups.

The withdrawal of staff raises a serious challenge for community residences. If staff in the community are faced with the same conflicts and frustrations as those in the institutions, if they are as stigmatized and isolated from the community patterns, they will be likely to exhibit the same pattern of withdrawal evidenced in this study. This suggests an unpleasant prospect: Alienated staff may use the control offered by community residences to withdraw, recreating mini institutions that are smaller but no less destructive than the present large asylums.

There are several ways to prevent this catastrophe. Firstly, direct-care staff themselves must be allowed control in a more systematic manner. They must have input in the full range of decisions that affect them, from scheduling to matters of local policy. They must be treated as professionals deserving physical and social control, such as time and space for uninterrupted one-on-one conversation. And of course, they must be salaried at the level that a professional would expect.

A second critical staffing issue is training. Just as residents need training in the appropriate use of normalized physical environments, so do the staff. Staff must be trained to allow residents to control their own space, allowing the residents to have messy, disordered rooms if that is their desire. The staff must understand that they too must be sensitive to the niceties of social intercourse: knocking before entering, being aware of when residents want solitude or companionship, not intruding into bathrooms. Staff can only teach and model appropriate behavior when they are trained to understand the full range of opportunities offered by the built environment. This training must occur within a work context in which administrated job requirements do not compel staff to limit residents' control to preserve their own independence and dignity.

Implications for Environmental Design

Environmental designers cannot simply rely on the same mechanisms of control from setting to setting. In the ELEMR Project the corridor design was the "best" design, because it provided an appropriate level of control for *the specific (low-functioning) residents involved*. For a more capable group the suite design might well emerge as the better setting. Designers must consider the full range of physical and social coping mechanisms available to users of environments before they design. For example, the designer may ask about the importance of symbols for a specific group. For instance, how potent are low partitions as indicators of an individual's territory? They may be very effective in an open-plan office, but useless in an institution. As we have seen, these mechanisms are determined by the physical form of the environment, by the background of the users, and by the social systems operating in a setting.

In a practical sense, this suggestion implies that important environmental interventions should be piloted or simulated in some way to understand how users actually use the choice and control provided in the setting.

In general, residents and staff need environments that will allow them to control their sensory and social experiences. This involves physical control of lights and sound, and social control of their exposure to large and small groups of people. However, developmentally disabled residents, especially those with institutional histories, have had very little opportunity to learn sophisticated social skills for manipulating social contact, discouraging interaction, or manipulating groups of people to meet their personal needs. Therefore, we have the following specific physical design suggestions for offering the opportunity for control:

1. *The arrangements of spaces should clearly define territorial and spatial hierarchies within the building.* Bedrooms should be spatially separated from public and social areas. Transition zones are particularly important: hallways, doorway alcoves, and so on.

a. *Within public areas, spaces should be designed to create alcoves and smaller sitting areas as well as larger living rooms.* These differentiated spaces, defined physically, can support a variety of activities that the residents might find difficult to coordinate within less clearly defined designs.

b. *Graphics, wall hangings, and area rugs may be used effectively to support physical designs for demarcating spaces and transition areas.* Although these solutions will probably not be sufficient in and of themselves, they may provide helpful support for changed definitions of spaces. In addition, these solutions can be very inexpensive.

2. *Designed environments should allow direct control:*

a. *Light switches, knobs, and windows-that-open must be available and designed for easy manipulation. They must be within a range of styles that are typically used in other homes.* Many residents have some difficulties with eye-hand coordination, and this should be kept in mind in the choice of furnishings. On the other hand, the selection of style should not be so outlandish as to serve as a symbol of stigmatization.

b. *Surface materials should provide opportunities for alteration and decoration.* It is important that residents be able to participate in changing and shaping their environment. Materials that are easily altered and realtered will facilitate this activity (e.g., corkboard). Surface treatments have been recently developed that can convert ceramic tile, cinder block, and other institutional surfaces into more homelike materials.

c. *Furnishings should be movable, comfortable, and well-designed, not overly heavy or dull.* Although it is important that furnishings be durable, an overconcern with this quality can easily lead to inflexibility if the resulting furniture is particularly heavy.

d. *Sound-absorbing materials should be well-used.* There is some evidence that developmentally disabled residents are especially handicapped by poor acoustical environments (Gentry & Zimring, 1979). A generous application of soft absorbing materials will help create sound environments that will allow residents to more successfully discriminate words and develop verbal skills. If need be, these materials can be quite unobtrusive, such as carpets and other sound baffles.

3. *Institutional environments should be comfortable and homelike.* For example, although specific recommendations concerning color and materials are not indicated, by all means avoid institutional pastels, ceramic tile, and walls painted in two tones with glossy bottom and flat paint top. These colors and materials have become symbols of institutional atmosphere. The danger in using them resides in their historic symbol and meaning: "This is an institution."

Directions for Future Research

Although the present findings and theoretical analyses suggest many directions for future research, several are of particular importance.

Further examination of the actual mechanisms employed by users to control their environment would be quite useful. In the present research it was not possible to record actual instances of environmental manipulation. It would be of considerable importance to see if and how doors to private rooms are used, or how moveable furniture is manipulated, and so on.

Similarly, whereas it is of importance to consider how environments are adjusted to fit behavior, it is of equal importance to see how behaviors are adjusted to fit situations. Raush, Dittman & Taylor (1959) suggested that the adjustment of behavior can be a major sign of therapeutic progress for disturbed individuals. The implication is that if private behaviors, such as masturbation, only occur in private spaces, the individual is responding to the expectations of the setting. Investigation of these adjustments is called for.

Tests of the importance of control in community settings would be useful. Whereas many developmentally disabled people are still housed in large institutions, it is widely recognized that a wide range of living facilities are needed that are well-integrated with the community. It seems likely that the "opportunity for control" would also operate in community settings.

Finally, further examination of the effectiveness of control as an explanatory heuristic is also called for. Efforts to compare the interpretations offered by the concept of "opportunity for control" with explanations using other heuristics would provide a test for the explanatory power of this heuristic. Although control played an influential role in the interpretation of the ELEMR project data, the application of this heuristic to other similar settings as well as other more diverse settings would serve to test for its durability and flexibility.

SUMMARY

The purpose of the ELEMR Project was to study the impacts of designed environments on people labeled "severely and profoundly retarded." Court-ordered renovations allowed the comparative study of three design schemes, all of which were loosely based on the normalization principle. These schemes included: the module design, suite design, and corridor design. Research methods included several quantitative and qualitative techniques, such as: direct observations of residents, direct observations of staff, structured and unstructured interviews, participant and nonparticipant observations, physical measurements of sound and acoustics, and experimental simulation of the impact of sound and acoustics on speech discrimination, and analysis of background and archival data.

Results indicated that the corridor designs had the most positive impacts on resident behavior. In the corridor design, residents used their own spaces more, interacted with other residents more, were more verbal, were more alert and less withdrawn. Similar, though less positive, changes occurred in the suite design. Few changes were recorded in the module design. Changes in staff behavior were somewhat antithetical to resident changes. Staff actually interacted less with residents in the corridor design and suite design than they did in the unrenovated setting or in the module.

The heuristic of "opportunity for control" serves as a useful explanatory concept for these findings. The corridor design offered the greatest opportunity for residents to directly control their situations and to exercise choice over varied rooms. This "opportunity for control" was a likely contributing factor in the differential effects of the design schemes. Moreover, the suite and corridor design also offered staff the greatest opportunity for control. Often, they exercised their control by withdrawing from what remained, in a wider context, very unpleasant working conditions.

ACKNOWLEDGMENTS

The research reported in this chapter was supported by a grant from the Developmental Disabilities Office of the U. S. Department of Health, Education, and Welfare (51-P-05374). Graphics and photographs are by Alyce Kaprow. Many of these results first appeared in the ELEMR Project final report (Knight, Weitzer, & Zimring, 1979). Requests for further information should be addressed to: Craig Zimring, College of Architecture, Georgia Institute of Technology, Atlanta, Georgia, 30332.

REFERENCES

Averill, J. R. Personal control over aversive stimuli and its relationship to stress. *Psychological Bulletin,* 1973, *80,* 286–303.

Barnes, R. D. Perceived freedom and control and the built environment. In J. Harvey (Ed.), *Cognition, social behavior and the designed environment.* Hillsdale, N. J.: Lawrence Erlbaum Associates, 1980.

Baron, R., & Rodin, J. Personal control as a mediator of crowding. In A. Baum, J. E. Singer, & S. Valins (Eds.), *Advances in environmental psychology* (Vol. 1). *The urban environment.* Hillsdale, N.J.: Lawrence Erlbaum Associates, 1978.

Baum, A., Singer, J. E., & Baum, C. S. Stress and the environment. *Journal of Social Issues,* 1981, *37.*

Baum, A., & Valins, S. *Architecture and social behavior: Psychological studies of social density.* Hillsdale, N. J.: Lawrence Erlbaum Associates, 1977.

Gentry, D. M., & Zimring, C. M. Effects of institutional room acoustics on speech discrimination of developmentally disabled residents and of staff. *Journal of Applied Psychology,* 1979, *64,* 541–546.

Knight, R. C., Weitzer, W. H., & Zimring, C. M. *Opportunity of control and the built environment: The ELEMR Project.* Amherst: University of Massachusetts Environmental Institute, 1978.

Knight, R. C., Zimring, C. M., & Kent, M. J. Normalization as a social–physical system. In M. J. Bednar (Ed.), *Barrier-free environments.* Stroudsberg, Pa.: Dowden, Hutchinson, & Ross, 1977.

Raush, H. L., Dittman, A. T., & Taylor, T. J. Person, setting and change in social interaction. *Human Relations,* 1959, *12,* 361–379.

Seligman, M. *Helplessness: On depression, development and death.* San Francisco: Freeman, 1975.

Steele, F. *Physical settings and organizational development.* Reading, Mass.: Addison-Wesley, 1973.

Viet, S., Allen, G., Chinskey, J., Dailey, W., Harris, J., & Corcoran, C. *The interaction recording system; Instruction manual.* Unpublished manuscript, University of Connecticut at Storrs, 1974.

Viet, S., Simon, J., & Billings, A. *Behavioral observation form.* Unpublished manuscript, Mansfield Training School, Mansfield, Conn., 1974.

Wolfensberger, W. *Normalization.* Toronto: Canadian Institute on Mental Retardation, 1972.

8 The Human in Extreme Environments

Arthur J. Bachrach
Naval Medical Research Institute
Bethesda, Maryland

In addition to the natives of extreme environments (Arctic dwellers, desert denizens, and the like), there are persons who enter these environments for a particular purpose. The major reasons appear to be military, scientific, commercial, and recreational. Fundamentally, the types of extreme environments can be described as hot, dry, wet, and cold (Pythagoras' four basic elements); to these may be added high (for altitude) and differential pressure (related to altitude on the one hand and underwater high pressure on the other).

In dealing with extreme environments, particularly in planning entries into such environments, the concept of hazard must be considered. As Kates (1970) observed: "natural events are indeed natural and . . . . hazards—the threat potential for man and his works—are by definition human phenomena [p. 404]." Kates divided hazards as environmental events into two types: *Intensive,* which are: "characteristically small in area extent, intense in impact, of brief duration, sudden onset, and poor predictability [p. 405]."; *Pervasive,* which are: "widespread in extent, have a diffuse impact, a long duration, gradual onset, ... predicted more accurately [p. 405]."

An example of an intensive hazard is a volcano or an avalanche; a pervasive hazard can be illustrated by drought, fog, or air pollution. A natural hazard that poses a serious threat to working skiers is an avalanche; avalanches are responsible for many, if not most, ski fatalities.

Any significant deviation from the accustomed normal environment will provide some measure of stress for the typical individual, a stress that follows a continuum going from discomfort → pain → injury → death. At any point along the continuum, an accident may result in marked discomfort or worse; therefore, emergency response training is a protective measure. By definition, an accident is an unforeseen, sudden event; as Licht (1975) has stated, there is no such thing as accident prevention; rather, we should speak of accident *mitigation* in the hope that the untoward results of an accident might be mitigated by planning for emergency response. Certainly, protective gear such as exposure suits for pilots who fly over water is a mitigating technique in the event of accident. Licht (1975) also suggests that an accident, again by definition, is not the end result of a series of events, but it is the event that results in the individual's loss of control. Hence, an accident occurs when a car begins to skid out of control. What happens to restore control determines not whether there is to be an accident—this has already occurred as an unforeseen, sudden event—but what the consequences of the accident will be. Diagrammatically, this may be expressed as follows:

EVENT   CONSEQUENCES

CONTROL IS REGAINED

ACCIDENT (LOSS OF CONTROL)   CONTROL IS NOT REGAINED
(DAMAGE, INJURY, DEATH)

An accident Waller (1977) describes as the "moment at which task demand exceeds the performance" of the individual or group. Because of the unforeseen nature of an accident, the individual must have certain capabilities of response so that control will not be lost. Waller (1977) suggests four crucial capabilities:

1. The knowledge that "one has about one's self in relation to different aspects of the environment," knowledge that depends on such factors as basic intelligence, education, experience, as well as attitudes and beliefs that are culturally determined.
2. The ability to "receive information about the environment through inherent senses," including sight, hearing, and so on.
3. "The ability to make rapid judgments about one's self in relation to the environment as a result of the combination of the information received through the senses and knowledge applied in interpreting such information."
4. "The capability to act in response to judgments that suggest danger may exist [p. 34]."

In sum, the individual must have the ability to obtain and receive information accurately, process the information in a timely fashion, and react with appropriate and effective response. Within this context, Waller's definition of an accident as the moment in which task demand exceeds performance is germane.

Hence, the effective completion of a task or mission in a potentially hazardous environment depends firstly on adaptation to the physical and physiological change to be encountered in the extreme environment, and secondly on accident mitigation in the form of emergency response and training as well as equipment preparation.

Why do individuals enter extreme and potentially hazardous environments? We stated earlier that a person entering an extreme environment is fulfilling a mission. Thus, we assume the individual going into such an environment has a goal such as adventure or thrill seeking (recreation), profit (commercial), defense purposes of salvage and rescue (military), or exploration (scientific). We also assume that the individual's purpose is not served by mere survival in such an extreme environment but necessitates the completion of a goal; hence, adaptation to the extreme and performance of the mission are essential to the analysis. One further requirement is that the individual enter the extreme environment willingly—not as a hostage, prisoner, or "remittance man."

By definition, the extreme environment is stressful—in varying degrees—to specific individuals. It must be perceived as markedly different from the environment in which the individual normally performs: It requires the person to adapt to an environmentally evoked imbalance of normal functions. Here, our model is that of Bernard (1856), Cannon (1939), and more recently, Selye (1971), which deals with homeostasis, the restoration of body balance in a stress situation. Restoration through adaptation is a physiological and behavioral response following stress; acclimation is a method of preparing the organism for the impending stressor encountered in the extreme environment.

THE CONCEPT OF ADAPTATION

Adaptation in the human is a remarkable process. Consider, for example, the ability of skin to adapt to severe extremes of heat and cold. Can you visualize any other insulating material that tolerates extremes in temperature and humidity with minimal problems, is self-lubricating, and repairs itself after puncture?

There is disagreement about the use of the terms *acclimatization* and *adaptation,* but a sense of meaning may be derived from a brief discussion of the concepts. Prosser (1964) defined a "stressor" as: "an environmental circumstance which induces adaptations [p. 11]" (very much in the Selye mode). And, in a reference to Adolph (1956), Prosser (1964) defined an *adaptate* as that: "increment of function that comprises adaptive response to a stressor [p. 11]." Further, he defined *acclimation* as the compensatory alterations occurring in an animal under laboratory conditions altered for one stressful parameter; the term *acclimatization* he reserves for the changes under "natural conditions" in a multiple stress exposure. Eagan (1963, p. 930) used adaptation as an overall term encompassing *genetic adaptation,* which favors a species surviving in an extreme environment. He considered "acclimatization" as the adaptation in the natural environment to a complex of factors, "acclimation" as the exposure to a single environmental stressor in a controlled laboratory situation, and "habituation'' as a change in physiological response that results from a diminution in central nervous system responsiveness to specific stimuli.

For example, preparing individuals to enter an extreme environment might involve controlling exposure to acclimate them for penetration into a hot, humid environment. Acclimatization would be expected to result in some measure of adaptation after the exposure penetration. The procedures to accomplish these conditions vary, and highly complex aspects of physiology are involved. Many investigators are convinced that physical fitness is a key factor in successful acclimatization or acclimation; other investigators are equally convinced that physical fitness is not sufficient to prepare an individual for the first impact of the extreme environment.

Bligh and Johnson (1973) define acclimatization as a physiological change occurring within a person's lifetime that reduces the strain caused by environmental stressors. Certainly, physiological adaptation as response to environmental stress is often found. For example, physiological change has been shown to take place in the diving women of Japan and Korea, known as the *Ama*. The Ama wear only a facemask for improved visibility and cotton clothing with an occasional wet suit; they dive for pearls to depths averaging 60 ft but at times dive as deep as 145 ft (Bachrach, 1975a).

When the physiological changes in the Ama were compared to a control group of nondiving women, the Ama showed a larger vital capacity (probably a result of development of inspiratory muscles) and an increase of 35% in the basal metabolic rate during the winter months. Hong (1963) reported modifications of the peripheral blood flow in the Ama (possibly in the counter-current heat exchange systems) that shift thermal insulation from the body core to the surface. Other reports of such changes in cold response are discussed by Cooper (1976).

When these physiological adaptations are viewed in the context of the whole body, they are relatively minor. What seems more important as we consider individuals penetrating extreme environments for brief periods is their *behavioral adaptation* (Sloan, 1979).

We use the term *adaptation* in a broad sense to cover, firstly, the means of preparing individuals to enter an extreme environment and, secondly, the changes that may occur after entry into such an environment, changes that will aid in the individuals' survival and performance.

We view adaptation as an effort to engineer the individual's personal or environmental situation to eliminate or minimize physiological change. Behavioral approaches to modify individuals to prepare for the extreme environments are represented by the development of protective clothing to insulate against heat or cold, the construction of pressure suits that may be used for space or ocean depth, the evaluation of effective diets for specific environment, and training. Similarly, the development of space vehicles, the architecture of housing, and the construction of submersibles represent the modification of the extreme environment to protect the individual. Such inventions and developments extend the entry of humans into such extreme environments; lacking such aids, life would be incapable of support. Further consideration of such conceptualizations of adaptation may be found in Follinsbee, Wagner, Borgia, Drinkwater, Gliner, and Bedi (1978), Sloan (1979), and Mount (1979).

Adaptation to Novel Stimuli

Another aspect of adaptation not clearly understood is the initial response to a stressor that we may consider to be a novel stimulus. Selye's (1971) General Adaptation Syndrome (GAS) depicts a stressor evoking an alarm with a decrement in response followed by a countershock that leads to an overcompensatory response, finally settling back to either normal behavior or to deterioration and death.

The initial response to a stress stimulus is dimunition, or near cessation of a response (e.g., as in the blocking of alpha rhythm). A novel stimulus can momentarily degrade performance. Although insufficient data regarding the mechanisms of adaptation are available, we may feel confident that enough information resides in learning theory (Bachrach, 1980a) to tell us that preparing a subject for a novel stimulus by exposure, such as would occur in a laboratory acclimation, can be useful.

THE COMPLEX NATURE OF STRESS

A discussion of stress is complicated by many factors: the definition of stressors, stimulus and response, the related individual nature of defining and responding to stress, and the wealth of contradictory research data.

We have extensive demonstration of the individual characteristics of stress response. Appley and Trumbull (1967) summed it up: "Different individuals respond to the same conditions in different ways. Some enter rapidly into a stress state, others show increased alertness and apparently improved performance, and still others appear to be 'immune' to the stress producing qualities of the environmental conditions [p. 11]." A clear example of an individual response to stress may be found in Fig. 8.1.

Lack of stimulation is in itself stressful as may be seen in cases of *ennui* or boredom. The literature is filled with the need for varied experience (Fiske & Maddi, 1961; Zuckerman, 1979) and examples of this need from Berlyne (1970). Furthermore, the stress picture is made complex by the fact that it is not necessarily a negative concept or experience. The human is unique within the animal kingdom in that he/she deliberately seeks body imbalance for the apparent pleasure of a "thrill" or the pleasure of imbalance and its restoration. Sex is com-

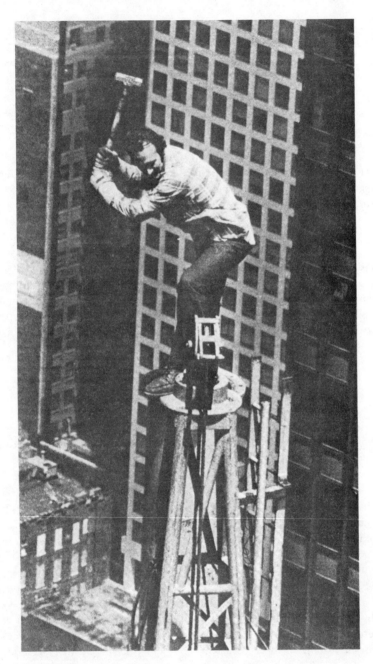

FIG. 8.1. An individual response to stress (Chicago Tribune photo).

monly sought as an imbalance among animals, but nowhere in the animal kingdom is the search for excitement more intense than in skiing, sky diving, or scuba diving.

A recent extensive survey of social trends relevant to consumer marketing (The Yankelovich Monitor, 1979) foresaw one trend described as "flirtation with danger," an eagerness to enter into high-risk situations for several apparent complex motives. Such motives include excitement and a self-worth component with a stated belief that mastering dangerous leisure activities can make one a better person and that: " 'driving yourself to the brink' is a path to better self-understanding [p. 56]." The predicted increase in risk-taking leisure activities foresees a trend toward more active involvement in high-risk recreation such as sky diving, hang gliding, scuba diving, and high-speed automobile racing. Of interest to social psychologists is the increase in illegal risk taking as well, with a trend toward such exciting and unlawful activities as shoplifting among classes of people who do not "need" the items illegally acquired.

One basic assumption in regard to these sought-after stress activities is that an element of risk exists, but participants are in control of their own behavior and the consequences; hence, there is a strong emphasis on training and physical fitness. In addition, participants in these sports are protected by a built-in safety factor engineered by equipment manufacturers, track owners, dive operators, and resort supervisors. The odd behavior of getting on a roller coaster for the thrill of it has an underlying belief that there is no *real* risk involved, that the structure is engineered and inspected, and that the mathematics of the transcended curves along the tracks have been thoroughly plotted. A paper in the German diving magazine *Tauchen* (Fritz, 1979) proposed the question via the title: *Sind Taucher Selbsmörder* (Are divers suicidal)? The question was prompted in large measure by the significant number of accidents to German scuba divers. We can only invoke the principle espoused by Durkheim (1951), who observed that if a person engages in high-risk behavior and believes there is a chance he will emerge alive then this is not defined as "suicide." Only when there is absolute certainty of death as a consequence of the behavior would such a definition be acceptable. Therefore, in the case of a scuba-diving fatality, we would assume that death is accidental.

Obviously, there is a marked, positive quality to adventure, to thrill seeking, to enlarging one's scope by going underwater to view different worlds, to schuss down a swift snowy slope, to exercise and tax one's abilities.

So, the penetration of extreme environments for individual reasons of adventure, and the like, is one motivation we can see as relevant to performance. The profit motive for activities such as a high-risk commercial diving enterprise is clear, but profit alone does not seem to account for the choice of such a profession—again, one fraught with danger, as evidenced by the number of fatalities in the oil fields of the North Sea. Commercial divers do relatively well financially, but their account of why they chose such a profession will probably evoke responses that suggest elements of focused machismo, strength, and the related feat of overcoming a dangerous obstacle.

METHODOLOGICAL PROBLEMS IN THE STUDY OF STRESS

Variability

The individual nature of stress response contributes to the problem of subject variability in stress research. In an analysis of underwater performance, Bachrach (1975b) found that *subject variability* along with *task variability* contributed toward an inability to compare experiments across studies. A classic example of subject variability comes from the studies reported by Case and Haldane (1941) on diving research in a chamber. They described their subjects:

> The majority are English, but two are Irish, one Spanish, one Czech, and one German. Their occupations had varied from prime minister to tailor, and loader for a transport company. The majority are, however, university graduates.

This charming subject description by Case and Haldane tantalizes: *Which* prime minister of England volunteered to be a subject in a chamber experiment? It is also illustrative of a wide range of cultural backgrounds; the stated age range was 23–47 years and two of the 17 subjects were female. This variation in sex and age is frequently encountered in studies and cannot help but contribute to subject variability. Given the individual nature of stress response, studies must be examined with care.

The other contributing aspect of variability that creates problems is *task variability*. In a study of underwater performance, Bachrach (1975b) found wide variations in experimental methods even when they were given by what appeared to be the same name. For example, choice reaction tests had different positions, different types of stimulus lights, different colors, differences in the response required, yet all were grouped under the term *choice reaction* and compared with each other, a questionable tactic at best.

That this problem is not unique to the undersea environment is seen in a cogent comment by Theologus, Wheaton, Mirabella, Brahlek, and Fleishman (1973):

> Examination of the literature on environmental stressors and their effects upon performance reveals a number of problems impeding the development of a systematic body of knowledge and the application of that knowledge. Within any particular study, environmental stressor variables and performance measures may be defined precisely, and employed effectively. However, it is often impossible to

relate them systematically to different variables from other studies. Various researchers have employed different measures of performance, different methods of testing and different data analysis techniques. Descriptive data relating to the values and ranges of environmental stressors employed, the intervals of exposure, and the characteristics of subjects indicate considerable variation from study to study. Until the relationships among these and similar components are established systematically, development of a cohesive body of knowledge may be impossible [p. 2].

This situation appears to obtain in different types of research into the effects of environmental stress. Tune (1964), for example, commented on research involving the effects of high altitude on performance; he found results either to be contradictory across studies or reported by the investigators with insufficient detail to permit conclusive interpretation. Techniques of research varied so much that Tune observed: "It is impossible to compare the performance of Ss in these studies because of a lack of standardization of the techniques used [p. 560]."

The very nature of combined stress research, wherein a number of relevant factors are studied, contributes to the problem. And experimental designs may not be sufficiently rigorous, as suggested by Rowell (1978) in a discussion of adjustments to heat stress: "Perhaps the biggest problem is the tendency to mix together findings from humid and dry environments in an effort to explain circulatory changes that appear to be unique in a particular environment [p. 23]."

Laboratory Versus Field Conditions

Perhaps even more crucial to the relevance of research studies to the understanding of stress and stress responses is the abiding problem of relating laboratory experiments to the "real world." Extrapolating from a controlled laboratory experiment to the field situation is, at best, a touchy issue, especially when one gets into the various aspects of simulation.

In a paper dealing with the relevance of laboratory studies to practical situations, Chapanis (1967) commented on the many problems. He noted that: "by their very nature, laboratory experiments are at best only rough and approximate models of any real-life situation [p. 557]." He stated that a laboratory experiment selects a few relevant variables for study, and even these selected variables will change when brought under laboratory control. Another concern of Chapanis' was that the control for precision in laboratory studies may create the risk of discovering effects so small that they are of no practical importance. Chapanis also suggested that "the methods used to present variables in the laboratory are sometimes artificial and unrealistic," and he noted that "the safest and most honest conclusion to draw from all these considerations is that one should generalize with extreme caution from the results of laboratory experiments to the solution of practical problems [p. 557]."

Another approach to this problem was that of Brunswik (1952) who proposed his "representative design," a design for an experiment that has a minimum of artificiality and a maximum of control. It is an "ideal" experiment in that it brings together the problems of the real world with the exacting methods of the experimental laboratory. Figure 8.2 is an illustration of this representative design from Bachrach (1980b).

Brunswik's model, the concept of a representative design, echoes Chapanis' concern. The model indicates that field research (studies accomplished in the actual environment) has higher reality but less control, whereas laboratory research (in which field conditions are assumed to be simulated insofar as is possible) has optimal control but greater artificiality. Both field and laboratory studies are necessary for a complete approach to a problem area. What is particularly risky is the extrapolation of findings from the laboratory to field conditions.

The methodological problem of extrapolation is found even in the most rigorously designed laboratory experiments. For example, in a long series of well-designed and executed studies of isolation and confinement (Haythorn, 1973), conditions presumed to be similar to those encountered in space flight and undersea-habitat living were simulated in isolation chambers in which subjects lived and worked for periods up to 10 days. In a number of the confinement experiments, expressions of hostility occurred, even to the point of an attempted stabbing. Mannerisms that would have been, at the most, mild irritants under nonisolation conditions took on highly irritating intensities—perhaps not too surprising in view of the diminished stimulus environment. Some of the experiments had to be aborted because of the potential for bodily harm to one or more of the subjects. These experiments were, indeed, well-designed and conducted by skilled researchers, but the problems encountered did not materialize to a

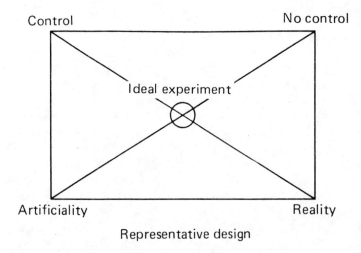

FIG. 8.2.   Illustration of representative design for an experiment (From Bachrach, 1980b).

significant degree in the real world of space and in the tens of thousands of hours in undersea-habitat dwelling and decompression chambers, where people were isolated and confined under conditions of hazard. We can only assume that the major elements missing in the simulated isolation/confinement situation were: (1) true stress in the sense of external danger; and (2) the inability to terminate the experience in space or in the undersea environment, where pressure and required decompression made aborting the mission impossible. In other words, the experiments simulating the space of undersea environment could simulate the isolation, and investigators could, if problems arose, abort the experiment, allowing the subjects to leave the isolation condition. Not so in space or undersea, where the subjects had to accomodate. To be sure, the mannerisms probably continued to irritate, but the inability to leave the field made it necessary to adapt. As one SEALAB II aquanaut observed, they worked hard at getting along during the 15-day undersea-habitat experience; "we were walking on eggs!"

In another excellent experiment simulating deep diving, a recent world-record dive was accomplished at Duke University's hyperbaric facility in which three subjects were pressurized in a hyperbaric chamber to a depth of 686 m (2250 feet).

The subjects were remarkably successful in completing tasks involving fine coordination, a finding different from similar deep chamber dives in which tremor and other neurophysiological signs indicated disorder of impaired function known as the *high pressure nervous syndrome* (Bachrach & Bennett, 1973; Hunter & Bennett, 1974). What differentiated this dive from similar dives was the addition of a percentage of nitrogen to the breathing mixture of helium and oxygen. According to Bennett (1975a), the addition occasions membrane permeability changes that damp out effects of the high pressure nervous syndrome. The accomplishment of such a deep dive without untoward results is, indeed, remarkable. Caution in extrapolating the data from this type of dive to an open-sea situation is strongly needed. The laboratory conditions of a chamber dive with a dry, temperature-controlled, land-based, and continually monitored dive do not duplicate deep dives in an ocean environment: There, in addition to the pressure (simulated effectively in the chamber), a diver would encounter cold water, current, turbidity and reduced visibility, reduced communication with personnel topside, and potential marine hazards, all of which represent real danger not encountered in a land-based simulation (Fig. 8.3). This comparison in no way detracts from the Duke dive; it simply underscores the need to exercise care when one suggests that divers may now safely operate at depths in the oceans approaching 686 m.

The example of the conditions a deep-sea diver could encounter suggests another problem area in the move from a simulation environment to a real world operational situation: the relationship between training and operational performance in an extreme environment. Training requirements are based on the assumption that the behaviors and skills developed in a training situation are the

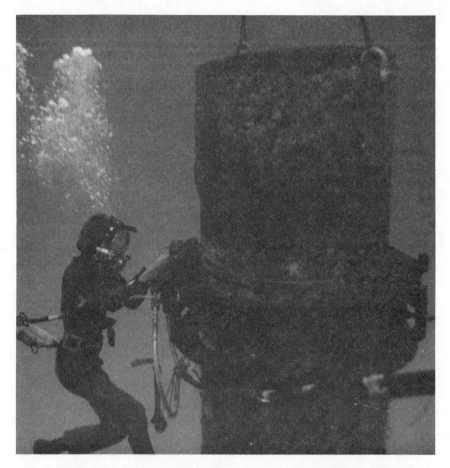

FIG. 8.3.   Diver working in the ocean (Courtesy of Santa Fe Diving Services).

relevant behaviors needed to perform tasks in the operational environment. An essential requirement in such situations is the precise definition of successful performance, which, if ideally conceived, should define the needed behaviors to perform. With precise criteria for successful performance, instructors could develop for the training situation more effective predictor variables related to the transfer of skills to the operational condition.

Biersner (in press) described two related studies on UDT (Underwater Demolition Team) candidates in a training program. The first study was conducted by Hertzka and Anderson (1956), who administered a set of personality tests and collected: (1) Navy Basic Test Battery (BTB) scores that measured general comprehension, arithmetic reasoning, mechanical aptitude, and clerical aptitude; (2) demographic information on age, number of years of education completed, pay grade (rank); and (3) scores on a series of physical fitness measures, which included swimming, pull-ups, squat-jumps, push-ups, sit-ups, and one-mile runs. These data were correlated with a pass–fail criterion. In commenting on this study, Biersner observed that: "These findings would establish a precedent that would later be repeated in other diver selection research—that noncognitive variables such as physical fitness and demographic information would predict performance substantially better than the more traditional cognitive measures, especially intelligence, aptitudes and personality." Noncognitive variables, Biersner observed, "appear to measure more validly the major dimensions necessary to perform well in the UDT training situation—vigorous physical performance and maturity (age)."

The second related study reported by Biersner was done by Alf and Gordon (1957) 15 months after the Hertzka and Anderson study; these investigators analyzed variables that accounted for UDT performance effectiveness in operational situations for 50 of the 64 UDT graduates from training programs. In this study executive officers of the commands to which these UDT personnel had been assigned were asked to rank order the graduates for overall operational effectiveness and for swimming skills. None of the measures of physical fitness obtained during the training programs was related to overall operational effectiveness.

All four of the Navy BTB scores were found to be significantly related to the criterion of overall operational effectiveness; in addition, two personality measures, "masculinity" and "objectivity," were related to effectiveness, as were swimming skills. Given the subjective nature of instructor and supervisor ratings of overall effectiveness in both training and operational situations, there remains an interesting finding: that success in training seems in this program, at least, to be not only unrelated but even opposed to success in performing the tasks for which the training presumably prepared the students. Biersner (in press) summed up the contrasting findings: "The unsettling conclusion from this research is that a large discrepancy exists between variables that account for success in training and those that are related to operational effectiveness."

THE UNDERWATER ENVIRONMENT

I continue to take as my model for an extreme environment the underwater world with its stressors of cold, pressure, turbidity, current, marine hazards, relative weightlessness, and task difficulty when compared to land performance. These major stressors will occur in varying combinations during the course of a diver's entry into the water. Scott Carpenter, who has performed as astronaut and aquanaut, has stated that he experienced the ocean bottom as being infinitely more hostile than space.

One of the favorite themes of science fiction writers who take as their subject the underwater world is the fantasy or prospect of humans living and working in cities beneath the sea, a theme that has much romance, evoking, as it does, images of golden people of Atlantis and pioneers for the last frontier of the ocean. What is frequently lacking in such romantic portrayals of human adventure and courage beneath the seas is the feasibility of such a concept. There are, basically, two ways in which the human enters and remains below the surface of the ocean. One is an *engineering* approach in which the earth's atmospheric pressure (1 ATA) is brought to the undersea environment (e.g., in submarines, where the outside ambient environment of cold, current, and pressure are kept from the human by the insulation of a steel hull). The other is a *physiological* approach in which the human is required to adapt physiologically to the external environment, carrying with him as personal gear the needed protection from cold but adapting physiologically to differential pressure. Our discussion of diving deals with physiological adaptation, recognizing that advances in diving technology including remote-controlled vehicles and "walking submersibles" such as the one-atmosphere diving system JIM, in which the operator can function at depths to 1780 feet of sea water (fsw), will make much of the human physiological adaptations obsolete in future years.

For the human entering the ocean as a diver there are four fundamental modes (Bachrach, 1975a).

1. *Free Diving or Skin Diving.* In this mode divers carry their own air inhaled at the surface for a breath-holding dive and are limited in depth only by their supply of air and their ability to equalize to the increased pressure as depth is achieved. Diving depth, using this mode, is usually limited to relatively shallow depths such as 60 fsw, but practiced skin divers such as the Ama of Japan and Korea (see page 214) have achieved depths to 145 fsw. The equipment usually consists of a face mask for improved visibility and a snorkel through which the surface air is inhaled and exhaled upon surfacing.

2. *Scuba Diving (Self-Contained Underwater Breathing Apparatus).* Scuba diving allows the diver to spend more time underwater because the air is not limited to the amount inhaled on the surface, as in skin diving, but is carried in tanks supplying compressed air, usually around 2500 pounds per square inch per tank. As a result of this carried air, diving depth is extended but limited to depths approaching 150 fsw. One limitation is the problem of nitrogen narcosis (Bennett, 1975b), a somewhat poorly understood and highly variable phenomenon in which a diver loses ability for speedy reaction, shows poor judgment, and appears "intoxicated," presumably as a function of nitrogen under increased pressure; this condition can occur at depths beginning around 100 fsw. Nitrogen has an anesthetic effect under pressure, and Workman (1966) describes nitrogen narcosis as "a state of light anesthesia," probably complicated by

carbon dioxide retention as a result of diminished pulmonary ventilation. Narcosis is not a major problem, particularly with experienced divers who apparently adapt; only experienced scuba divers should be going to those depths. Scuba divers carry their own compressed air in tanks; they have a regulator with a mouthpiece that controls the flow of the air, which reduces the pressure through stages of filter reduction; they wear a weight belt for buoyancy control. In cold waters a diver would be protected by a neoprene wet suit for insulation.

3. *Helmet Diving.* Helmet, or hard-hat diving, is a system through which the diver is encased in a protective suit and receives a steady supply of air via a hose from topside. Depending on the diving conditions, several types of diving suits are used; a dry suit in which air is the insulating mode, a wet suit with a layer of water within, or a hot-water suit in which heated water is forced through the suit by a hose from topside control aboard ship, the hot water acting as a heating mechanism. For deep dives (greater than 200 fsw) the air mode can be replaced with a mode of supplying helium/oxygen mixture for breathing, a mix that is less stressful on pulmonary function and less toxic under pressure than air. Helmet diving is the most frequently used working mode for divers in commercial applications of underwater activity. Gases such as nitrogen go into solution in the body under pressure to reappear as bubbles, when the pressure is reduced upon rising to the surface. The usual cliché to illustrate this is opening a bottle of a carbonated beverage and observing the CO_2 under pressure in solution begin to bubble as the pressure is released. Bradley (1981) has observed that divers, like good vintage wines, should not be shaken. The process by which the reabsorption of gases under pressure is accomplished without risk to the diver is called *decompression* and is the debt the diver pays for deeper diving. If a diver ascends too rapidly, the gases that have gone into solution can be hazardous as gas bubbles enter areas of the body such as the joints; this disorder commonly is referred to as "the bends," with knee and elbow joints frequently affected. Central nervous system "hits" can also occur: the penetration of bubbles into the central nervous system can result in neurological disorders. Slow ascent, timed for reabsorption, is essential.

4. *Saturation.* In the late 1950s many investigators, principally a group of U. S. Navy researchers, experimented with saturation diving. The concept was based on decompression problems and, simply stated, noted that gas went to solution under pressure, and the diver was not at risk until surfacing when the differential pressure would allow the bubbles of gas to reappear. The reasoning went, once a diver is completely saturated with the solution of gas, where further tissue intake is not possible, it does not matter how long the diver remains under pressure. It is only when the ascent occurs that decompression becomes necessary. Saturation diving is a frequent mode of working dives in which divers are kept under pressure in a chamber aboard a ship, lowered to the working level in a

pressurized diving bell, raised in the bell, and locked back into the pressurized chamber. Ocean floor saturation dives such as SEALAB II are better known as long habitat operations in which the divers, in teams, stayed below the surface at a depth of 205 fsw for a period of 15 days. It is in such undersea living operations that psychologists have a marked interest, particularly the social interactions under stress and confinement. And, it is in such events that the necessity of working together because one cannot leave the situation produces such adaptation.

The cost of decompression, as noted, occurs at the end of the saturation; as a general rule a diver once saturated must undergo decompression in a surface chamber at the rate of 1 day for each 100 feet of depth in the operation. An example of a controlled saturation dive is the Duke 686-m dive, discussed earlier, which required a decompression period of almost 3 weeks of slow ascent because a depth of over 2000 fsw was achieved.

Casualties in the Underwater Environment

The number of fatalities is proportionally higher for persons entering the underwater environment than those entering other extreme environments, particularly environments that are cold or hot. Cold and heat stress are two important environmental stressors that need evaluation to insure effective entry into areas that are important to the commercial, military, and recreational communities. But, the hazards attendant upon entering the underwater environment allow much less recovery in the event of accident. The problem of recovery under rapid conditions of change is similar in aviation where pilots have to respond with speed in emergencies (Dean & Thatcher, 1975). As another example, fatigue is a common response to stress and energy expenditure. On dry land, the fatigued individual probably may create an opportunity for rest, a feat at best difficult, if not impossible, for the person underwater.

Let us elaborate on the observation that there are more casualties in the diving environment than in the extreme environments of cold and heat. I use the term *casualties* because there are no statistics regarding the number of accidents in diving (nor for that matter, any other environment), if we keep to the definition of an accident as an unforeseen event in which there is a loss of control. The numbers of accidents in which control was regained, the so-called "near drownings" or "near-misses" in the air, can only be estimated. What is usually termed accident statistics, are, in reality, *casualty* statistics in which injury or death will be documented. And even here, the accuracy of reports on known injuries or deaths is questionable because of the anecdotal nature of much of the reporting.

Nonetheless, the casualty statistics in diving suggest that underwater is an extreme and hazardous environment. In sports diving in the United States, there were 175 deaths in the water reported in 1976 (Schenck & McAniff, 1978). (Comparable figures were obtained in West Germany and France, where the waters are substantially colder than in many of the diving areas in the United States.)

Although it is difficult to estimate the number of active divers in the U. S., we know that the various training agencies that certify scuba divers list approximately a quarter of a million trained divers a year. What percentage of these 250,000 become active divers we do not know, but it is known that attrition occurs. The number of fatalities when evaluated against the number of exposures (dives per year) is probably not great, but in comparison with other recreational activities—even high-risk activities—it appears high.

With regard to commercial diving fatalities, fully accurate statistics are, once again, difficult to obtain. And, again, the estimation of accidents in which control was regained and a casualty averted is only a guess but is probably much higher than the fatalities would suggest. Bradley (1981) reports around 905 commercial divers working mostly on oil exploration in the Gulf of Mexico and a similar population of 700 in the British Sector of the North Sea. The diving fatality rates for the Gulf of Mexico from 1968 to 1975 were 2.49/1000 working divers per year; for the British Sector of the North Sea between 1971 and 1978 a higher rate of 4.82/1000 working divers per year was obtained. In the Gulf the fatalities occurred between 0 and 340 fsw, with a mean of 136 fsw; in the North Sea the mean depth of fatalities was 223 fsw, with a range of 0 to 500 fsw.

Comparing commercial diving with Navy diving is not an effective analysis because the character of the diving is so different. The U. S. Navy casualty record is extremely low, but Navy diving operations are mainly shallow. Berghage, Rohrbaugh, Bachrach, and Armstrong (1975) analyzed a total of almost 130,000 U. S. Navy dives logged from January 1972 through December 1973 and found that 99% of these dives were done in less than 200 fsw, with a mean of 47 fsw and an average bottom time of 31 minutes. Dives were made in waters above 50°F in temperature. The commercial diver works deeper, longer, and in waters often much colder than those encountered in Navy diving. As Navy ocean dives become deeper, and if operational needs so demand, it is probable that higher casualty rates will be experienced.

Environmental Factors in Diving Accidents Which May Lead to Casualties

The underwater environment is a complex set of variables. Patently, we cannot discuss more than a few of them, and even those in brief. We discuss the more salient ones.

Cold. In 11% of the North Sea casualties, Bradley (1981) describes cold as a factor contributing to the accident and consequent fatality. No casualties were mentioned in the Gulf of Mexico. Hayward and Keatinge (1979), in discussing the 42 cases of loss of consciousness reported by Childs and Norman (1978), suggest the cause of loss of consciousness in these North Sea divers was a progressive "silent" hypothermia, not normally detected during routine dives. They suggest a gradual, unnoticed cooling that leads to physiological dysfunction. Hayward and Keatinge (1979) list as one dysfunction an: "unexplained confusion and bad judgment leading to diving accidents [p. 1182]," attributed in large measure to the effects of cold. This is interesting in the light of Bradley's (1981) note that 15% of the North Sea fatalities were largely a result of poor diver judgment.

Cold also adversely affects performance underwater primarily in a loss or degradation of manual dexterity. Gloves may provide protection, but they necessarily interfere with manipulation. Childs (1978) suggests that performance degradation and discomfort resulting from cold may contribute to divers being less aware of possible threats to safety.

How does cold affect the sports diver? The commercial diver is provided with more efficient thermal insulation than the average sports diver. Dry suits for deep cold diving and suits through which hot water is forced are standard for commercial diving. The sports diver in cold water normally relies on a neoprene wet suit, which is effective only in shallow water; the suit loses a great deal of its protective capability under pressure. At best it is a time extender, for the ocean is a heat sink. With a body core of 37°C and an ocean of, let's say even 32°C, the second law of thermodynamics dictates that heat transfer will move from warm to less warm, through the insulating layer of the skin to the water encased in the wet suit, and through the insulating layer of the wet suit to the outer ocean water. Because this occurs, Egstrom (1976) suggests that even in tropical waters some form of thermal protection in a wet suit is desirable.

Again, progressive hypothermia appears to be a major problem in sports divers as it was in commercial divers. The gradual cooling described by Hayward and Keatinge (1979), noted earlier in this section, occurs in sports divers and is also likely to be unnoticed. The problem here, as it is with commercial divers, is that the gradual "silent" hypothermia is made more pronounced by in-water exercise and is followed by fatigue. In sports divers, where the supply of air is limited to the amount carried in the tanks, the progression of gradual hypothermia → fatigue → low air supply can be extremely hazardous. At a point in time when good judgment, good physical condition, and an adequate supply of air are crucial, the diver is apt to be cold and fatigued and concerned about the availability of air. Such circumstances are likely to set the stage for an accident and possible casualty.

Cold has been implicated in a number of deaths among scuba divers in recent years in California waters. These divers, males whose ages ranged from the mid 30s to the mid 50s, had been perceived by their buddies as being "calm," but they sank below the surface in a matter of moments. Eldridge (1979), in reporting on the postmortems in these diver deaths, said that the divers apparently lost consciousness and rapidly disappeared below the surface. Most of the victims had previous cardiovascular symptoms such as hypertension or arrhythmias and/or showed significant coronary artery stenosis (narrowing) on autopsy. All were experienced divers, but the risk of diving was exacerbated by factors such as cold and fatigue.

Cold water is a particularly powerful stimulus for changes in cardiac rhythms. Water immersion in itself evokes what is called the "dive reflex," found in all diving animals. Immersion of the face in water, even with the remainder of the body out of water, results in this reflex, which is characterized by a slowing of the heart (bradycardia), a peripheral vasoconstriction, and a marked reduction in oxygen consumption. The increased slowing of the heart in man increases as the water temperature decreases. Hong (1976) observed that: "the cutaneous cold receptors on the face play a very important role in the development of diving bradycardia" [p. 280]; this statement again reiterates the importance of cold stimuli. When a diver is fatigued, already hypothermic and running low on (or out of) air, problems can occur. The diver may be resting on the surface with the flotation device inflated, as seems to be the case in the deaths reported in Eldridge's study. It is possible that cold water slapping at the exposed portions of the face might engender further cold stimuli and a response akin to the diving reflex, which would further create cardiac arrhythmias that might have been induced in the susceptible diver by cold, fatigue, and exercise, as well as possible stress stimuli. Childs (1978) observed: "The possibility exists that maximal thermal shivering may require an increase in cardiac output that can only be met by a fit myocardium; if further stresses are applied, for example, by frantic swimming efforts, or if the myocardium is unfit for any reason, high output cardiac failure may follow [p. 9]." This appears a probable condition in Eldridge's cases where prior cardiac problems, of varying degrees, produced a circumstance in which the stressors of cold and exercise taxed the physical condition of the divers to a point of collapse. A further discussion of psychophysiological factors in diving and the phenomenon of "sudden death" appears in Bachrach (1978).

Exercise.   As a factor in diver fatigue we should briefly consider the complex variable of exercise. The human is not efficient in propelling himself through the water. Kidd (1969) observes from the standpoint of an engineer that the efficiency of propulsion expressed as a function of fuel consumed for velocity achieved is very uneconomic in underwater swimming. He further notes that an Olympic standard swimmer can achieve an efficiency of slightly better than 2%, which can be improved with swim fins to around 6–8% with scuba; time on bottom is extended but the drag is increased by the tanks and other gear by around 30%. Add cold and salinity, and efficiency is further reduced. In a viscous medium, swimming is clearly hard work.

We are aware that physical exercise is one of the most stressful conditions imposed on the cardiovascular system of man. The diver entering the underwater environment is heavily taxed, but even before he enters the water he is stressed. The equipment needed to penetrate the ocean is in itself a stressor as well as a protection. As Egstrom (1970) has observed, a diver in a summer dive in cold water is on a boat donning equipment that consists of a 43-lb tank, and 16–18 lb of lead weight (to allow him or her to remain underwater without floating to the surface), with a ¼" neoprene wet suit for protection against the cold. Before entering the water the heart rate of this diver has been measured at 160 beats/ minute, a rate indicating a moderate to heavy work load. These reasons lead most diving physiologists to state that physical fitness is an essential for entering the extreme environment of the underwater world.

Pressure.   The exercise of swimming demands, among other costs, increased respiratory exertion. Hydrostatic pressure results from the weight of water and increases (in sea water) at a rate of 0.445 psi per foot of descent. Increased pressure produces some decrease in ventilation that is made worse by diving equipment. Edmonds, Lowry, and Pennefather (1976) stated that, when a subject is on the surface breathing air through minimal resistance, the maximum ventilation that can be maintained for longer than a few minutes is approximately 40% of the maximum breathing capacity. If one adds resistance in the form of breathing equipment, which includes a regulator placed in the mouth to provide air from the tanks, and a face mask, the maximum ventilation over a period of longer than a few minutes will be about 25% of the maximum breathing capacity. Water immersion to the neck can lower vital capacity by about 10%. This is a result of the hydrostatic pressure compressing the thorax, as well as gravitational effects (lowering limb blood flow and increasing thoracic volume) (Edmonds, et al., 1976).

Marine Hazards.   It is likely that if you interrogated a nondiver as to what might be the greatest hazard underwater he or she would respond "sharks!" There is undoubtedly a mystique about sharks abetted by exotic TV coverage of ravenous great white sharks and slightly hysterical motion pictures. The fact is that the ratio of shark sightings to shark attacks is highly favorable to the diver, although Baldridge (1974) noted divers constitute a significant (approximate 25% of victims) group. Especially vulnerable are divers out from shore (76% of 115 attack cases were greater than 200 feet from shore) and spearfishermen. Of the free divers (skin divers) who were attacked, 86% of 103 victims were spearfishing and in 72 cases had a captive fish when attacked. Provocation of attacks, either unwitting or otherwise, is frequent. Certainly, a speared fish is an invitation to problems. Unwitting provocation appears to be related to territoriality in some cases. We have largely assumed sharks to be nomads that did not establish territories. Recent work by investigators such as the shark biologist Nelson (personal communication) suggests sharks may be territorial, and so-called "unprovoked attacks'' by sharks may be not unlike the territorial defense behavior of other species. Another hypothesis that Nelson suggests is that attacks may be defense against a possible predator. Nelson himself has been attacked in his small submersible a number of times.

Despite these statistics and the chill a shark can produce underwater, the fatality statistics are not frightening. Approximately, one fifth of attack victims die from a shark attack, a total of 15–20 deaths a year in all the sea of the world (Baldridge, 1974, p. 252). Baldridge suggested that this number compares favorably with the estimate by the American Medical Association that a minimum of 17 fatalities each year occur in the United States alone from bee or wasp stings.

It is obviously the fear of a threat that is exaggerated by humans entering the underwater environment, a fear based on the knowledge that the human underwater is not in his natural environment and is, therefore, not as much in control.

Factors in the Loss of Control Underwater

In evaluating the accidents that occur underwater, many leading to casualties, certain factors appear to be most significant and frequent. In earlier discussions, the loss of judgment resulting, perhaps, from environmental factors such as hypothermia has been discussed. A most significant factor, associated with diving problems in sports and commercial divers as well, is the loss of control represented by the experience of panic. Bradley (1981) states in his survey of diving casualties in commercial diving populations that: "anxiety and panic have been recognized as important contributions to fatal diving accidents." In the Gulf of Mexico, he observes, 17% of the accidents leading to casualties involved the citation of "poor judgment or panic on the part of the diver," and a similar percentage of 15% was noted in the North Sea casualties. An even higher percentage is assumed by investigators in recreational casualties, although this is clearly inferential from a reconstruction of the accident and consequences leading to the casualty. Almost universally, those that investigate scuba-diver deaths find that the tank has some air remaining, the mask is intact, the flotation device uninflated, and the weight belt is still attached to the body (Bachrach, 1970). These findings support the hypothesis that there was no fault with the equipment, but that human error, loss of judgment, and panic caused the casualty. The antecedent conditions appear to be those discussed, with cold leading to gradual hypothermia and its attendant problems, including loss of judgment; fatigue resulting from exercise; the physiological cost of other factors such as the equipment required to dive; and the possible appearance of a marine hazard such as a shark or other novel stimulus. These events coupled with the probable lowering of the air supply can set the occasion for an apprehensive response that can lead to a full loss of control manifested by panic (Bachrach, 1979; Bachrach & Egstrom, 1977).

The Centrality of Breathing

There are many elements in common across the varying extreme environments. What makes the underwater environment unique is that it is the only one in which, at deep levels of diving, the human is breathing a mixture that is not air. Helium/oxygen as a breathing mix is essential for deep diving; heat loss in helium is approximately seven times that of air; heat is lost through body areas, but it is also lost in the breathing mix upon expiration, where warmed, moistened gas is vented into the environment. To begin, heat loss in water is 25 times that of air. Compound that with such factors as helium, and problems increase. But this breathing problem is also found in sports divers whose regulators require effort, particularly on exhalation, that can be stressful. Breathing problems appear in virtually all stress situations, land and sea, and the changes in respiratory rate and pattern appear to be common to stress responses. As long ago as 1953, Ross McFarland (McFarland, 1953) noted that persons under stress appear to: "sigh more frequently as well as breathe more rapidly and irregularly than normal conditions [p. 119]." This has been commented upon by Bachrach and Egstrom (1977), who observed that agitation is the first sign of impending stress, and that a frequent (if not universal) sign of stress is a change in breathing rate and pattern from smooth and regular to rapid, shallow, and irregular. The physiological consequences of such rapid and shallow breathing are complex, but, at its simplest, the problems in oxygen and carbon dioxide exchange resulting from a probable hypoventilation can be important, particularly in the underwater environment where ventilatory exchange is crucial. Another aspect is that less lung intake necessarily alters buoyancy.

Breathing changes as a problem and indication of impending problems have also been observed in the North Sea commercial diving population. Childs and Norman (1978) in an analysis of 42 diving fatalities associated with loss of consciousness, all in the North Sea sector, noted: "The commonest problems associated with all incidents were related to breathing, and included breathlessness, hyperventilation, and difficulty in breathing. Hyperventilation, which may be noticed over the communications system, is the most accurate indicator at present available of a potentially dangerous situation [p. 128]."

These authors use the term *hyperventilation* as it is commonly used to describe rapid breathing. The term, so used, is not entirely appropriate, for hyperventilation implies an excess of ventilatory exchange, whereas, as noted, it is probable that the rapid, shallow breathing is more likely to produce hypoventilation. The proper term for rapid breathing, obviously more difficult to pronounce, would be *tachypnea*. Dyspnea, marked difficulty in breathing, is known to be one of the most important medical problems in diving, particularly deep diving. In a review of the problem, Fagraeus (1981) discusses the problems of pressure and breathing mixtures in deep diving, coupled with exercise observing: "by penetrating into the deeper regions of the underwater environment man is exposed to a combination of physiological stresses which has no equal in the history of human exercise [p. 141]." He defines dyspnea as a shortness of breath or a feeling of breathlessness or an awareness of difficulty in breathing and recognizes its subjective nature. Like pain, it is difficult to measure and, also like pain: "can only be identified and graded by the individual suffering from it." It has also been described as a subjective "air hunger," a sense of not being able to obtain enough air. The emotional components of such an experience can be devastating. In a colorful account, Lanphier (1963), a respiratory physiologist, describes dyspnea as: "a period of terror that has no equal in my experience [p. 130]."

The diver is performing in a strange and extreme environment, somewhat exposed to cold, working often in conditions of reduced visibility with a lack of normal cues (tactile, visual, and auditory), breathing an unusual mixture of gases, and subjected to great hydrostatic pressure, all of which further exacerbate the exertion needed to handle the task as well as the encumbrance of gear in the underwater environment. To me, this underwater world stands apart as the epitome of an extreme environment.

ACKNOWLEDGMENT

Naval Medical Research and Development Command, Work Unit No. MF58524.023.2018. The opinions and assertions contained herein are the private ones of the writer and are not to be construed as official or reflecting the views of the Navy Department or the Naval Service at large.

REFERENCES

Adolph, E. F. General and specific characteristics of physiologic adaptations. *American Journal of Physiology*, 1956, *184*, 18-28.

Alf, E. F., & Gordon, L. V. *A fleet validation of selection tests for underwater demolition team training*. San Diego, Calif.: U. S. Naval Personnel Research Field Activity, 1957 (Memo 57-3).

Appley, M. D., & Trumbull, R. *Psychological stress*. New York: Appleton-Century-Crofts, 1967.

Bachrach, A. J. Diving behavior. In *Human performance in scuba diving*. Proceedings of the symposium on underwater physiology. Chicago: The Athletic Institute, 1970, 119-138.

Bachrach, A. J. A short history of man in the sea. In P. B. Bennett & D. H. Elliott (Eds.), *The physiology and medicine of compressed air work* (2nd ed.). London: Baillière Tindall, 1975. (a)

Bachrach, A. J. Underwater performance. In P. B. Bennett & D. H. Elliott (Eds.), *The physiology and medicine of diving and compressed air work* (2nd ed.). London: Baillière Tindall, 1975. (b)

Bachrach, A. J. Psychophysiological factors in diving. *Weekly Update: Hyperbaric and Undersea Medicine*, 1978, *1*(29), 2-7.

Bachrach, A. J. Diving stress. *The Undersea Journal*, 1979, *12*(4), 14-15.

Bachrach, A. J. Learning theory. In *A. M. Freedman, H. I. Kaplan, & B. J. Sadock (Eds.), Comprehensive textbook of psychiatry, III*. Baltimore: Williams & Wilkins, 1980. (a)

Bachrach, A. J. *Psychological research* (4th ed). New York: Random House, 1980. (b)

Bachrach, A. J., & Bennett, P. B. The high pressure nervous syndrome during human deep saturation and excursion diving. *Forsvärsmedicin*, 1973, *9*, 490–495.

Bachrach, A. J., & Egstrom, G. H. Apprehension and panic. In *British Sub-Aqua Club diving manual*. London: British Sub-Aqua Club, 1977, 40–45.

Baldridge, H. D. *Shark attack*. Anderson, S. C.: Droke House, Hallux, 1974.

Bennett, P. B. Elucidating anesthesia mechanisms: Current concepts and problems. *Anesthesiology*, 1975, *5*, 1ff. (a)

Bennett, P. B. Inert gas narcosis. In P. B. Bennett & D. H. Elliott (Eds.), *The physiology and medicine of diving and compressed air work* (2nd ed.). London: Baillière Tindall, 1975. (b)

Berghage, T. E., Rohrbaugh, P. A., Bachrach, A. J., & Armstrong, F. W. *Navy diving: Who's doing it and under what conditions*. Project MPN10.03.2040DAC9, Naval Medical Research Institute, Bethesda, Md., 1975.

Berlyne, D. E. Novelty, complexity, and hedonic value. *Perceptual Psychophysiology*, 1970, *8*, 279–286.

Bernard, C. Leçons de physiologie experimentale à appliquée à la médecine. *Cours du semestre d'ete* (Vol. II). Paris: Baillière, 1856.

Biersner, R. J. Psychological evaluation and selection of divers. In C. W. Shilling & C. B. Carlson (Eds.), *Physicians guide to diving medicine*. Bethesda, Md.: Undersea Medical Society, in press.

Bligh, J. & Johnson, K. G. Glossary of terms for thermal physiology. *Journal of Applied Physiology*, 1973, *35*, 941–961.

Bradley, M. E. An epidemiological study of fatal diving accidents in two commercial diving populations. In A. J. Bachrach & M. M. Matzen (Eds.), *Underwater physiology* (VII). Proceedings of the seventh symposium on underwater physiology. Bethesda, Md.: The Undersea Medical Society, 1981; 869–875.

Brunswik, E. The conceptual framework of psychology. *International Encyclopedia of Unified Sciences*, 1952, *6*, 659–751.

Cannon, W. B. *The wisdom of the body*. New York: Norton, 1939.

Case, E. M., & Haldane, J. B. S. Human physiology under high pressure (1). Effects of nitrogen, carbon dioxide and cold. *Journal of Hygiene (Cambridge)* 1941, *41*, 225–249.

Chapanis, A. The relevance of laboratory studies to practical situations. *Ergonomics*, 1967, *10*, 557–577.

Childs, C. M. Loss of consciousness in divers—a survey and review. In *Proceedings of medical aspects of diving accidents congress*. Luxembourg/Kirshberg, October 12–13, 1978, 3–23.

Childs, C. M., & Norman, J. N. Unexplained loss of consciousness in divers. *Médecine Aéronautique et Spatiale, Médecine Subaquatique et Hyperbare*, 1978, *17*, 127–128.

Cooper, K. E. Hypothermia. In R. H. Strauss (Ed.), *Diving medicine*. New York: Grune & Stratton, 1976.

Dean, P. J., & Thatcher, R. F. Analysis of human factors in aircraft accidents. *Aviation, Space, and Environmental Medicine*, 1975, *46*, 1260–1262.

Durkheim, E. Suicide (Book II) (Trans. by J. A. Spaulding & G. Simpson). Glencoe, Ill.: Free Press, 1951 (1st ed., 1897).

Eagan, C. J. Introduction and terminology. Symposium on temperature acclimation. *Federation Proceedings*, 1963, *22*, 930–933.

Edmonds, C., Lowry, C., & Pennefather, J. *Diving and subaquatic medicine*. Mosman N. S. W., Australia: Diving Medical Centre, 1976.

Egstrom, G. H. Effect of equipment on diving performance. In Human performance and scuba diving. *Proceedings of the symposium on underwater physiology*. Chicago: The Athletic Institute, 1970, 5–16.

Egstrom, G. H. Diving equipment. In R. H. Strauss (Ed.), *Diving medicine*. New York: Grune & Stratton, 1976.

Eldridge, L. Sudden unexplained death syndrome in cold water scuba diving. In Program and abstracts, Undersea Medical Society, Annual Scientific Meeting. *Undersea Biomedical Research*, 1979, *6*(Suppl.), 41.

Fagraeus, L. Current concepts of cardio-respiratory responses to exercise. In A. J. Bachrach & M. M. Matzen (Eds.), *Underwater physiology* (VII). Proceedings of the seventh symposium on underwater physiology. Bethesda, Md.: The Undersea Medical Society, 1981; 141–149.

Fiske, D. W., & Maddi, S. R. *Functions of varied experience*. Homewood, Ill.: Dorsey Press, 1961.

Follinsbee, L. J., Wagner, J. A., Borgia, J. F., Drinkwater, B. L., Gliner, J. A., & Bedi, J. F. (Eds.). *Environmental stress: Individual human adaptations*. New York: Academic Press, 1978.

Fritz, M. Are divers suicidal? *Tauchen*, 1979, *2*, 24–25.

Haythorn, W. W. The miniworld of isolation: Laboratory studies. In J. E. Rasmussen (Ed.), *Isolation and confinement*. Chicago: Aldine, 1973.

Hayward, M. G., & Keatinge, W. R. Progressive symptomless hypothermia in water: Possible cause of diving accidents. *British Medical Journal*, 1979, *6172*, 1182.

Hertzka, A. F., & Anderson, A. V. *Selection requirements for underwater demolition team training*. San Diego, Calif. U. S. Naval Personnel Field Activity, 1956 (Memo 56-4).

Hong, S. K. Comparison of diving and nondiving women of Korea. *Federation Proceedings*, 1963, *22*, 831–833.

Hong, S. K. The physiology of breath-hold diving. In R. H. Strauss (Ed.), *Diving medicine*. New York: Grune & Stratton, 1976.

Hunter, W. L., Jr., & Bennett, P. B. The causes, mechanisms and prevention of the high pressure nervous syndrome. *Undersea Biomedical Research*, 1974, *1*, 1–28.

Kates, R. W. Experiencing the environment as hazard. In H. M. Proshansky, W. H. Ittelson, & L. G. Rivlin (Eds.), *Environmental psychology: Man and his physical setting*. New York: Holt, Rinehart, & Winston, 1970.

Kidd, D. J. Underwater activities—physiology. In *Conference on man in cold water*. Ottawa: Canadian Society of Oceanology, 1969.

Lanphier, E. Influence of increased ambient pressure upon alveolar ventilation. In C. J. Lambertsen & L. J. Greenbaum (Eds.), *Second symposium on underwater physiology*. Washington, D. C.: National Academy of Sciences/National Research Council, 1963, 124–133.

Licht, K. F. Safety and accidents—a brief conceptual point of view. *Journal of School Health*, 1975, *45*(9), 530–534.

McFarland, R. *Human factors in air transportation*. New York: McGraw-Hill, 1953.

Mount, L. E. *Adaptation to thermal environment. Man and his productive animals*. Baltimore, Md.: University Park Press, 1979.

Nelson, D. R. *Personal communication*, 1980.

Prosser, C. L. Perspectives of adaptation: Theoretical aspects. In D. B. Dill (Ed.), *Adaptation to the environment* (Sect. 4), *Handbook of physiology*. Washington, D. C.: American Physiological Society, 1964.

Rowell, L. B. Human adjustments and adaptations to heat stress—where and how? In L. J. Folinsbee, J. A. Wagner, J. F. Borgia, B. L. Drinkwater, J. A. Gliner, & J. F. Bedi (Eds.), *Environmental stress. Individual human adaptations*. New York: Academic Press, 1978.

Schenck, H. V., Jr., & McAniff, J. J. *U. S. underwater diving fatality statistics, 1976*. Rockville, Md.: U. S. Department of Commerce, 1978 (Report No. URI-SSR-78-12).

Selye, H. The evolution of the stress concept—stress and cardiovascular disease. In L. Levi (Ed.), *Society, stress, and disease—the psychosocial environment and psychosomatic diseases*. London: Oxford University Press, 1971.

Sloan, A. W. *Man in extreme environments*. Springfield, Ill.: Charles C. Thomas, 1979.

Theologus, G. C., Wheaton, G. R., Mirabella, A., Brahlek, R. E., & Fleishman, E. A. Development of a standardized battery of performance tests for the assessment of noise stress effects. Washington, D. C.: NASA, 1973, 2 (Report CR-2149).

Tune, G. S. Psychological effects of hypoxia: A review of certain literature from the period 1950 to 1963. *Perceptual and Motor Skills Research,* 1964, *19,* 551-562 (Cited in Theologus et al., 1973, p. 560).

Waller, J. A. Epidemiologic approaches to injury research. In V. J. Pezoldt (Ed.), *Rare event/ accident research methodology*. Washington, D. C.: National Bureau of Standards Special Publication 482, 1977.

Workman, R. D. Other medical problems associated with exposure to pressure. In Committee on hyperbaric oxygenation: *Fundamentals of hyperbaric medicine*. Washington, D. C.: National Academy of Sciences, 1966, 110-114.

Zuckerman, M. *Sensation-seeking: Beyond the optimal levels of arousal*. Hillsdale, NJ: Lawrence Erlbaum Associates, 1979.

The Yankelovich Monitor. Trend No. 44, Flirtation with danger. New York: Yankelovich, Skelly, & White, Inc., 1979.

9 Behavioral Responses to Air Pollution

Gary W. Evans
Program in Social Ecology and
Public Policy Research Organization
University of California, Irvine

Stephen V. Jacobs
Department of Psychology and Social Relations
Harvard University

Neal B. Frager
School of Medicine
University of California, Los Angeles

The aspect of the problem of adaptation that is probably most disturbing is paradoxically the very fact that human beings are so adaptable. This very adaptability enables them to become adjusted to conditions and habits which will eventually destroy the values most characteristic of human life.
                                                    —Dubos, 1965, p. 278

There are many ways to porvent Paluicon such as us the Kind of gasolien that Does not let out Paluicon, or enstead of rideing in a car ride a Bicecle or another way of getting around . . . . Paluicon we should fit agenst. it is worth it. many people are very Ill and unhappy and it is all becase of that Teribal thing PALUICON.
                                                    —Kari Greenberger, 1971, Age 8

Whereas there is an extensive literature on the physiological and health effects of air pollution on humans, there is a marked paucity of psychological theory and data on human responses to air pollution. This chapter has three purposes. Firstly, we review the survey literature on human responses to air pollution, noting areas where further research is necessary. Secondly, recent research on air pollution and overt behavior is discussed. Thirdly, we describe two preliminary studies on human adaptation to air pollution.

SURVEY LITERATURE

Unfortunately, there is a relatively large but unsystematic survey literature on human responses to air pollution. This literature suffers from several problems. Firstly, few researchers have conceptually organized human reactions to air quality. For example, many studies intermix attitudinal components with other aspects of human responses to air pollution such as awareness, knowledge, or behavioral intentions. In addition, many survey studies provide scant statistical information, rarely even analyzing bivariate responses. Moreover, most studies do not provide basic psychometric data on scale construction, reliability, or validity of instruments. Finally, nearly all the surveys have taken place at one point in time and space without any comparison groups. Therefore, the basic experimental design of most survey studies of air pollution and human behavior precludes hypothesis testing. The research program on adaptation to air pollution that we present in the latter part of this chapter is offered, in part, as a preliminary model of more rigorous, conceptually based research on human responses to air pollution.

Recently, Evans and Jacobs (1981) reviewed the literature on air pollution and human behavior. They used an attitude–behavior framework to organize the literature into three major categories: cognitive, affective, and conative. The cognitive component can be subdivided into awareness and knowledge. We highlight some of the major findings on cognitive and affective components of human behavior and air pollution and describe in more detail recent work on overt behavior.

Cognitive Responses to Air Pollution

Approximately 80% of individuals interviewed in air pollution areas note the presence of air pollution if they are directly probed about air quality, whereas considerably fewer persons mention air pollution as a problem if indirectly queried (e.g., Please list the five most serious problems in your community, Creer, Gray, & Treshow, 1970; Rankin, 1969). Public awareness of air pollution is effected primarily by the physical parameters of air quality and mass media publicity about air quality (Barker, 1976). The strongest physical stimuli influencing awareness are sensory cues such as visibility, odor, and dustfall (filth). Publicity about air-quality issues generally increases public awareness of air pollution.

Knowledge and beliefs about air pollution are similar to the awareness data. Generally, people define air pollution in terms of its sensory effects (reduced visibility, odor), and few mention either health impacts of pollution or the causes of air pollution (Crowe, 1968; Medalia, 1964). Interestingly, experts define air pollution more in terms of causal agents than laypersons do (Barker, 1976). Experts use causes like the presence of cars or industry rather than poor visibility to gauge air quality.

Affective Responses to Air Pollution

Whereas studies between 1960–1970 generally found increasing concern about air pollution over time, recent national surveys indicate a lessening of public concern about environmental problems including air pollution (Dunlap, Van Liere, & Dillman, 1979). These trends probably reflect two factors. Firstly, interest in ecology and political action in general that were at a height in the late 60s (eg., Earth day) may explain the strong rise in concern about air pollution during the previous decade. Subsequent reductions in political activity and increasing concern about economic issues may account for the decline of concern about air pollution during the 1970s.

Like the awareness findings, direct probes of concern about air pollution yield greater concern than indirect queries. Furthermore, concern is also directly related to sensory components of air quality, particularly visibility and odor (Barker, 1976). Recently, researchers have begun to investigate how particular components of air quality influence perceived air quality. Flachsbart and Phillips (1980), for example, derived an observer-based air quality index in the Los Angeles area using a large sample of residents. The best combination of predictor variables in predicting perceived air quality consisted of visibility, ozone, and sulfur dioxide, measured as the number of days per year that state standards are exceeded for each index. Publicity can also increase concern about air pollution, although some studies have found that extensive publicity about cleanup efforts of one pollutant (eg., coal soot in England) is associated with greater complacency about other, remaining air pollutants (Wall, 1974).

Various personal characteristics of respondents are correlated with concern about air pollution. Concern is positively related to higher socioeconomic status, political liberalism, and degree of preexisting respiratory problems. In addition, females and whites tend to view air pollution as a more serious problem (Evans & Jacobs, 1981).

Individuals have also been surveyed about their attitudes toward control over air pollution. While many people believe air pollution can be controlled, most individuals are unaware of existing air quality management efforts. Furthermore, most people feel that "someone else" such as the government should do something about air pollution. Very few respondents acknowledge any personal role in air pollution control. Several studies have examined in more detail the relationship between attitudes toward air pollution and individual control over air quality.

Employees of a local industry that was a major polluter were significantly less bothered by air quality in their city than other town residents not employed by the polluter. In addition, employees of the company were also more aware of pollution abatement activities (Creer et al., 1970). Consistent with these findings, other researchers have shown that persons with high concern about air pollution are much more likely to ask elected officials for air pollution controls. Conversely, persons with low levels of concern about air quality tend to ignore existing air pollution (Medalia, 1964). Similarly, Rankin (1969) found that persons feeling the least control over air pollution also rate it as a relatively unimportant community problem. Finally, individuals who perceive air pollution as a serious problem report that they use mass transportation more and maintain their cars better than do persons less concerned about air quality (Hohm, 1976).

A few investigators have examined air pollution complaint data, attempting to determine why most people do not complain. Although approximately 20–25% of persons in high-air pollution areas feel like complaining, only about 5% actually do so. When asked why they do not complain, individuals typically respond: (1) They do not know where to complain; and (2) they feel that their complaints will not do any good (Rankin, 1969). Several other surveys have uncovered high levels of cynicism in the public about the efficacy of complaining to authorities about air pollution.

OVERT BEHAVIOR AND AIR POLLUTION

Until recently, few investigators have analyzed air pollution and overt human behaviors with the exception of human performance studies on carbon monoxide (see Evans & Jacobs, 1981, for a review of this literature). We focus our discussion here on two areas of behavior and air pollution, outdoor recreation patterns and social behaviors such as aggression and altruism.

Outdoor Recreation Behavior

Some investigators have asked persons what behavioral changes they make when air pollution is bad. A majority of respondents from several industrial towns in England report that they restrict their outdoor activity if possible during pollution alerts (Kirkby, 1972). Similar data have been reported in Southern California (Gold, 1970). It is important to examine actual outdoor behavior in addition to self-reported changes in activity. Two epidemiological studies have linked photochemical smog in the Los Angeles area with driving behavior and athletic performance. Ury (1968) found a moderate, aggregate level correlation between ozone levels and auto accidents in Los Angeles. In addition, running times of Los

Angeles high school cross-country runners increase with increments in ozone over a certain threshold (Wayne, Wehrle, & Caroll, 1967). Both of these behavioral findings should be interpreted cautiously, however, because aggregate level data were used and many potentially confounding variables could not be controlled for.

Three studies have directly examined individual levels of outdoor behavior under varying air quality conditions. In an early study, both the frequency and type of outdoor activity in New York City were not correlated to air-quality levels (Rivlin, 1974, p. 526). Because no data are available on this preliminary study, these findings are difficult to evaluate. One possible explanation for the absence of any association between air quality and recreation behaviors may be insufficient variability in air quality and the inability to use a within-subjects design. Daily fluctuations in air quality are relatively small and highly correlated. In order to capture variation in most air-quality parameters, sampling over large periods of time is necessary. Between subjects, designs examining recreation behavior undoubtedly have large error terms due to the substantial amount of variance due to individual differences in recreation behavior preferences. Chapko and Solomon (1976) in a similar study found, however, small but statistically significant correlations between air quality and daily attendance at some outdoor recreation sites in New York City.

In a more extensive study of outdoor recreation patterns and air quality, Peterson (1975) monitored the number of people participating in 39 recreational activities at 13 different sites over a 2½-month period in Southern California. The sampling period she chose included periods during which major fluctuations in photochemical smog and other oxidants occurred. Moreover, Peterson observed outdoor activities that vary considerably in energy-expenditure requirements (e.g., running versus sitting) in both indoor and outdoor settings.

Peterson's data contrast with Rivlin's equivocal findings. Air pollution indices significantly correlated with recreation behavior of Southern Californians. Furthermore, this overall conclusion is conservative, because the effects of air pollution held after partialling out variance due to sunlight, temperature, and visibility, which are all correlated with oxidant levels in Southern California. Peterson also found, as predicted, that the effects of poor air quality on outdoor recreation behaviors are stronger than on indoor behaviors. A final hypothesis of Peterson's that high-energy-expenditure activities would be curtailed more than low-energy activities during poor air-quality periods was not supported.

Social Behavior

Affect. Air pollution may also effect interpersonal affect and related behaviors such as altruism and aggression. Several epidemiological studies reveal moderate correlations among various air pollutants such as ozone and sulfur dioxide with eye irritation, headaches, and fatigue (Evans & Jacobs, 1981). Recent experimental investigations of cigarette smoke as a pollutant have found that when nonsmokers are exposed to secondary cigarette smoke they become annoyed, irritated, and tired, in comparison to their feelings during clear, ambient air conditions (Jones, 1978). Stone, Breidenbach, and Heimstra (1979), however, report a more complex relationship between nonsmokers' behaviors and exposure to cigarette smoke. In two laboratory studies in which individuals were exposed to both smoke and noise, there were no main effects of smoke or interactions with noise on subject ratings of affect. The strong effects of noise on affect may have masked any effects of smoke. A third study without noise found that smoke increased annoyance, but only under certain task conditions. When individuals worked on tasks under low-motivation conditions (reward not contingent upon performance), smoke heightened annoyance. Paradoxically, when rewards were dependent on performance, individuals felt slightly better in smoke versus clear conditions.

In another study, Rotton and his colleagues found that the presence of malodor significantly depressed subject's ratings of photographs and paintings in a laboratory setting (Rotton, Yoshikawa, Francis, & Hoyler, 1978). Thus, several findings indicate that, under some conditions at least, air pollution in the form of cigarette smoke or malodor can increase annoyance and negative affect. Given the effects of air pollution on affect, other interpersonal behaviors like aggression and altruism may also be affected by air quality. Recently, some preliminary research on these interpersonal behaviors has begun.

Aggression.   One behavioral manifestation of greater annoyance or irritation between two persons is greater interpersonal distance (Evans & Howard, 1973). Bleda and Bleda (1978) tested whether cigarette smoke would influence proxemic behavior by invading the personal space of individuals sitting on a bench in a public shopping mall. When the invader smoked a cigarette, subjects were more likely to leave and left the bench where they sat faster. Aggressive behaviors are also effected by air quality. When nonsmokers are exposed to cigarette smoke, they are more likely to agress toward an experimental confederate in a laboratory setting (Jones & Bogat, 1978). Aggressive behavior was operationalized as the intensity of noise bursts a subject was willing to use to negatively reinforce a confederate "learning a task." An anger provocation manipulation did not interact with air quality.

More complex effects of air quality on aggression have been found by Rotton and colleagues (Rotton, Frey, Barry, & Fitzpatrick, 1979). Subjects were placed in a situation where they believed they were delivering shocks to another subject (confederate) for making errors on a learning task. One half the subjects were previously exposed to an aggressive model. In addition, three levels of air quality were created: unpolluted, moderately malodorous, extremely unpleasant odor. Air quality had no effects on aggressive behavior when an aggressive model had been presented. When no model had been present, the authors found a curvilinear function between aggression and air pollution; shocking was highest during the moderate malodor condition and uniformly low for both control- and high-pollution conditions. Research on other environmental stressors such as heat (Bell, 1981) has also found similar inverted U-shaped functions between stress and aggression. One explanation for this nonlinear effect is that under high, noxious conditions individual's main concern is to escape the situation as soon as they can. Less shocking occurs to reduce the amount of time spent in the experimental setting.

In the second portion of this chapter, we argue that the behavioral effects of air pollution can be conceptualized from a psychological stress perspective. Rotton and his colleagues have independently pursued a similar approach in their work on air quality. Because air pollution can affect aggression and negative affect in a manner similar to several other environmental stressors (Evans & Jacobs, 1981), Rotton, Yoshikawa, and Kaplan (1979) reasoned that individual control might mediate some of the negative effects of air pollution. Previous research with noise (Glass & Singer, 1972) and crowding (Sherrod, 1974), for example, revealed the ameliorative effects of subject's instrumental control over environmental stressors. Thus, Rotton et al. (1979) applied the Glass and Singer (1972) aftereffect and perceived control paradigm to air pollution.

Individuals were placed in one of three conditions: no odor, malodor, malodor with perceived control. Perceived control was induced by informing subjects they could place a cork in a bottle of foul-smelling liquid if they wanted to. In the malodor with no control condition, subjects were instructed to leave the open bottle alone. Immediately following exposure to the stressor, subjects were given several puzzles to solve, of which half were impossible to complete. Frustration tolerance was measured by persistence on the impossible puzzles. Persons in the malodor with no control condition had significantly less frustration tolerance than individuals in either the odor with control or the no-odor condition. The latter two groups did not differ from one another.

Mental Health.   Thus, several studies show that poor air quality can increase negative affect and heighten negative interpersonal behaviors. Air quality may also influence mental health. Recent preliminary findings indicate moderate correlations between some air pollution indices and admissions of psychiatric patients into hospitals in the St. Louis area (Strahilevitz, Strahilevitz, & Miller, 1979). Daily carbon monoxide concentrations correlated ($r = .25$) with admissions of all psychiatric patients, and nitrogen dioxide levels correlated ($r = .22$) with admissions of alcoholic patients and patients with organic brain damage ($r = .20$). Unfortunately, very little research has systematically examined the effects of ambient pollutants on mental health and other stress-related disorders. Given the preliminary findings that poor air quality can effect annoyance, irritability, and perhaps interpersonal relationships, it seems reasonable that in addition to the impact of air quality on physical health, mental health may also be negatively affected by air pollution. We are currently engaged in an epidemiological study examining the effects of smog on the mental health of persons living in the Los Angeles metropolitan area. Four hundred persons are being interviewed twice over a 3-month interval across a 3-year span. Mental health data being collected include standardized measures of depression, mental status, anxiety, and use of mental health facilities. In addition, information is collected on occurrence of recent stressful life events, social support networks, and basic sociodemographic data. Air quality data are supplied by the Southern California Air Quality Management District. At this time no data are available, but the two principle hypotheses we are testing are: (1) Persons who have recently moved into the Los Angeles area will be most susceptible to the negative health effects of smog because they have not adapted to the poor air quality of the region; and (2) individuals experiencing a high level of stressful life events will be most vulnerable to negative physical and mental health effects of smog. Hopefully, our study that includes more rigorous controls than the Strahilevitz et al. (1979) study and a repeated measures design reveals important data on the relationship between air pollution and mental health.

Prosocial Behavior.   Air pollution may also affect more positive social behaviors such as attraction and altruism. When individuals are exposed to an attitudinally similar stranger, poor air quality can actually *increase* attraction for that person (Rotton, Barry, Frey, & Soler, 1978). No effects of air quality were noted when attraction toward a markedly, attitudinally dissimilar stranger was measured. Under the latter conditions, attraction was consistently low in both malodorous and control conditions. Attitudinal similarity was manipulated by giving subjects false feedback from another subject (confederate) answering an identical set of questions given to the subject. Attraction was measured on a rating scale. Rotton and his colleagues conjectured that the increased attraction in odor conditions was due to the subject's empathy for the "liked stranger." Thus, they designed a second experiment where it was clear to the subject that the other subject (confederate) was not also exposed to the same malodor that he or she was. Under these conditions, malodor depressed attraction for the stranger.

Because interpersonal attraction may be affected by air pollution, it is possible that behaviors reflecting positive affect such as altruism may also be affected by air pollution. Recent field work has found small but significant correlations between ambient air pollution levels and individuals' willingness to fill out a questionnaire for a stranger (Cunningham, 1979). Stronger effects of sunshine and temperature on altruism were not partialled but, however, from the association between air quality and helping behavior.

Unfortunately, many of the behavioral studies on air pollution are either conducted under field conditions, where little control over other variables is possible and random assignment of subjects is impossible, or are conducted under laboratory conditions, where the pollutants used (cigarette smoke, malodor) may not realistically model ambient effects in the community. In addition, subjects know their exposure is temporary. Furthermore, as noted earlier, most behavioral studies on air pollution have been atheoretical. One purpose of the two preliminary studies in the following sections is to illustrate how conceptually derived, quasi-experimental field studies of air pollution and human behavior can be conducted. Hopefully, these studies demonstrate that it is possible to conduct relatively controlled, careful research on air pollution and human behavior in a meaningful, community context. A second purpose of our two studies is to examine the process of physiological and psychological adaptation to a chronic environmental stressor, air pollution.

STUDY I: HUMAN ADAPTATION TO AIR POLLUTION

One perspective that may provide some insight into people's reactions to such chronic environmental conditions as air pollution comes from Helson's (1964) adaptation-level theory. According to this theory, individuals who are continuously exposed to a particular stimulus use it as a standard against which they judge other similar stimuli. Applying adaptation-level theory to environmental quality, Wohlwill suggests that people who habitually experience a particular pollutant (such as air pollution) use a different standard for assessing it than do people who have little or no experience with the same environmental pollutant (Wohlwill, 1974; Wohlwill & Kohn, 1976).

Drawing from Wohlwill's extension of adaptation-level theory, we address the following question in this study: Will people perceive and react to air quality differently as a function of their experience with air pollution? In order to investigate this issue, we compare long- and short-term residents of the Los Angeles Air Basin on their attitudes and responses to photochemical smog.

Wohlwill found that residents of a medium-sized city who had migrated from low-air pollution areas judge air pollution in their new city as more severe than other residents who had previously lived in high-air pollution areas (Wohlwill & Kohn, 1973, 1976). Furthermore, in their ground-breaking studies of human adaptation to stress, Glass and Singer (1972) demonstrated that human responses to noise generally diminish with repeated exposure under short-term, laboratory conditions.

Lipsey (1976) argues against an adaptation-level explanation of human responses to air pollution. Instead of habituating to air pollution, he suggests that the longer people are exposed to air pollution, the more exasperated they will become with the problem. His conclusion is based on two areas of research on attitudes toward air pollution. Firstly, he notes that many air pollution surveys find moderate to high correlations between concern about air pollution and physical indices of pollution. Lipsey reasons that once a certain amount of stress accumulates from continued exposure to poor air quality, individuals will not continue to tolerate poor air quality but will express increasingly negative reactions to it.

Lipsey's second source of support comes from an empirical study in which exacerbation rather than habituation apparently results from continued exposure to air pollution (Medalia, 1964). Residents of a town who had lived there prior to and after the construction of a foul-smelling paper mill were interviewed. Awareness and negative attitudes toward air pollution were greater the longer people had lived in the town. These data are not strong evidence against the adaptation position, however, because residents living in the town prior to the mill were compared to those moving there after its construction. Thus, only the long-term residents could compare present ambient air quality to prior premill conditions. Furthermore, whereas newer residents chose to live in the town with knowledge of the poor air quality, older residents did not have that choice.

Consistent with Wohlwill's application of adaptation-level theory to environmental quality assessment, we predict that long-term residents, as compared to new migrants of the Los Angeles air basin, will estimate lower levels of ambient smog. Moreover, we hypothesize that long-term residents will use higher response criteria in detecting smog than new migrants; that is, long-term residents will be less likely than new migrants to report seeing smog when it is present at low concentrations. We do not anticipate any differences in the relative abilities of our two groups of residents to detect the presence of smog. Rather, we expect an adaptation-level shift in response bias. In order to test this hypothesis, we use signal detection techniques that allow us to separate response bias from detection sensitivity (see Baird & Noma, 1978, for an excellent discussion of signal detection).

In addition to viewing air pollution from an adaptation-level perspective, we consider it to be a stressor. A predominant psychological perspective on stress emphasizes individual's cognitive assessment of environmental conditions (Lazarus, 1966; Lazarus & Cohen, 1977; Lazarus & Launier, 1978). Lazarus and his colleagues suggest that there are two major modes of coping with a stressor—instrumental and palliative. Instrumental coping entails active attempts to deal with a stressor. Modes of instrumental coping with smog might include acquiring more information about smog, behavioral changes such as curtailment of outdoor activities to lessen negative health impact, or by taking action to lower smog levels such as using mass transit. Palliative coping with smog might include exaggerated self-assessment of knowledge about smog, or failure to acknowledge the negative effects of smog on one's health. Interestingly, several air pollution attitude surveys have found that residents living in poor air-quality areas consistently judge (incorrectly) air quality to be worse in neighboring communities than in their own (DeGroot, 1967; Rankin, 1969). This finding may be a form of denial, perhaps caused by dissonance reduction. The role of denial as a coping device for dealing with stress has been discussed using medical settings as an example by Janis (1977).

Adaptation processes are amenable to Lazarus' framework of coping with stressors. Adaptation to a chronic stressor like air pollution may reflect a shift from predominantly instrumental to palliative coping mechanisms. Thus, we expect recent arrivals to the Los Angeles air basin to manifest greater instrumental coping with smog than long-term residents. Conversely, long-term residents will exhibit more palliative forms of coping with smog. In addition, we hypothesize that recent arrivals to the Los Angeles air basin who are more internal will be most likely to curtail outdoor activities when smog levels rise. External, recent migrants are not expected to alter their outdoor, recreational behaviors as much as internal, recent migrants in the presence of smog. The utilization of such preventative behaviors in response to a stressor presupposes that the individual believes he/she can effect life outcomes by his/her own efforts. We believe that those persons who have not habituated to smog and who are more self-efficacious are most likely to engage in preventative, recreational behaviors to reduce the negative effects of smog on their health.

Photochemical smog may also affect human physiological mechanisms as a function of amount of previous exposure to ozone, the major toxic component of photochemical smog. Preliminary laboratory studies have shown effects of ozone on human biochemical responses in the blood and lung tissues, pulmonary reactivity, and other respiratory-related discomfort (Coffin & Stokinger, 1977; National Academy of Sciences, 1977). Ozone exposure may cause biochemical changes reflecting response to oxidant challenge; that is, they measure how the blood reacts to reductions in oxygen intake. These changes include increased red blood cell fragility, serum Vitamin E levels, and lipid peroxidation, and reduced acetylcholinesterase and glutathione levels in the blood. However, subsequent investigations of human biochemical reactivity to ozone have had mixed results (Hackney, Linn, Buckley, Collier, & Mohler, 1978). Changes in pulmonary function under controlled, chamber exposure to ozone have included reduced air-flow rate and forced vital capacity, and increased respiratory air-flow resistance. Other respiratory effects include chest tightness or soreness, cough, shortness of breath, and nose and throat irritation. Nausea, anorexia, and headache have also been noted. Finally, eye irritation is caused by PAN that covaries with ozone under ambient conditions.

Epidemiological studies of ozone and human health have generally found little or no association between fluctuations in ambient ozone levels and changes in health indicators. Existing data indicate that there is no substantial relationship between ambient ozone and human mortality; weak association for respiratory-related hospital admissions and respiratory infection rates; and moderate evidence for aggravation of preexisting respiratory diseases (Goldsmith & Friberg, 1977; National Academy of Sciences, 1977). Epidemiological evidence for a link between ambient ozone and human discomfort is much stronger. As discussed earlier, ozone has been linked to athletic and automobile driving performance. Furthermore, numerous studies have associated increased ozone levels with eye irritation, cough, chest discomfort, and fatigue (Goldsmith & Friberg, 1977; National Academy of Sciences, 1977).

Two important limitations of toxicology studies on ozone are their use of single air pollution constituents and short-term exposures. Ambient exposures to pollutants occur over a longer period of time and include ozone as well as other gases and particulates. Although epidemiological studies have greater generalizability than toxicology research, their use of static, correlational designs and aggregate levels of analysis generally precludes causal analysis at the individual level.

Some biochemical research on adaptation to toxic pollutants has examined tolerance in animals. Tolerance is measured by preexposing animals to low levels of toxic substances for some fixed time period. Subsequently, these animals are exposed to larger doses of the toxin that normally would be debilitating or lethal. If tolerance to the toxin has developed, preexposed animals will better withstand exposure to large toxic dosages than will control animals, not preexposed to low levels of the toxic (Coffin & Stokinger, 1977; Frager, Phalen, & Kenoyer, 1979; National Academy of Sciences, 1977).

Preexposure of rodents to low levels of ozone allows them to subsequently tolerate ozone levels that would normally be lethal (Coffin & Stokinger, 1977; National Academy of Sciences, 1977). More recent work suggests that preexposure to approximate ambient ozone levels induces attentuated biochemical responses and diminishes effects on the respiratory tract mucociliary clearance system (Frager et al., 1979) that are normally associated with ozone exposure. Very recently, environmental toxicologists have examined biochemical, adaptation responses in human beings.

Hackney and colleagues in an important series of laboratory studies have begun to examine whether human biochemical and pulmonary responses adapt to ozone. In one study, six hypersensitive volunteers were exposed to ozone in a control chamber 2 hours per day for 4 successive days. Five of the subjects evidenced less reactivity in pulmonary function on the last day than on the previous 3 (Hackney, Linn, Mohler, & Collier, 1977). In a second study, six long-term residents of Los Angeles were compared with nine recent arrivals to Los Angeles ($\leq$ 5 days) in a controlled laboratory chamber during the high smog season. The new arrivals had significantly greater pulmonary function reactivity but similar biochemical reactivity to ozone (Hackney, Linn, Buckley, & Hislop, 1976). In a third study, Hackney and associates compared the relative reactivity of four Los Angeles residents and four Northern Canadians to ozone, again in a laboratory chamber. The Canadians experienced more respiratory discomfort and had larger decrements in pulmonary function in comparison to their performance in filtered air. Unlike the previous study, greater biochemical reactivity was found for the new arrivals' erythrocyte fragility and serum Vitamin E levels (Hackney, Linn, Karuza, Buckley, Law, Bates, Hazucha, Pengelly, & Silverman, 1977). Therefore, there is mixed evidence for biochemical adaptation to ozone in human beings, but consistent reports of pulmonary adaptation.

We hypothesized that long-term Los Angeles residents would biochemically adapt to photochemical smog in comparison to new migrants to the area. The present study extended previous research on human adaptation to smog by providing a broader perspective on health. Firstly, we examined not only physiological reactivity to smog but self-report measures of health and personal evaluations of the effects of smog on individual health. Secondly, unlike previous experimental research on ozone, we examined the effects of ambient smog conditions on health.

Summarizing, we hypothesized that long-term residents of the Los Angeles air basin would differ in four aspects of their responses to photochemical smog from recent migrants to the basin who had lived in previously low-air pollution areas. We predicted that long-term residents in comparison to new migrants would: (1) Assess smog as less of a problem; (2) use a higher response criterion to determine if smog is present in a signal detection paradigm; (3) cope in a more palliative, less-instrumental manner with smog as a stressor, with recreational, behavior changes in response to smog mediated by locus of control; and (4) show reduced biochemical sensitivity to oxidant challenge.

METHOD

Subjects

Forty college students were randomly selected from a prospective pool of individuals signing up to participate in a study on migration behavior. Subjects were unaware that the research was on smog prior to the experimental session. All subjects were paid for their participation. In order to be a subject in the experiment, each person met the following criteria: (1) lived in the Los Angeles air basin either 5 years or more, or less than 3 weeks; (2) moved to the test site within the previous 3 weeks; (3) spent summer vacation in home areas; (4) had no previous history of respiratory, allergy, or cardiac problems and generally were in good overall health (determined by self-report); (5) did not smoke. In addition, recent migrants must have lived in previously low smog areas (e.g., New York, Denver, San Francisco were eliminated; Portland, Vancouver, Honolulu were acceptable). Note that all subjects had recently moved to the test site. Long-term residents had previously lived in smoggy conditions; new migrants had previously lived in low-air pollution conditions.

The two groups, long-term residents and recent migrants, did not differ in age, gender, family income, parental occupation, or average number of hours spent outside during the week prior to the study. One older subject (greater than 55 years) was dropped from the long-term sample to equate the two groups on age and income. The exclusion of this subject had no effect on the results reported here. The response rate for the new migrants was 88% and 86% for long-term residents.

Dependent Measures

Problem Assessment.   Individual's assessment of the extent of the smog problem in their community was measured in three ways. Firstly, prior to any other data collection, participants rank ordered the five most negative aspects of living in their community. Secondly, individuals estimated the amount of smog in their community on a 1–100 absolute-magnitude estimation scale. Test–retest reliability over a 5-day interval revealed acceptable stability for the smog estimation procedure on a different group of individuals, $r = .78$. Finally, participants rated their current respiratory health on a standardized respiratory-symptoms checklist (Hackney, Linn, Buckley, Pederson, Karuza, Law, & Fischer, 1975). Subjects rated 10 symptoms (chest tightness, wheezing, shortness of breath, etc.), ranging from one indicating no symptoms to 40 indicating the symptom was incapacitating.

Signal Detection.   Participants viewed several slides of two different, unfamiliar Southern California scenes. One of the scenes depicted a small valley with foothills in the background, whereas the second was of a city skyline. Subjects were informed that one half the slides from each scene were clear and one half contained some smog. Their task was to judge whether or not smog was present in each picture. Each slide was shown for 20 seconds, 10 feet directly in front of the subject. Subjects were shown three different smog slides for each scene plus the clear slide. Each slide was presented six times; thus, subjects saw 18 smog slides and 18 clear slides for each of the two visual scenes. The order of slides was randomized across subjects.

The clear slide and low-smog slide were constructed as follows. For each of the two scenes, the identical view was photographed using a mounted tripod with fixed stops. A series of shots were taken at various times of the day over a 5-week period. The clearest day for each set was determined both by physical composition of the air and the visual quality of the slide. Low-smog slides with similar cloud coverage and sun angle were picked using a just noticeable difference procedure (Baird & Noma, 1978). Simultaneous slide comparisons were made by three observers. The three slides in each set that were closest to the clear slide were used as the low-smog slides.

Hit rate, false-alarm rate, *d* prime, and beta were calculated on the basis of group totals for new migrants and long-term residents, respectively. Statistical analyses used slides within each scene as the unit of analysis. Thus, the two scenes were analyzed separately in order to achieve a replicated data set. More information on signal detection analysis can be found in Baird and Noma (1978).

Coping.   Participants were questioned about palliative and instrumental coping. One measure of palliative coping included a comparison of subject's actual knowledge about smog to their perceived level of knowledge. Prior to actual knowledge assessment, the subjects were asked to rate their knowledge of smog on a five-point scale. Each participant was also asked to define three terms related to smog—ozone, smog alert, and inversion layer that were scored as; 0 = incorrect, .5 = partially correct, 1.0 = correct. Coping was measured by the difference between each person's actual and perceived knowledge in standardized units. Construct validity of the knowledge test was measured by comparing the scores of environmental scientists (graduate students in ecology), $M = 2.75$ to scores of graduate students in the social sciences ($M = 1.85$), $t(19) = 4.50$, $p < .01$. Secondly, palliative coping was measured by subject's ratings of the relative effects of smog on themselves in comparison to other healthy young adults in their community. The scale ranged from 1 = smog has a much greater negative effect on me than others to 7 = smog has a much less-negative effect on me than others (test–retest reliability, $r = .82$).

Three modes of instrumental coping were also assessed including information seeking, beliefs about taking direct action to reduce smog, and behavioral changes to alleviate smog effects on health. Information seeking was measured by self-reports of how often in the last 2 weeks individuals had sought information about smog from friends, relatives, media sources, the library, etc. As a second measure of instrumental coping, participants rated how much using mass transportation/car pooling would reduce the smog problem in Southern California (reliability for test–retest, $r = .90$). The scale ranged from 1 = smog will be greatly reduced to 5 = smog will not be reduced at all.

Finally, as a measure of behavior change to ameliorate the health effects of smog, each participant was asked to rate how much smog affected his/her participation in outdoor and indoor activity. Each response was scaled according to how much outdoor activity was curtailed (1) to increased (5). Separate probes were conducted for vigorous outdoor activities (e.g., sports) and for moderate outdoor activities (e.g., walking). Participating in indoor activity was also rated. The mean of the three scales was used as a behavioral adjustment measure. Cronbach's alpha for the three activity scales was .54.

Locus of control that was used in conjunction with the behavioral adjustment scale was determined by a median split on Rotter's scale (Rotter, Chance, & Phares, 1972). Furthermore, in accordance with Rotter's discussion of the proper assessment of locus of control (Rotter, 1975), measures of specific expectancy, the reinforcement value of the behavior, and the psychological situation were included as controls (covariates). Specific expectancy was measured by the individual's rating of the utility of curtailing physical activity to reduce the effects of smog on health. Reinforcement value was determined by assessing the value of physical health to each person. The psychological situation was measured by counting the number of available behavioral options, other than reducing outdoor physical activity; subjects said they had to reduce the effects of smog on their health.

Biochemical. Biochemical analyses were conducted by an independent laboratory. These assays as discussed previously measure the reactivity of the blood to oxidant challenge. Red blood cell fragility was measured by colormetric evaluation of hemoglobin release following osmotic infusion in a buffered saline solution (Williams, Beutler, Erslev, & Rundles, 1972). Red blood cell acetylcholinesterase activity was determined by an electrometric method (Michel, 1957). Serum Vitamin E levels were measured by a fluorimetric technique (O'Brian, Ibbott, & Rogerson, 1968).

Procedure

All testing occurred under ambient conditions in a high-smog area southeast of Los Angeles, California, during the second and third weeks of September, Wednesday through Saturday, between 2:00 and 5:00 PM. Air-quality conditions were moderately severe but typical for that time period and location (South Coast Air Quality Management District, 1978).

Upon arrival at the testing site, subjects went indoors and completed the open-ended question about problems in their community. Subjects then filled out a brief sociodemographic questionnaire and the locus of control scale. This was followed by the signal detection task. Of the total 40 subjects, 20 then had biochemical testing and filled out questionnaire items on health effects and attitudes toward smog. Twenty other subjects filled out the same questionnaires but did not undergo biochemical testing. This was done because of biochemical testing costs. Subjects who had biochemical testing (10 recent arrivals, 10 long-term residents) went outside for a 45-minute time period after the signal detection task. During the 45-minute period they rode exercise bicycles at 250–300 ergs for 15 minutes, rested for 15 minutes, and then rode again for 15 minutes. During the 15-minute break the respiratory-symptoms checklist was completed by each subject. Immediately after the exercise period, .7 oz. of blood was drawn from the nondominant arm by a nurse while the subject rested indoors. The biochemical subjects returned the next day to complete the questionnaire items on health effects and attitudes toward smog. The 20 subjects who did not have biochemical testing completed the health-symptoms checklist immediately after the perception task and then completed the questionnaire items on health effects and attitudes about smog.

RESULTS

As a partial check on the independent variable (extent of previous exposure to smog), subjects rated the amount of smog in the area where they had lived before moving to the test site, where 1 = the area in the U. S. with the least smog, and 100 = the area with the most smog. New migrants to the Los Angeles basin rated their previous home area significantly lower in smog ($M = 13$) than did the

TABLE 9.1
Signal Detection Results

Scene One				
	HIT RATE	FALSE ALARM	d'	
Longterm	.88	.18	2.171	.709[1]
New Migrants	.97	.24	2.751	.211
Scene Two				
Longterm	.89	.21	2.052	.637[2]
New Migrants	.95	.31	2.340	.276

[1] $t(4) = 2.42$, $p < .05$.
[2] $t(4) = 2.67$, $p < .05$.

long-term residents ($M = 69$), $t(37) = 8.38$, $P < .001$.[1] In order to examine the potential effects of the physiological testing procedures on the problem assessment and coping data, a 2×2 factorial analysis of variance was conducted (long/short-term resident—physiological/no physiological testing). There were no main effects of physiological testing status or significant interactions or residential status and physiological testing group. Thus, we report overall long-term—new migrant differences.

Problem Assessment

Long-term residents in comparison to new migrants judged that smog was less of a problem in their community. In an open-ended question, new arrivals ranked smog 1.4 on the average and long-term residents, 1.9, $U(19, 20) = 78$, $p < .05$. New arrivals also spontaneously mentioned smog more frequently than long-term residents, $\chi^2 = 4.26$, $p < .03$. Furthermore, on a scale where 1 = area in the U. S. with the least smog and 100 = the area with the most smog, recent arrivals estimated the amount of smog in their community as 84, and long-term residents placed it at 64, $t(37) = 2.91$, $p < .003$. Finally, recent migrants to Southern California had significantly greater respiratory symptoms ($M = 83$) than long-term residents did ($M = 69$), $t(36) = 2.86$, $p < .005$.

Signal Detection

The signal detection results are shown in Table 9.1. As predicted, long-term residents used a higher response criterion (beta) to report smog in the slides. Inspection of Table 9.1 reveals that this difference in beta was replicated for both sets of visual scenes, whereas d prime remained stable for the two groups. Thus, both groups of participants were equally sensitive in detecting the presence of

---

[1]All significance tests are one tailed. Degrees of freedom vary because of missing data.

smog. The significant beta differences indicate, however, that for low levels of smog, long-term residents in comparison to new migrants are less likely to report that smog is present.

Coping

Palliative modes of coping were found more frequently in long-term residents. Long-term residents have more actual knowledge about smog ($M = 1.29$) than recent arrivals ($M = .95$), $t(37) = 1.72$, $p < .05$. Of particular interest here is the difference between standardized scores of perceived knowledge and actual knowledge that varied considerably for the two groups of subjects, $M = .49$ for long-term residents, $M = -.17$ for recent arrivals, $t(37) = 1.98$, $p < .05$. The difference between *standardized* scores rather than *raw* scores is used because the two groups differ in their actual knowledge scores. New migrants knew little about smog and correctly assessed their low level of knowledge. Conversely, long-term residents exaggerated their levels of perceived knowledge in comparison to their actual knowledge. As another indication of palliative coping, the long-term residents felt that smog had a less-negative effect on them than other healthy young adults ($M = 4.7$), whereas the new arrivals felt that smog had a more negative effect on them than others ($M = 3.6$), $t(37) = 2.57$, $p < .01$.

Three measures of instrumental coping were also assessed. As a measure of information seeking, participants were asked how many times in the past 2 weeks they had actively sought information about smog. New migrants sought out information significantly more, 4.9 times, than long-term residents, 1.3 times, $t(37) = 2.43$, $p < .01$. As a second index of instrumental coping, participants rated how much using mass transportation/car pooling would reduce smog in Southern California. Recent arrivals felt that using mass transit/car pooling would reduce smog more, $M = 1.7$ than long-term residents did, $M = 2.2$, $t(37) = 1.62$, $p < .05$.

As a third measure of instrumental coping, individuals were asked how much smog affected their participation in indoor and outdoor activities. As inspection of Table 9.2 indicates, our hypothesis that locus of control would interact with residential status was supported, $F (1,21) = 3.99$, $p < .05$ with more internal, new migrants most likely to engage in more preventative behaviors in the pres-

TABLE 9.2
Behavior Changes in Response to Smog

	Longterm	New Migrant
Internal	2.78	1.42
External	2.67	2.47

The lower the total, the more preventive behaviors taken to reduce negative impacts of smog.

TABLE 9.3
Biochemical Assay

	Red Blood Cell Fragility	Vitamin E	Acetylcholinesterase
Longterm	.567%	1.14% mg	.655 Delta p^H Units
New Migrants	.556%	1.03% mg	.620 Delta p^H Units
	t^*_{12} <1.0	t_{17} <1.0	t_{18} <1.0

*Degrees of freedom vary because of missing data due to laboratory accidents.

ence of smog. There were no main effects for locus of control or experience with smog.

Biochemical

The results of the biochemical assays are shown in Table 9.3. As is readily apparent, there were not significant differences for any of these measures between long-term residents and recent residents of the Los Angeles air basin. Further, all these values fall within normal limits.

DISCUSSION

Most of our results are consistent with the adaptation hypothesis. Long-term residents of the Los Angeles air basin, in comparison to new migrants, are generally less sensitive to photochemical smog. Converging evidence from three sets of measures supports this conclusion. The major exception to this conclusion is the biochemical data.

Firstly, long-term residents mention smog less frequently than new migrants do when asked to rank order community problems. Long-term residents also rank smog lower among community problems and have fewer respiratory symptoms than new migrants do.

Secondly, the signal detection results reveal a shift in response criteria for judging the presence of smog in a visual scene. Long-term residents have significantly higher betas than the new arrivals for two different visual scenes; yet, there are no differences between the two residential groups in d prime. Thus, both groups are equally sensitive in detecting the presence of smog, but the long-term residents employ a systematically greater response criteria to affirm that smog is present; that is, for low levels of smog, long-term residents of the Los Angeles air basin are less likely to say that smog is present than are new migrants to the air basin. This finding is due to differences in response bias, because both groups are equally accurate in visually detecting low levels of smog. The direction of the difference in response bias is consistent with our adaptation hypothesis.

Thirdly, the coping data suggest that new arrivals are more likely to employ instrumental modes of coping with smog. New migrants are more likely to seek out information about smog and favor the use of mass transportation as a partial remedy for smog. Furthermore, a significant locus of control by residential status interaction indicates that new arrivals who are internal are more likely to make preventative changes in their behavior when smog is present. Internal, new migrants to the Los Angeles air basin are most likely to restrict outdoor activities and spend more time indoors when smog conditions are prevalent.

The significant interactive effects of locus of control and previous residential history with air pollution on outdoor behaviors is consistent with a previous study by Trigg and her colleagues on locus of control and anti-pollution activities (Trigg, Perlman, Perry, & Janisse, 1976). They found that locus of control affected political activism toward water pollution. Internally oriented individuals who were also optimistic about future levels of pollution engaged in more political, anti-pollution activities than did externally oriented persons. Interestingly, there was no effect on locus of control among pessimistic respondents. This interaction of locus on control with optimism about future pollution levels is similar to one explanation of our adaptation findings.

Conceivably one reason why individuals with greater exposure to air pollution become less reactive to poor air quality is because they feel over time more pessimistic and helpless to do anything about the problem. As you may recall, we found that long-term residents of the Los Angeles air basin in comparison to new migrants to the basin were more pessimistic about the utility of mass transportation as an effective means of air pollution control. It is possible that optimism about future pollution conditions changes as a function of one's perceived ability to impact environmental quality. We suspect that attributions of self-efficacy with respect to air quality probably diminish with continuous exposure to ambient environmental pollutants.

In contrast to the instrumental behaviors of new migrants, long-term residents engage in more palliative coping. Long-term residents exaggerate their perceived knowledge of smog and feel they are more immune to the effects of smog relative to other healthy young adults. New arrivals accurately assess their own knowledge of smog and rate themselves as more negatively affected by smog in comparison to other healthy young adults.

The biochemical data are equivocal in terms of our adaptation hypothesis. As discussed earlier, the effects of ozone exposure on oxidant reactions in human blood are not definitive. Whereas some studies show effects on erythrocyte fragility, others find no effects (Hackney et al., 1978). Similarly, the ability of humans to biochemically adapt to oxidant challenge is also questionable at this time. Hackney and colleagues, for example, noted shifts in biochemical sensitivity to ozone in adapted persons in the Los Angeles area in one study (Hackney et al., 1977) but did not replicate these data in other studies (Hackney et al., 1976, 1978).

Two important differences in our experimental procedures and Hackney's work on biochemical adaptation to photochemical oxidants are noteworthy. Firstly, we used a between-subjects design, comparing the levels of two groups. Hackney and colleagues compared base line data in filtered, clean air and then analyzed difference scores between pure air and air with specified ozone levels. Because there are large individual differences in the biochemical indices, a between-subjects design is much less statistically powerful than a within-subjects design.

The second important difference is our use of ambient photochemical smog exposure. Previous researchers have used filtered air with controlled ozone exposure under air-chamber conditions. Ambient smog contains ozone plus other pollutants. Furthermore, the time course of actual, daily individual exposure to ozone is more gradual than in chamber studies, where the toxic is either absent or presented immediately at full dose. Under natural conditions, human exposure to pollutants builds up gradually over the day, reaching a peak in our geographic location between 12 and 3 PM. In conclusion, our biochemical data add to the largely equivocal set of findings on human biochemical adaptation to photochemical oxidants.

The pattern of behavioral results supports the adaptation-level perspective on attitudes toward environmental pollution offered by Wohlwill. Furthermore, the coping data fit into Lazarus' analysis of coping with stressors; that is, one means of adapting to a chronic environmental stressor such as air pollution is to adopt more palliative coping mechanisms. Further research is needed to examine this process more closely. For example, does palliative coping result from unsuccessful instrumental coping strategies that are initiated upon early contacts with a stressor?

Because our experiment does not conform to a true experimental design, some caution is necessary in evaluating our findings. Because our subjects are not randomly assigned to conditions, the possibility of self-selection arises. As reported previously, however, both groups had comparable socioeconomic status, age, gender, and previous health status. Nevertheless, some selection issues are inevitable in a field study such as this one.

For example, it is conceivable that the most smog-sensitive persons move out of the Los Angeles area as soon as possible, thus biasing the remaining population available for sampling. We can offer some preliminary arguments against this interpretation. Firstly, because our sample was college students, it is less likely that they could freely choose to leave or stay in the Los Angeles area relative to their parent's decisions to do so. Related to this argument are data from our second study presented later, suggesting adaptation in grade school children who have even less control over where they live. Secondly, we interviewed a sample of 50 Los Angeles adults planning to move out of the area.

None of them cited smog or poor air quality as a major reason for their move; nearly all persons were moving for economic reasons. Realistically, most adults and especially young adults and children do not have that much flexibility in choosing where to live.

A second problem related to the basic design of our study is the effects of moving per se. Whereas all our subjects had moved to the test site within the previous 3 weeks, the new migrants had moved from farther distances (mainly the Pacific Northwest and parts of Northern California); the long-term residents had all moved to the test site from within the Los Angeles air basin (i.e., within a 50-mile radius of Los Angeles). Therefore, the amount of previous exposure to smog (our independent variable) is confounded with extent of moving. Because moving is a stressful experience, it is possible that given the greater distances the new migrants had to move, they were suffering greater stress in general and thus were more susceptible to smog as well as a multitude of other environmental sources of discomfort. The best solution to this potential confound would be to include a third comparison group in our experimental design of new migrants to the Los Angeles area from previously high smog areas. Nevertheless, it is unlikely that this potential confounding can explain our findings. Firstly, subjects were given the opportunity to mention various community problems in an initial, open-ended question. The only factor that differed between the long-term and new-migrants groups was mention of smog. Secondly, it seems highly unlikely that so many of our specific probes about health and smog could be altered by a general level of greater discomfort engendered from moving a greater distance.

Probably the best analytic solution to the design issues inherent in this field study would be a longitudinal design that included new migrants to high and low smog areas crossed with previous residences in high and low smog areas. If the problems of retesting sensitivity could be solved, the longitudinal design would allow for a more fine-grained analysis of the time course of adaptation using a within-subjects design. This design would also control for the effects of moving per se and would also allow us to examine the adaptation process in the opposite direction. Namely, what happens when an individual moves from a highly polluted setting to a clear one?

Whereas the cautions we have raised about our design are appropriate, we feel that the converging evidence justifies support for our adaptation hypothesis. Furthermore, our study illustrates the usefulness of the stress construct in studying environmental pollution. In addition, our experimental design, though imperfect, represents an important adjunct to the more traditional epidemiological and toxicological paradigms prevalent in research on air pollution. This is the first study to examine individual, human reactions to air pollution with a broad array of health indices. Furthermore, from a broader theoretical perspective, our data reiterate the critical role of psychological factors in the human-environment interface. Individuals with differential experience with air pollution react in predictably different ways to current air-quality levels.

In addition to the use of a more sophisticated, longitudinal design in future research, we also wanted to examine the ontogeny of human attitudes toward air pollution within the adaptation framework developed here. Do children also adapt to air pollution, and if so at what age does this pattern emerge? The purpose of our second study was to examine developmental trends in human, behavioral adaptation to air pollution.

STUDY II: CHILDREN'S RESPONSES TO AIR POLLUTION

Current air-quality standards are based on adverse health effects of air pollutants upon healthy adults, not children who are more sensitive to air pollutant than adults are. One reason children are especially sensitive to air pollution is because their lungs are developing. Some immature pulmonary tissue contain cells that are more reactive to various atmospheric pollutants. Children also have a much greater air-exchange volume per unit body weight and have a higher respiratory rate than adults do. In addition, children are generally more physically active outside than adults are and thus have greater penetration of pollutants into lower air cavities (Kane, 1976; State of California Air Resources Board, 1977).

The focus of our study on children and air pollution is on psychological aspects of their responses. In examining the existing literature on children's behavior and air pollution, one is immediately struck by the absence of data on the topic. We have been able to locate only four studies related to children and air pollution.

Bartnik and Wall (1975) asked kindergartners through eighth graders of Harlan County, Kentucky to write essays and draw pictures about coal mining in their community. Until the sixth grade, there was no mention of environmental problems, but 57% of the older children mentioned environmental issues including destruction of plant life, water pollution, and air pollution. Nearly two thirds of the children mentioned safety problems that seemed to be their major concern about the mines.

When children are directly probed about environmental problems, most of them are concerned (approximately 65% say they are concerned), and levels of concern rise with age (Holloway, 1972; Horvat & Voelker, 1976; Miller, 1975). Of particular interest here, Horvat and Voelker found that fifth and eighth graders in southern Wisconsin respond that air pollution is the most serious of environmental problems (40%), followed by water pollution (20%).

Researchers have also measured children's knowledge and attitudes about pollution and its control. Out of a possible score of 50, fourth through sixth graders averaged about 30 on a pollution knowledge test (Holloway, 1972). Reliability was adequate, but insufficient validity data were provided. Holloway also probed where children learn about pollution, finding that most children learn about pollution from their teachers or television. Teachers reported, in this same study, that they discussed environmental issues, ranging from 1 to 4 weeks, during the school year. Miller (1975) also asked children from second through eighth grade about the causes of pollution. Most children felt that air pollution is caused by people littering, factory smoke, and smoke from cars and trucks. With increasing age, more sophisticated answers followed attributing pollution to human choices. Horvat and Voelker (1976) also found that older children are more likely to recognize the central role of human behavior in environmental problems.

Summarizing, existing research on children's behavior and pollution has been limited to survey research on children's opinions about environmental problems. Children are concerned about pollution if directly probed but up until sixth grade or so indicate little spontaneous awareness of pollution problems. Younger children mention the visual aspects of pollutants in responding to questions about causes of air pollution. Around junior high age, children begin to attribute pollution to human use of automobiles and other technology.

Similar to most of the survey research on adults and air pollution, research on children's attitudes about environmental problems is largely atheoretical and methodologically unsophisticated, without comparison groups, with limited statistical analyses and with little psychometric data. The purpose of our study was to take a preliminary look at young children's attitudes about, and reactions to, smog within the stress and adaptation perspective we developed in the adult study. We viewed this children's study as preliminary and largely descriptive in nature. Our basic goals were to see what children thought about smog and to determine if any similar adaptation processes were occurring.

METHOD

Subjects

Seventy-seven children in grades three through six were randomly selected from a prospective pool of children whose parents completed permission slips for a study on air pollution. Both the parents and their children knew the research topic was on smog but were not aware of the adaptation issue. In order to be a participant in our study, each child met the following criteria: (1) lived in the Los Angeles air basin either 3 years or more, or less than 5 weeks; (2) moved to the test site within the previous 5 weeks; (3) spent summer vacation in home areas; (4) had no previous history of respiratory problems, allergy, or cardiac problems and generally were in good health (all information determined by parental report and/or school records). In addition, recent migrants must have lived in previously low smog areas. Note that all children had recently moved to the test site. Long-term residents had previously lived in smoggy conditions; new migrants had previously lived in low-air pollution conditions.

The two groups of children, long-term residents and new migrants, did not differ in gender, socioeconomic status, or race. The long-term residents groups consisted of 16 third graders, 12 fourth graders, 12 fifth graders, and 11 sixth graders for a total of 51 children. The new-migrants group included 7 third graders, 5 fourth graders, 8 fifth graders, and 6 sixth graders for a total of 26 children. The new-migrants group is smaller because the pool of eligible children for the category was more limited. The response rate for the new migrants was 82%, and 79% of long-term residents.

Dependent Measures

Problem Assessment.   Children's assessment of the extent of the smog problem was measured in four ways. Firstly, prior to any other data collection, children listed and then ranked problems in their town. Then, children were directly asked if they had ever heard of smog and what it meant to them (i.e., to define it). Finally, children rated their respiratory health for the previous week. A standardized respiratory-health checklist (Hackney et al., 1975) was modified to enhance children's comprehension. Children answered questions about symptoms (e.g., 'during the past week, that is since _____ has your throat hurt, if yes—how bad was it, was it very bad, bad, hardly noticeable?').

Coping.   Children were asked several questions about their responses to smog. Questions measured either palliative or instrumental forms of coping. Firstly, children were asked to compare the effects of smog on themselves to the health of other same-aged children in their neighborhood. They were asked if smog affected them more, about the same, or less than others. If the child responded more or less, they were then asked if it effected them a lot more (less) or a little more (less). The scale was scored from 1 = a lot less to 5 = a lot more. Children were also asked how long they believed smog had existed in their neighborhood (1 = 1 month to 5 = greater than 5 years), and how important they thought the automobile was as a cause of smog.

More active forms of coping were also measured. Children were asked if they felt they had any control over smog (Do you feel you can do anything about the amount of smog in your neighborhood?), and whether they thought adults in their community could do anything about smog there (1 = a lot of control to 3 = no control). Children were also asked what they thought people could do to reduce smog in their community. They chose from a list of six alternatives including: don't know, smoke less, drive cars less, use less electricity, litter less, and stop making campfires. Finally, children were asked to what extent their indoor behavior was affected by smog (1 = no to 3 = yes, spend a lot more time indoors).

Procedure

All testing occurred under ambient conditions in a high smog area southeast of Los Angeles, California, during the second and third weeks of September, Tuesday through Friday, between 11:00 AM and 2:00 PM. Air-quality conditions were comparable to those reported by the South Coast Quality Management District (1978). Children were interviewed individually inside their school. Children from five elementary schools were interviewed for a period approximately 15 minutes per interview.

After introducing him/herself, the interviewer (college undergraduates) explained that the purpose of the interview was to find out what the child thought about his/her community. We emphasized the anonymity of their responses (no names were recorded) and the fact that there were no wrong or right answers to any questions; what we cared about was their opinions. Children were encouraged to ask questions at all times. As each question was read, the children followed along on their own copy of the questionnaire. All responses were coded by the interviewer.

All children answered the questions in the same order. After the initial open-ended probe about community problems, children's respiratory-health symptoms for the previous week were coded. Then children were asked several questions about their attitudes and responses to smog. After getting the child's description of what smog was, we defined smog as the type of air pollution that existed in their community. All children were asked if they know what we meant by smog and to describe it if any uncertainty was apparent. None of the children interviewed appeared to have any difficulty understanding what was meant.

The interview schedule went through several stages of development. Two child psychologists reviewed a draft for readability and comprehension for children as young as 7. A second draft was then pretested with a group of third and fourth graders in another community. The pretesting included followup questions for each interview item, asking the child if he/she understood the question and to restate it in his/her own words. Only questions that all children readily comprehended were included in the final instrument. Test–retest reliability on the various items was established over a 3-day period for another group of children. Scores ranged from .52 for perceived adult control over smog to .79 for the respiratory-health checklist.

RESULTS

There were no grade differences in any of the results nor significant grade by residential-length status interactions with the exception of a couple of grade main effects that are noted in the following.

Problem Assessment

In sharp contrast to the adult findings in our earlier study, hardly any of the children spontaneously mentioned smog as a problem in their neighborhood, with only one long-term resident and one new migrant listing smog. However, when directly asked if they had ever heard of smog, all children but one said yes. Fifty percent of the long-term residents and 88% of the new migrants described smog in terms of its physical characteristics (e.g., some comment about visibility), $\chi_3^2 = 8.25$, $p < .05$, with remaining responses scattered evenly among health effects (e.g., makes me cough), causes of air pollution (e.g., pollution from cars), and "don't know" responses. There was a significant grade effect on this question with more sixth graders defining smog in causal terms. Finally, there was no difference between long-term residents, $M = 23.34$ and new migrants, $M = 22.71$, on respiratory symptoms, $t(75) = 1.0$.

Coping

Several measures suggest greater palliative coping in the long-term residents. There was no difference in children's ratings of the effects of smog on their health relative to other children, $M = 3.02$ long-term residents, $M = 2.92$ new migrants, $t(75) < 1.0$. New migrants judged that smog had existed in their neighborhood for a significantly longer period of time, $M = 3.69$ than long-term residents did, $M = 2.71$, $t(75) = 1.95$, $p < .05$. The two groups also differed in the role of the automobile as a cause of smog. New migrants were more likely to attribute smog to cars 50% more than long-term residents were, 19% with other responses evenly distributed among factories, fires, heat, and don't know, $\chi_4^2 = 9.86$, $p < .05$.

Some differences in instrumental coping were also apparent between the two groups of children. There was no difference in children's perceptions of their own control over the amount of smog in their neighborhood that were uniformly low, $M = 2.45$ long-term residents, $M = 2.42$, new migrants, $t(75) < 1.0$, but new migrants did feel that adults could do more to reduce smog, $M = 1.76$ than long-term residents felt they could, $M = 2.12$, $t(75) = 1.89$, $p < .05$. When asked what people could do to reduce smog, new migrants chose reduce car driving most frequently (60%), compared to 25% or long-term residents. Interestingly, long-term residents most frequently chose "don't know" (58%), compared to 18% of the new migrants $\chi_5^2 = 15.29$, $p < .05$. Sixth graders were also more likely to choose cars as the preferred method and less likely to state don't know than younger children. There was no difference in the amount of time spent indoors during smog periods between the two groups, $M = 2.37$ long-term residents, $M = 2.39$ new migrants, $t(75) < 1.0$.

DISCUSSION

The children's data are more equivocal on the adaptation question than the adult findings are. Whereas the adult data indicate solid support in favor of an adaptation hypothesis, the children's data are only suggestive. Children as a group are considerably less aware of smog as a community problem than adults are. Few children spontaneously mentioned smog when asked to list problems in their neighborhoods. When directly probed about smog, however, nearly all children had heard of it and could define it. These findings are consistent with previous research on children's attitudes about smog as reviewed earlier. Generally, children are less aware of environmental pollution than adults are unless directly probed about it, in which case comparable levels of adult and child concern emerge.

Only when asked to define smog did any differences in problem assessment emerge between the new-migrant children and the long-term-resident children. A larger proportion of new migrants defined smog in terms of its physical characteristics, principally visual. This finding may relate to the signal detection findings in the adult study. Children less familiar with smog may respond differently to visual cues of smog, as was found in the adult study. As you may recall, we found that long-term adult residents of areas with smog were much less likely to report the presence of smog in low-level smog scenes. Conceivably, the finding that most long-term children do not define smog in terms of its visual characteristics may reflect a similar response bias. Whereas this interpretation is clearly speculative, the data are potentially important and worthy of future study. We did not use a signal detection task in the child interview because of time limitations placed on the interview by the schools involved. Our final measurement of problem assessment, respiratory-health symptoms, revealed no differences in respiratory complaints between the two groups of long-term and new-migrant resident children. The absolute levels of symptoms reveal, however, that both groups are experiencing respiratory difficulties.

It is difficult to draw any definitive conclusions from this set of findings on children's assessment of smog as a problem. The data do not provide as much evidence in favor of the adaptation hypothesis as was found in the adult study. Children may not adapt as readily to air pollution as adults can, at least in terms of problem assessment. The absence of any apparent adaptation effects in respiratory-health symptoms may reflect a ceiling effect, because both groups of children are bothered by the poor air quality present at the time of testing. This finding is consistent with the research discussed earlier that has shown that children's health is more severely affected by air pollution than adults is (Kane, 1976; State of California Air Resources Board, 1978).

Alternatively, our interview may not have been understood by the children and/or been sensitive enough to detect subtle differences between the two groups.

It is unlikely that the instrument was not understood by the children given the thorough pretesting we conducted, but this alternative is difficult to rule out in self-reported measures with young children. The other option of insensitive response formats is more likely, because many of our scales from the adult study were reduced from five- and seven-point alternatives to three-point scales. The respiratory-health checklist used with the adults, for example, has six alternatives for each symptom, whereas the child's version has three.

Findings on children's responses to smog are also less clear than the adult data, although some trends suggest, as in the adult data, greater palliative coping in the long-term-resident children and more instrumental coping among the new-migrant children. Both groups judged that smog affected their own health about the same as it affected other children. This finding markedly contrasts with the adult data, where long-term residents judged that smog had a more negative effect on others and new migrants felt the opposite. On the other hand, new migrants in comparison to long-term children estimated that smog had been present in the area for a much longer time period. New-migrant children also place more blame on cars as a cause of smog. Long-term children seem less aware of the causes of photochemical smog and less cognizant of how long it has been present. The latter findings are particularly interesting, because long-term residents have lived with smog for at least 3 years, yet children newly exposed to smog say it has been present for a longer period of time. Both groups underestimate how long smog has been present in their community.

Whereas both groups of children felt little personal control over the amount of smog in their community, new migrants felt that adults in their community could do more about it than the long-term children felt adults could. New-migrant children also felt that people could reduce smog by driving less, whereas long-term-resident children did not know how smog could be reduced. Both of these findings may suggest new migrant's greater belief in more active modes of coping with smog. They feel adults can do something about controlling smog, and that driving cars less will help reduce smog. Children of long-term residents do not know what will reduce smog and are relatively pessimistic about adult's controlling it.

Both groups of children changed their patterns of indoor play as a function of high ambient smog levels, which is encouraging because health advisories in Southern California recommend reduced, outdoor physical activity during peak smog periods. The lack of any long-term—new-migrant differences may reflect children's general inability to control their play activities. California law, for example, mandates restricted outdoor play in elementary schools during high smog periods.

Summarizing, there are some indications of different coping styles between the two groups of children with slightly more active coping on the part of the new migrants and more palliative coping among the long-term residents. New migrants may also be more reactive to the visual characteristics of smog. Support for both of these conclusions is not strong, and more research on children's attitudes and responses to air pollution is necessary.

CONCLUSIONS

Our review and discussion of behavioral research on air pollution has hopefully demonstrated that environmental problems are not the exclusive province of biology and medicine. Human behavior plays a central role in the condition of our physical surroundings, and the effects of nonoptimal environmental conditions include both physical and psychological health outcomes. Human beings can apparently accomodate considerable change and disruption in their environments that may be facilitated by psychological adaptation to pollution. Important research issues are raised on how humans adapt to pollution, and what the costs and benefits of adaptation are for human health and well being.

ACKNOWLEDGMENTS

Preparation of this chapter was supported by The Southern California Edison Company, Contracts No. B-2058902, J-1909902, and the Focused Research Program on Stress, University of California, Irvine. We thank Andrew Baum, Edward Faeder, Jack Hackney, Richard Lazarus, Sally Shumaker, and Daniel Stokols for critical comments on earlier drafts, and Jeff Abramowitz, William Banks, Lauren Nowels, Martha Moreno and Anna Marie Schmidt for assistance running the studies reported.

REFERENCES

Baird, J. C., & Noma, E. *Fundamentals of scaling and psychophysics.* New York: Wiley, 1978.

Barker, M. Planning for environmental indices: Observer appraisals of air quality. In K. Craik & E. Zube (Eds.), *Perceiving environmental quality.* New York: Plenum, 1976.

Bartnik, G., & Wall, G. Children's perceptions of environmental problems. *Proceedings of the Association of American Geographers,* 1975, *7*, 36–39.

Bell, P. Physiological, comfort, performance and social effects of heat stress. *Journal of Social Issues,* 1981, *37*, 71–94.

Bleda, P., & Bleda, S. Effects of sex and smoking on reactions to spatial invasion at a shopping mall. *Journal of Social Psychology,* 1978, *104*, 311–312.

Chapko, M., & Solomon, H. Air pollution and recreational behavior. *Journal of Social Psychology,* 1976, *100*, 149–150.

Coffin, D., & Stokinger, H. Biological effects of air pollutants. In A. C. Stern (Ed.), *Air pollution* (3rd ed., Vol. III). New York: Academic Press, 1977.

Creer, R., Gray, R., & Treshow, M. Differential responses to air pollution as an environmental health problem. *Journal of the Air Pollution Control Association,* 1970, *20*, 814–818.

Crowe, J. Towards a 'definitional model' of public perceptions of air pollution. *Journal of the Air Pollution Control Association,* 1968, *18,* 154–158.

Cunningham, M. Weather, mood and helping behavior: Quasi-experiments with the sunshine samaritan. *Journal of Personality and Social Psychology,* 1979, *37,* 1947–1956.

De Groot, I. Trends in public attitudes toward air pollution. *Journal of the Air Pollution Control Association,* 1967, *17,* 679–681.

Dubos, R. *Man adapting.* New Haven, Conn.: Yale University Press, 1965.

Dunlap, R., van Liere, K., & Dillman, D. Evidence of decline in public concern with environmental quality: A reply. *Rural Sociology,* 1979, *44,* 204–212.

Evans, G. W., & Howard, R. B. Personal space. *Psychological Bulletin,* 1973, *80,* 334–344.

Evans, G. W., & Jacobs, S. Air pollution and human behavior. *Journal of Social Issues,* 1981, *37,* 95–125.

Flachsbart, P., & Phillips, S. An index and model of human responses to air quality. *Journal of the Air Pollution Control Association,* 1980, *30,* 759–768.

Frager, N. B., Phalen, R., & Kenoyer, J. Adaptation to ozone in reference to mucociliary clearance. *Archives of Environmental Health,* 1979, *34,* 51–57.

Glass, D., & Singer, J. *Urban stress.* New York: Academic Press, 1972.

Gold, D. Public concern and beliefs about air pollution in California: A statewide survey. *Project Clean Air, Research Project S-11,* University of California, September 1970.

Goldsmith, J., & Friberg, L. Effects of air pollution on human health. In A. C. Stern (Ed.), *Air pollution* (3rd ed., Vol. III). New York: Academic Press, 1977.

Greenberger, K. This is an article about Paluicon and how to stop it. *Phi Delta Kappan,* October 1971, 14.

Hackney, J., Linn, W., Buckley, R., Collier, C., & Mohler, J. Respiratory and biochemical adaptations in men repeatedly exposed to ozone. In L. Folinsbee, J. Wagner, J. Burga, B. Drinkwater, J. Gliner, & J. Bedi (Eds.), *Environmental stress.* New York: Academic Press, 1978.

Hackney, J., Linn, W., Buckley, R., & Hislop, H. Studies in adaptation to ambient oxidant air pollution: Effects of ozone exposure in Los Angeles residents versus new arrivals. *Environmental Health Perspectives,* 1976, *18,* 141–149.

Hackney, F., Linn, W., Buckley, R., Pederson, E., Karuza, S., Law, D., & Fischer, D. Experimental studies on human health effects of air pollutants. *Archives of Environmental Health,* 1975, *30,* 373–378.

Hackney, J., Linn, W., Karuza, S., Buckley, R., Law, D., Bates, D., Hazucha, M., Pengelly, L., & Silverman, F. Effects of ozone exposure in Canadians and Southern Californians. *Archives of Environmental Health,* 1977, *32,* 110–116.

Hackney, J., Linn, W., Mohler, J., Collier, C. Adaptation to short-term respiratory effects of ozone in men exposed repeatedly. *Journal of Applied Physiology,* 1977, *43,* 82–89.

Helson, H. *Adaptation level theory.* New York: Harper & Row, 1964.

Hohm, C. A human ecological approach to the reality and perception of air pollution. *Pacific Sociological Review,* 1976, *19,* 21–44.

Holloway, M. Cognitive and affective orientations of elementary school children toward air, water, and soil pollution. *Dissertation Abstracts International,* 1972, *32,* 6836-A (University Microfilms No. 72-17, 107).

Horvat, R., & Voelker, A. Using a Likert scale to measure "Environmental Responsibility." *The Journal of Environmental Education,* 1976, *8,* 36–47.

Janis, I. Adaptive personality changes. In A. Monat & R. Lazarus (Eds.), *Stress and coping.* New York: Columbia, 1977.

Jones, J. Adverse emotional reactions of nonsmokers to secondary cigarette smoke. *Environmental Psychology and Nonverbal Behavior,* 1978, *3,* 125–127.

Jones, J., & Bogat, G. Air pollution and human aggression. *Psychological Reports,* 1978, *43,* 721–722.

Kane, D. N. Bad air for children. *Environment*, 1976, *18*, 26-34.

Kirkby, A. Perception of air pollution and individual adjustments in Edinburgh, Exeter and Sheffield. In I. Burton (Ed.), *Selected social aspects of air pollution in the United Kingdom*. International Geographical Union Commission on Man and Environment, Calgary, Canada, July 1972.

Lazarus, R. *Psychological stress and the coping process*. New York: McGraw-Hill, 1966.

Lazarus, R., & Cohen, J. Environmental stress. In J. Wohlwill & I. Altman (Eds.), *Human behavior and environment*. New York: Plenum, 1977.

Lazarus, R., & Launier, R. Stress-related transactions between person and environment. In L. Pervin & M. Lewis (Eds.), *Perspectives in interactional psychology*. New York: Plenum, 1978.

Lipsey, M. W. Attitudes toward the environment and pollution. In S. Oskamp (Ed.), *Attitudes and opinions*. Englewood Cliffs, N. J.: Prentice-Hall, 1976.

Medalia, N. Air pollution as a socioenvironmental health problem: A survey report. *Journal of Health and Human Behavior*, 1964, *5*, 154-165.

Michel, H. Cholinesterase in human red blood cells and plasma. *Standard Methods of Clinical Chemistry, III*. New York: McGraw-Hill, 1957.

Miller, J. The development of preadult attitudes toward environmental conservation and pollution. *School Science and Mathematics*, 1975, *8*, 729-737.

National Academy of Sciences, *Ozone and other photochemical oxidants*. Medical and Biological Effects of Environmental Pollutants. Washington, D. C., 1977.

O'Brien, O., Ibbott, F., & Rogerson, D. *Laboratory manual of pediatric micro-biochemical techniques* (4th ed.). New York: Harper & Row, 1968.

Peterson, R. L. *Air pollution and attendance in recreation behavior settings in the Los Angeles basin*. Chicago: American Psychological Association, 1975.

Rankin, R. Air pollution control and public apathy. *Journal of the Air Pollution Control Association*, 1969, *19*, 565-569.

Rivlin, L. Personal communication. In R. Baron, D. Byrne, & W. Griffitt, *Social psychology*. Boston: Allyn & Bacon, 1974.

Rotter, J. Some problems and misconceptions related to the construct of internal versus external control of reinforcement. *Journal of Consulting and Clinical Psychology*, 1975, *43*, 56-67.

Rotter, J., Chance, J., & Phares, E. *Applications of a social learning theory of personality*. New York: Holt, Rinehart, & Winston, 1972.

Rotton, J., Yoshikawa, J., Francis, J., & Hoyler, R. *Urban atmosphere: Evaluative effects of malodorous air pollution*. Atlanta, Ga.: Southeastern Psychological Association, 1978.

Rotton, J., Yoshikawa, J., & Kaplan, F. *Perceived control, malodorous air pollution and behavioral aftereffects*. New Orleans: Southeastern Psychological Association, 1979.

Rotton, R., Barry, T., Frey, J., & Soler, E. Air pollution and interpersonal attraction. *Journal of Applied Social Psychology*, 1978, *8*, 57-71.

Rotton, R., Frey, J., Barry, T., Milligan, M., & Fitzpatrick, M. The air pollution experience and physical aggression. *Journal of Applied Social Psychology*, 1979, *9*, 397-412.

Sherrod, D. Crowding, perceived control and behavioral aftereffects. *Journal of Applied Social Psychology*, 1974, *4*, 171-186.

Stone, J., Breidenbach, S., & Heimstra, N. Annoyance response of nonsmokers to cigarette smoke. *Perceptual and Motor Skills*, 1979, *49*, 907-916.

South Coast Quality Management District. Vol XXIII (9), September, 1978, El Monte, California, 91731. Ozone ranged from a one-hourly maximum of .34-.17 ppm during the study; NO_2 from .37-.17 ppm, SO_2 from .05-.03 ppm, and CO from 12-7 ppm.

State of California Air Resources Board. Air pollution health effects on children. Staff Report 77-20-1, September 23, 1977.

Strahilevitz, M., Strahilevitz, A., & Miller, J. Air pollution and the admission rate of psychiatric patients. *American Journal of Psychiatry*, 1979, *136*, 205-207.

Trigg, L., Perlman, D., Perry, R., & Janisse, M. Anti-pollution behavior: A function of perceived outcome and locus of control. *Environment and Behavior*, 1976, *8*, 307–314.

Ury, H. Photochemical air pollution and automobile accidents in Los Angeles. An investigation of oxidant and accidents, 1963 and 1965. *Archives of Environmental Health*, 1968, *17*, 334–342.

Wall, G. Public response to air pollution in Sheffield, England. *International Journal of Environmental Studies*, 1974, *5*, 259–270.

Wayne, W., Wehrle, P., & Carroll, R. Oxidant air pollution and athletic performance. *Journal of American Medical Association*, 1967, *199*, 901–904.

Williams, W., Beutler, E., Erslev, A., & Rundles, R. *Hematology*. New York: McGraw-Hill, 1972.

Wohlwill, J. F. Human response to levels of environmental stimulation. *Human Ecology*, 1974, *2*, 127–247.

Wohlwill, F., & Kohn, I. The environment as experienced by the migrant: An adaptation level view. *Representative Research in Social Psychology*, 1973, *4*, 135–164.

Wohlwill, J. F., & Kohn, I. Dimensionalizing the environmental manifold. In S. Wapner, S. Cohen, & B. Kaplan (Eds.), *Experiencing the environment*. New York: Plenum, 1976.

10 The Relationship Between Crowding and Health

Verne C. Cox, Paul B. Paulus, Garvin McCain
University of Texas at Arlington

Marylie Karlovac
Southern Methodist University

It has long been known that crowding promotes transmission of infectious agents. However, only recently has it become evident that there is significant psychological stress associated with crowding that can contribute to the increased incidence of *both* contagious and noncontagious illnesses. We evaluate the evidence for this relationship by reviewing pertinent animal and human studies and discussing at length our research during the last decade on the health-related consequences of prison crowding. We conclude by considering the theoretical and practical implications of these findings.

CONCEPTUAL AND METHODOLOGICAL CONSIDERATIONS

The investigation of the effects of crowding has produced a bewildering array of often conflicting conclusions. The fact that the research involves many disciplines including psychologists, sociologists, biologists, and epidemiologists has no doubt slowed the emergence of consensus. There have been wide-ranging differences regarding definitions, choice of dependent variables, statistical techniques, sample selection, and crowding measures (Baldassare, 1979; Gove, Hughes, & Galle, 1979; Sengel, 1978).

A positive outcome of earlier confusion has been an increased emphasis on differentiating between physical density and the experience of crowding as well as greater precision in defining dimensions of crowding (Rapoport, 1975; Stokols, 1972). For example, the distinction between spatial density (space per person) and social density (number of people in a unit area) has proved important

(Baum & Koman, 1976; Paulus, McCain, & Cox, 1973), as has that between internal and external density (Stokols, 1976; Zlutnick & Altman, 1972). Internal density refers to the density characteristics of the primary living environment (e.g., apartment or room), whereas external density refers to the density characteristics of other environments outside of this one (e.g., the neighborhood, hallway, or institution).

We believe that the term crowding should be reserved for those levels of density that are *aversive*. Thus, we conceptualize crowding as involving one or more of the following variables: *aversive* amount of space per person in dwellings (proximal spatial crowding) or in more extensive surrounds such as neighborhoods (distal spatial crowding), and *aversive* levels of social interaction in dwellings (proximal social crowding) or in more extensive surrounds (distal social crowding). Undoubtedly, there are other determinants of the psychological experience of crowding in addition to the preceding factors, as well as individual differences in responses directed toward attenuation of the crowding experience. Ideally, we would like to describe the relative contribution of all these factors to variations in physical and mental health. This task is complicated by the fact that social and spatial factors are usually inextricably confounded in nonlaboratory environs. Nevertheless, there are a number of studies that we review that have examined occasional independent variations among these components.

CROWDING AND HEALTH: A STRESS PERSPECTIVE

Crowding As A Stressor

The contention that crowding can have a negative impact on health rests in part on direct evidence, but also on the assumption that crowding induces psychological stress. This assumption is evident in the common use of crowding in animal studies as a convenient stressor in investigating the relationship between health and psychological stress (Cassel, 1974; Rogers, Dubey, & Reich, 1979). Both animal and human studies provide plentiful evidence that crowding induces psychological stress, as expressed in autonomic nervous-system sympathetic activity and elevations in adrenocortical hormones. For example, crowding has been shown to elevate blood-pressure levels in mice (Henry, Meehan, & Stephens, 1967), as well as adrenocortical hormones (Christian, 1968) and adrenal medullary hormones (Welch, 1964). Furthermore, D'Atri (1975) and Paulus, McCain, & Cox (1978) have reported elevated blood pressure in some crowded prison housing, and Gruchow (1974) has found adrenal medullary activity to be elevated in individuals living in crowding households. Even relatively short-term crowding may have a stressful impact on humans. For example, Singer, Lundberg, and Frankenhaeuser (1978) found elevated catecholamine levels for commuters traveling by train under crowded conditions.

Mediating Factors.   Why would crowding be a source of stress? Some explanatory concepts that have appeared in the literature are stimulus overload, interference, and negative social interactions. Although there is some imprecision in these terms, they have proved to have heuristic value. Having to deal with too many others in a crowded setting increases the level of stimulation and may result in stimulus overload (Milgram, 1970; Saegert, 1978). Relative to rural settings, social interference is also more likely in crowded urban settings where one is more likely to bump into others, have to wait in lines, confront traffic jams, wait for elevators, be distracted by noises, and experience reduced privacy. Crowding may also increase the number of negative social interactions because one may be more likely to encounter social situations that are dangerous, unpredictable, uncomfortable, or otherwise undesirable in crowded environments than uncrowded ones (Paulus, 1980).

Moderating Factors.   There are a number of factors that may determine the extent to which these variables will result in stress (Lazarus & Cohen, 1977). These factors include the nature of the social stimuli, personal characteristics, and physical features of the environment. For example, positively valued social stimuli such as friends, familiar people, and cooperation have been shown to reduce the negative impact of crowding (Baum & Valins, 1977; Seta, Paulus, & Schkade, 1976). Individuals who have a sense of control over their environment or a high need for social stimulation should be less vulnerable to the potential negative effects of crowding (Duke & Nowicki, 1972; Sales, Guydosh, & Iacono, 1974). Physical features of the environment such as partitions, barriers, and queuing devices that regulate social behavior should reduce the experience of crowding (Baum & Davis, 1980; Stokols, Smith, & Proster, 1975; Wicker & Kirmeyer, 1977).

Crowding, Stress, and Health

There is abundant evidence indicating that psychological stressors are associated with illness (Gunderson & Rahe, 1974; Henry, Meehan, & Stephens, 1977; Rogers et al., 1979; Weiner, 1977). The effects of crowding on the adrenocortical system are particularly pertinent to this problem. Elevated adrenocortical activity is associated with suppression of immune systems and no doubt accounts in part for poor health associated with psychological stress, including crowding-induced stress (cf. reviews by Christian, 1968; Rogers et al., 1979). Not only does a suppression of immune systems result in susceptibility to contagious disease, but it may also encourage susceptibility to microorganisms already being harbored by the body. Microorganisms involved in disease ordinarily exist everywhere in the environment, including the body, and disease may manifest itself when the balance between these microorganisms within the body and host is disturbed (Dubos, 1965). It is possible that as a stressor crowding may play a role in disturbing this balance and leading to physical pathology. Thus, crowding may have a double impact on health because it makes the individual vulnerable due to stress as well as providing opportunities for the transmission of illness.

Interpreting Illness Complaints

A common measure of health status in crowding research is the illness complaint. Undoubtedly, the relationship between health and illness complaints is complex. As Mechanic and his coworkers have indicated, illness complaints can reflect psychological factors as well as actual alterations in physical health (Mechanic, 1976; Tessler & Mechanic, 1978). For example, exposure to stress may increase one's sensitivity to internal states and in this way increase the likelihood of detection of physical symptoms (Mechanic, 1980; Pennebaker, Burnam, Schaeffer, & Harper, 1977). Illness complaints may in some instances simply be one manifestation of general irritability. Some illness-complaint behavior may even be viewed as an attempt to cope behaviorally with a stressful environment. For example, visiting a clinic may involve an attempt to assert control, escape one's environment, or obtain desired drugs.

From these various perspectives it can be seen that the meaning of a reported symptom may be difficult to ascertain, especially if it is not objectively verifiable (e.g., back pain, nausea, headaches). Even if one considers only verifiable symptoms, a higher complaint rate by one group could mean either increased physical pathology or merely increased sensitivity.

ANIMAL RESEARCH

The relationship between crowding and health has been examined in numerous animal experiments. Unfortunately, most pertinent animal studies have not systematically examined variations in levels of components of crowding in relation to health because their principle objective was investigation of relationship of stress and health. Some of these animal studies have demonstrated crowding-induced cardiomyopathy (Weber & Van Der Walt, 1973), parasite retention (Brayton & Brain, 1974), fetal malformations (Hamburgh, Mendoza, Rader, Lang, Silverstein, & Hoffman, 1974), and susceptibility to infection (Plaut & Grota, 1971).

A few animal studies of crowding and health have systematically varied crowding variables. For example, Myers, Hale, Mykytowycz, and Hughes (1971) examined variation in group size with space per rabbit constant and variation in space per rabbit with group size constant. These investigators found that variation in space per animal and total living area did have a negative impact on health status. In another study, Brayton and Brain (1974) reported that parasite retention increased as crowding of mice increased from single housing to groups of two, four, and six with cage size constant. Edwards and Dean (1977) examined mice in groups of 2, 10, 30, and 60. Differences in antibody response were evident when they compared the two smallest groups with the two largest groups. The failure to find differences among all four groups suggests substantial changes in group size may have been necessary for their subjects to display measurable changes in health status. One should exercise caution in drawing conclusions from animal studies of crowding. For example, Brain and Benton (1979) have noted that many studies assume that single housing is less stressful than group housing; yet the species typically used in such studies live in groups in their natural environs. It may well be that some group sizes actually represent less stress than single housing. Brain and Benton lament the lack of systematic variations in a wide number of pertinent variables such as sex, strain, prior housing history, and duration of exposure to housing. We would add age and degree and type of social organization as other factors that have received insufficient attention. In summary, most animal studies support the contention that crowding has a negative impact on health. However, it should be noted that in a recent provocative article based on animal findings Freedman (1979) has argued that crowding has no deleterious effects. Freedman's arguments rested on a narrow definition of crowding that involved only space per animal.

HUMAN RESEARCH

Many studies of the effects of crowding on human health have been nonexperimental field studies of individuals or statistical analyses of aggregate data from demographic units such as census tracts. We first discuss studies employing aggregate data.

Aggregate Data

A number of studies of urban crowding have demonstrated a statistically reliable relationship between some measures of crowding and mortality independent of socioeconomic variables (Galle, Gove, & McPherson, 1972; Levy & Herzog, 1974; Manton & Myers, 1977). For example, Galle et al. (1972) compared a number of measures of both proximal and distal crowding with mortality rates, mental hospital admissions, delinquency, public assistance, and fertility. These measures of crowding were persons per room, rooms per housing unit, housing units per structure, residential structures per acre, and persons per acre. All measures except persons per acre correlated significantly with the measures of pathology independent of socioeconomic variables. Levy and Herzog (1974) analyzed the relationship of household (persons per room) and neighborhood crowding (persons per square kilometer) in the Netherlands to measures of pathology such as mortality and hospital admissions. Whereas they found no consistent relationship between household crowding and pathology, a finding they explained in terms of Dutch family structure, neighborhood crowding was found to be strongly related to both overall mortality and deaths due to heart disease for males. In a study involving urban districts in Hanover, Germany, Manton and Myers (1977) found a positive association between mortality and number of measures of crowding, including both spatial and social measures of household crowding and crowding external to the home (e.g., housing units per dwelling structure).

The three previous studies yielded different conclusions regarding which aspects of crowding are related to pathology. Galle et al. (1972) concluded that crowding within homes was related to poorer health. However, housing units per structure and structures per acre bore no significant relationship to health. Manton and Myers (1977) found a positive association between household crowding and mortality, as well as association of deaths and some crowding measures reflecting spatial and social variables outside homes. In contrast, Levy and Herzog (1974) concluded that persons per acre was significantly related to overall death rate and even more strongly related to male death rates. However, within-dwelling measures of crowding were not related to poor health.

These conflicting findings are not surprising because of the wide variety of potentially confounding factors, the number of different measures used, and the differing levels of actual crowding involved. One major problem with the aggregate-demographic approach is the fact that the measures employed such as persons per room and number of buildings per acre may only superficially tap the degree of crowding experienced. The arrangement of the space within and outside of a housing unit and the interaction patterns of the inhabitants may be important contributing factors. For example, a high degree of comradery among members of large families or densely populated neighborhoods may mitigate the potential effects of such dense conditions. Sengel (1978) has recently proposed a model that may account for the inconclusiveness of findings resulting from analyses that attempt to separate crowding from socioeconomic variables. Sengel maintains that a simple two-variable linear causal model is inappropriate for analysis of the consequences of crowding that depend on a complex interplay between crowding and socioeconomic and personal characteristics.

Several studies involving urban areas claim to have found no evidence of crowding-health relationship. Factor and Waldron (1973) examined a number of cities throughout the world and found no consistent positive relationships between crowding and mortality, morbidity, mental hospital admissions, or delinquency. In a study of over 200 American cities, Dye (1975) found only neighborhood crowding to be positively related to death rate. A methodologically stronger study by Freedman, Heshka, and Levy (1975) measured the effects of household and neighborhood crowding in New York City on a number of health-related measures including infant mortality, and psychiatric admissions and terminations. They found that many simple correlations existed between the pathologies and both measures of crowding, but crowding had little independent effect on pathology when income and ethnicity were controlled statistically.

In sum, the weight of the evidence supports a relationship between crowding and health. However, there are differing views regarding the relevant factors mediating crowding effects on health.

Individual Data

A second approach to the study of crowding and health involves individual subject characteristics as measured by questionnaires, interviews, physical examinations, and analysis of medical records. Extensive projects of this nature have been conducted in a number of settings, including urban areas (Booth, 1976; Booth & Cowell, 1976; Booth & Johnson, 1975; Duvall & Booth, 1978; Gove, Hughes, & Galle, 1979; Johnson & Booth, 1976), naval vessels (Dean, Pugh, & Gunderson, 1975, 1978), and prisons (Cox, Paulus, McCain, & Schkade, 1979; D'Atri, 1975; Karlovac, Paulus, Cox, & McCain, in prep; McCain, Cox, & Paulus, 1976, 1980a, b). A number of these studies have indicated that crowding in urban settings may be related to health problems.

In an extensive study of Toronto residents, Booth and his colleagues found that under some conditions crowded households were related to health problems (Booth & Cowell, 1976). They examined individual subjects, employing comprehensive physical examinations by a physician, as well as interviews and questionnaires related to health status, such as physiological indices of stress, stress-related diseases, infectious disease, and uterine dysfunction. Whereas Booth and his colleagues found crowding to be unrelated to such measures as pregnancy history (Johnson & Booth, 1976), childhood illness, height, and school performance (Booth & Johnson, 1975), household crowding was found to have a very modest, statistically reliable impact on other measures of health. Females seemed less vulnerable to crowding-induced health changes than did males in these studies; however, Szklo, Tonascia, & Gordis (1976) found myocardial infarctions to be related to household crowding for women with existing biologic risk factors for coronary disease. Gove et al. (1979) also found strong evidence for a relationship between crowding and health for Chicago residents. They interviewed residents of census tracts and found household crowding, as it was related to "felt demands" and lack of privacy, to affect self-assessments of both physical and mental health. Consistent with Booth and Johnson's (1975) findings for childhood health, Essen, Fogelman, and Head (1978) failed to find a relationship between childhood illness and household crowding. Giel and Ormel (1977) failed to find health-related consequences for household crowding for a sample of married respondents in the Netherlands.

Health-related consequences of crowding have also been found in a number of settings other than the urban environment. For example, Dean and his colleagues have studied the effects of crowding on naval vessels. Findings from two of their studies substantiate a relationship between perceived crowding, space per person, and illness rates (Dean et al., 1975, 1978). In addition, D'Atri (1975) found higher blood pressure in more socially crowded prison housing. Our own prison research, to be discussed later, also has demonstrated substantial relationships between crowding and measures of health. Whereas field studies employing individual data in some cases present conflicting findings, evidence for a relationship between crowding and illness is much more consistent in this body of research than in studies of aggregate data.

Crowding and Infectious Disease

Thus far, we have considered the role of crowding in inducing various physical pathologies, including illness and death. We have not yet specifically considered the potential role of crowding-induced stress in infectious disease. The most obvious role for crowding in contagious illness simply involves disease transmission, where crowding may increase opportunities for contact. Most research linking crowding and infectious illness has emphasized this role (Jacobson, Chester, & Fraser, 1977; Koopman, 1978; McGlashan, 1977; Monto, 1968; Naggan, Morag, Bar-Shany, Egoz, & Brachott, 1976; Sims, Downham, McQuillin, & Gardner, 1976). However, there is considerable evidence linking crowding in its role as a stressor to both infectious and noninfectious disease. As indicated earlier, microorganisms involved in disease are ubiquitous and found within the body as well as external environment, and stress-induced suppression of immune systems may promote infectious illness.

The relationship between crowding and infectious disease has been studied for a wide range of illnesses, including meningitis (Jacobson et al., 1977), streptococcis (Quinn, Lowry, & Van Der Zwaag, 1978), hepatitis (McGlashan, 1977), vomiting, colds, and diarrhea (Koopman, 1978), conjunctivitis (Arnow, Hierholzer, Higbee, & Harris, 1977), and respiratory illnesses (Cassel, 1973; Fanning, 1967; Sims, Downham, McQuillin, & Gardner, 1976; Stewart & Voors, 1968; Wyndham, Gonin, & Reid, 1978; Yarnell, 1979; Yodfat, Fidel, Cohen, & Eliakim, 1979). A number of these studies have found evidence for a correspondence between crowding and infectious illness (Arnow et al., 1977; Fanning, 1967; Jacobson et al., 1977; Koopman, 1978; McGlashan, 1977; Sims et al., 1976; Wyndham et al., 1978; Yarnell, 1979).

Respiratory diseases comprise one group of infectious illnesses that has received particular attention with regard to its association with crowding. A number of field studies have found a relationship between respiratory illnesses in children and crowding (Fanning, 1967; Sims et al., 1976; Yarnell, 1979). For example, Yarnell (1979) collected census data on respiratory illnesses for children admitted to hospitals in Wales. He did not find bronchitis or pneumonia to be related either to number of persons per hectare or to percentage of houses with more than one person per room. He did find that whooping cough correlated strongly with number of persons per hectare and slightly with percentage of houses with more than one person per room. Asthma, on the other hand, was negatively correlated with both measures.

Sims and his colleagues (1976) compared census records of population figures, information on housing, and social conditions with data from medical records of children during an epidemic of respiratory syncytial virus infections. They found significant correlations between the diseases and two of five measures of crowding percentage of the population with over one person per room or with over six persons per household. Fanning (1967) compared the health of mothers and children in houses and four apartment buildings. He found that the incidence of respiratory disease was twice as high for apartment-dwelling children. Wyndham et al. (1978) studied hospital records of the incidence of acute respiratory disease, pneumonia, and meningitis among miners housed in large hostels. Over a 4-year period there was a pattern linking monthly rates of illnesses with fluctuations both in temperature and in the number of miners being housed in the hostels. Whereas seasonal drops in air temperature were the most important determinants of increases in respiratory diseases and pneumonia, seasonal increases in the number of miners were also influential.

In a study of patterns of transmission of viral hepatitis in Tasmania, McGlashan (1977) found that, whereas the population at large averaged .79 persons per room, residences of those afflicted had an average of 1.43 persons per room. Similarly, Jacobson et al. (1977) studied a 1975 epidemic of neisseria meningitis in Alabama and found that those not afflicted averaged .80 persons per room in the households, whereas afflicted households averaged 1.16 persons per room.

Whereas considerable research suggests a link between crowding and infectious disease, some studies have failed to find such a relationship (Cassel, 1973). Stewart and Voors (1968) noted that, whereas the incidence of respiratory illness and sick calls tended to be higher during the first 4 weeks of basic military training, these rates followed a cyclical pattern independent of crowding conditions. Yodfat et al. (1979) found no evidence for a relationship between household crowding and chronic bronchitis and asthma in a rural community in Israel.

In sum, there is abundant evidence that crowded environments can have a significant impact on health. This contention finds support from both human and animal studies. Nevertheless, those studies have some limitations. The animal studies provide greater control of variables and allow for systematic variation in degree of crowding; however, generalizing from animals to humans is not without risk. Human studies are plagued by potentially confounded variables and limited range of crowded conditions. To circumvent some of these problems we have turned to studies of crowding in prison environments.

Prison Research Findings

The greater portion of our research has been done in prisons, although we have also conducted human and animal laboratory studies and worked in V.A. hospitals, offshore oil rigs, and public schools. In the course of research-site selection, we have visited, in a period of 9 years, 40 correctional institutions ranging from city jails to large maximum security prisons. Within individual institutions we found wide ranges of housing conditions. Variations of housing types within prisons ranged from 3 to 8. Housing included units with 1, 2, 3, 4, 5, 6, 12 inmates and dormitories ranging from 20 to 74 inmates. Space per person ranged from 19 to 108 square feet.

We chose U. S. Federal prisons as our primary research sites for a number of reasons including accessibility (Cox, Paulus, McCain, & Schkade, 1979). In the U. S., Federal Prison System records are well-organized and detailed and contain a wide variety of background information and test data. Medical care, diet, disciplinary procedures, and schedules are also largely uniform within these institutions. Voluntary inmate participation was high, and administrative cooperation was excellent. Housing conditions in prisons are relatively free of confounding with socioeconomic factors. Crowding in prisons can be intense, prolonged, and generally inescapable. Any negative effects of crowding should be evident in such an environment.

There are potential limitations regarding the generality of prison data. Firstly, crowding in prisons is usually much more severe than typically encountered in nonprison housing in the United States. Secondly, the vast majority of inmates are male. However, in our one limited opportunity to examine an institution with both men and women, we did not find any substantial sex differences in reactions to housing (McCain, Cox, & Paulus, 1980a). Thirdly, prison life is associated with many stressors such as restrictions of activities, a boring environment, regimentation, the absence of family, and the presence of potentially dangerous individuals. Fourthly, in comparison to the general population prisoners are quite homogenous with regard to age and urban and socioeconomic background. Finally, a large percentage of inmates have a history of adjustment problems related to limited education, alcohol and drug abuse, unemployment, and racial discrimination. Characteristics such as these should be cause for caution in extrapolation from prison to nonprison populations. However, the comparability of our findings with those obtained from college dormitory studies (Baron, Mandel, Adams, & Griffen, 1976; Baum & Valins, 1977) suggests that our prison results have substantial generality.

Our use of illness complaints as a dependent variable is related to other findings indicating that stress, including that induced by crowding, is associated with indices of poor health. We have recently examined the relationship between housing and illness complaints in six federal prisons with a wide range of housing arrangements, security levels, administrations, facilities, etc. (McCain et al., 1980a; McCain, Cox, & Paulus, 1980b). We have examined over 1500 individual medical records to assess the relationship between illness complaints and crowding. We are primarily concerned with the effects of amount of sleeping unit space, number of inmates in a sleeping unit, and various design features on illness-complaint behavior. In each institution we recorded individual illness complaints during the period (up to 6 months) the inmate was in the housing quarters in which he or she resided on the days of our data collection visits. We recorded by date and nature of complaint all volitional visits to a medical facility except those associated with serious injury, emergency-illness conditions, and physician-scheduled visits such as x-rays, prescription renewals, and work-related physicals. The complaint dates allowed us to relate the complaints to both housing condition and length of time in that housing. The nature of the complaint allowed us to consider different subsets of the data. In some analyses we excluded colds and flu. In other analyses we examined contagious and noncontagious illnesses separately. All these measures have yielded very similar results.

During the first 6 weeks following the transfer to new housing, illness complaints were high and less related to crowding variables as compared to later time intervals. Consequently, many of our analyses focused on the period of time after the initial 6 weeks in a particular housing condition. Our analyses of illness-complaint data included examining the potential contribution of variables such as age, length of stay in current housing, and racial or ethnic identification.

The results of our prison studies have been quite consistent, both within and across institutions (McCain et al., 1980a,b). The findings from the Atlanta Penitentiary are typical of our results regarding illness-complaint rates. We examined one-man cells with 54 square feet and larger cells with 177 square feet that contained three to six inmates. As may be seen in Figure 10.1, there was an orderly increase in illness-complaint rates as number men per cell increases. It is interesting that in spite of the advantage in space per person, the three man cells had higher illness complaint rates than the one man cells.

Figures 10.2 to 10.6 illustrate some housing quarters at another institution (Texarkana Federal Correctional Institution). Housing consisted of single cells (54 sq. ft. per person), large single cells (66 sq. ft. per person), double cells (27 sq. ft. per person), large open dormitories (34–45 sq. ft. per person), and two more spacious dormitories providing from 42 to 51 sq. ft. per person. The two spacious dormitories consisted of three open bays each containing from 10 to 20 occupants.

Figure 10.7 illustrates the findings for the five types of housing. As can be seen, the dormitory housing yielded higher illness-complaint rates than single or double occupant housing. Furthermore, the spacious dormitories had 35% lower illness-complaint rates than open dormitories.

We have found that some architectural arrangements can reduce illness complaint behavior. In two prisons, we found that providing inmates with cubicles consisting of partitions greatly reduced the negative reactions to crowding and illness-complaint behavior. In a third prison, perception of crowding was reduced by cubicles but illness complaints were not.

Analyses both within and across institutions have indicated that amount of space is not as important a predictor of illness-complaint rate as number of residents. It seems reasonable to assume that space does play some role at least at extreme values. A principal problem has been finding situations where number of

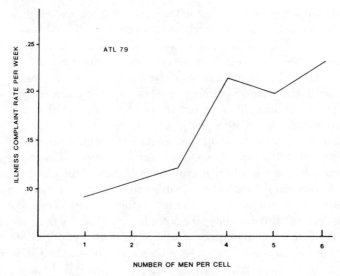

FIG. 10.1.   Illness-complaint rates at Atlanta Penitentiary plotted by number of inmates per cell.

occupants is held constant, but space per person varies. We suspect space does play a role in crowding effects, but the nature and dimension of that role remains to be established.

As discussed earlier, illness-complaint behavior cannot be viewed exclusively as a reflection of physical health status. Our illness-complaint data were obtained from official medical records and probably reflect physical health status to a greater degree than illness measures based solely on self-assessment. Regardless of the interpretation of illness-complaint behavior, this variable can have a significant impact on health services and is clearly related to variations in crowding in prison housing quarters.

We have also examined archival data in two different state prison systems regarding population levels and natural deaths, suicides, and psychiatric commitment rates (McCain et al., 1980a, b; Paulus et al., 1978). Both systems had experienced increases in population levels that were not accompanied by commensurate increases in housing facilities. Consequently, inmates experienced simultaneous intensification of spatial and social crowding. Our analyses indicated that increases in inmate population without concomitant increases in housing facilities produces a number of very undesirable effects, including a disproportionate increase in suicide rates and death rates of inmates over 50.

In our analyses we also examined the health-related effects of institutional size. Large prisons (1500 plus inmates) yielded more undesirable effects than small prisons (less than 1100 inmates), as indicated by higher psychiatric commitment rates, death rates, and suicide rates. Suicide rates for large institutions were approximately 10 times that of small institutions. Thus, in addition to space

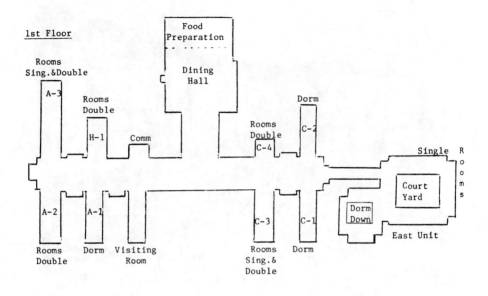

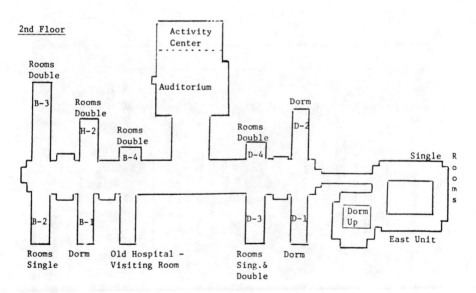

FIG. 10.2. Floor plan for Texarkana FCI. Note the bays in the East Unit spacious dormitories.

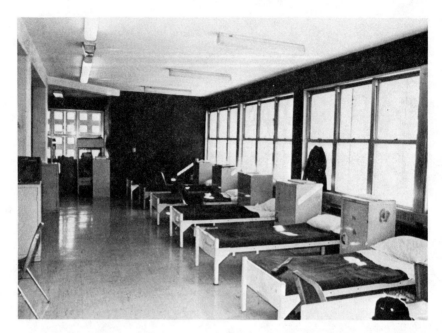

FIG. 10.3.   A bay in the East Unit (spacious) dormitory.

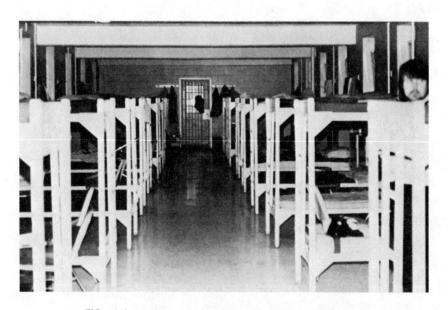

FIG. 10.4.   A large open dormitory with double decked bunks.

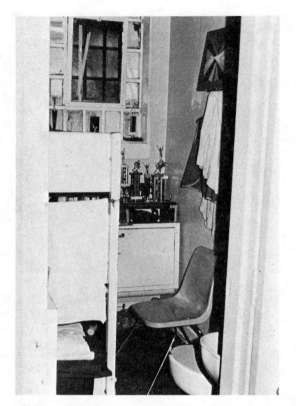

FIG. 10.5. A typical double cell.

per person and number of occupants in housing quarters, sheer population size of the institution is important.

Archival data can be difficult to interpret because of the potential contribution of confounded variables. Whereas we were able to examine the influence of age and race, we did not have information on other variables that might be important. Nevertheless, it seems plausible to attribute at least part of the differences in nonviolent death, suicide, and psychiatric commitment rates to intensification of one or more components of crowding.

We examined the effects of crowding on blood pressure (McCain et al., 1980a; Paulus et al., 1978), as have other investigators (Booth & Cowell, 1976; D'Atri, 1975). Blood pressure findings have been used in these studies primarily as an index of stress but also have implications for health. Some investigators believe that stress-induced elevations in blood pressure may lead to chronic hypertension in some individuals (Henry & Stephens, 1977). Whereas we found no reliable relationship between housing and blood pressure in six federal prisons (McCain et al., 1980a), we did find a significant relationship in an intensely

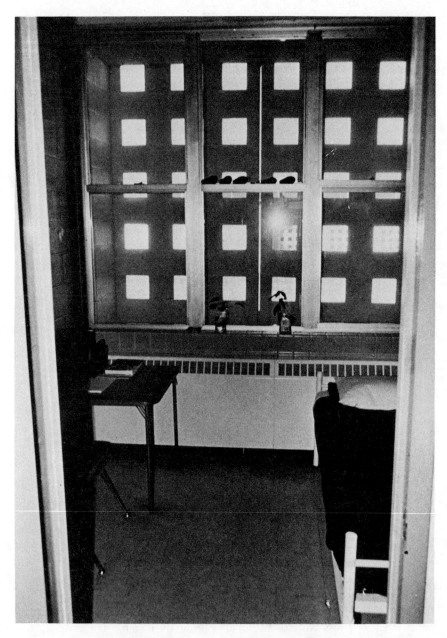

FIG. 10.6. A large (66 sq. ft.) single cell in East Unit.

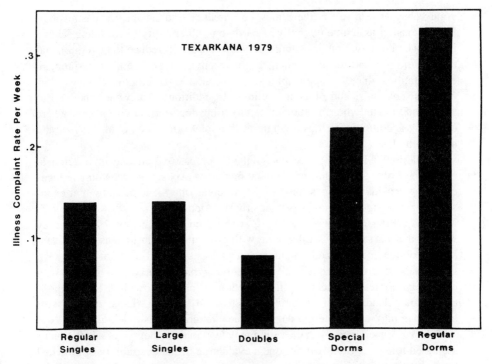

FIG. 10.7. Illness-complaint rates at Texarkana FCI plotted by types of housing.

crowded state prison (Paulus et al., 1978). We found significantly lower systolic pressure in two-man cells providing 29 square feet per occupant than in either three- or six-man cells providing 19 square feet per person. D'Atri (1975) had also found lower blood pressure in single rooms as compared to dormitories, even though the dormitories provided more space per person. Thus, stress induced by crowding under some circumstances may be reflected in heightened blood pressure and may have negative consequences for health.

THEORETICAL AND PRACTICAL IMPLICATIONS

We would expect individuals who cope with other stressors effectively would typically cope effectively with crowding as well. However, there may be unique biological and experiential factors that would enhance or diminish vulnerability to stress induced by crowding. The existence of individual differences in reactivity to crowding would have important implications for the organization and management of various work and institutional environments. For example, in prisons, assignment to less-crowded housing is typically based on seniority and good behavior. However, there may be unrealized advantages in basing individual housing assignment wholly or partly on vulnerability to crowding. Housing assignment based on crowding tolerance could well reduce the overall negative reactions to stress obtained in a prison environment. Similar assignment considerations may be applicable to work situations, schools, college dormitories, hospitals, and other institutions. In addition, it may be beneficial to select individuals who are tolerant of crowding for work environments where crowding is common such as offshore drilling platforms (Cox et al., 1979), and space vehicles.

Of particular interest is the potential role of past experience in reaction to crowding. Some studies have found that increased exposure to crowding reduces crowding sensitivity (Sundstrom, 1978), whereas other studies show that exposure to crowding increases one's sensitivity (Aiello, Epstein, & Karlin, 1975; McCarthy & Saegert, 1979; Paulus, Cox, McCain, & Chandler, 1975). It may well be that past unsuccessful coping with crowding would increase one's sensitivity or fear of crowded conditions. Thus, one should avoid housing such individuals in crowded housing. On the other hand, successful coping with crowding may reduce one's negative reaction or fear of crowding. Such experience should lead to more tolerance of crowded housing. Thus, type of past experience may determine the degree of adaptation or sensitization.

Whereas experiences with crowding may lead to some degree of adaptation or increased tolerance of crowding, one's evaluation of the desirability of crowded conditions may remain quite low. For example, someone who has lived under very crowded conditions may be better able to tolerate and cope with crowded living conditions in other environments such as camps, prisons, and college dormitories. However, such an individual may also place great value on living under uncrowded or private conditions because of past negative experiences. Thus, one might find such people showing low evidence of behavioral or physiological stress in crowded environments but negative evaluations of these environments.

The preceding possibilities suggest the need for assessment of actual tolerance of crowding. We have worked with three assessment devices. One involved the placement of model figures in a model room until it appeared crowded (Desor, 1972). This test has not proved useful. A second one consisted of drawings of various degrees of dormitory crowding. A third task involved having inmates choose between a series of two representations of housing arrangements that varied in number of bunks and amount of space per bunk. This task was designed to determine the degree to which people were averse to social density and spatial density. Although we have not had the opportunity to relate the results of these latter two tasks to our various stress-related measures, they may provide some basis for the development of an effective and valid crowding-tolerance measure.

Coping strategies may also be important in determining the magnitude of negative health consequences due to crowding. Coping can occur at many levels—behavioral, psychological, physiological, and environmental (Altman, 1975; Lazarus, 1966; Selye, 1956). Lazarus (1966) has focused on various psychological techniques such as reappraisal or avoidance. Altman (1975) has highlighted the use of various psychological, behavioral, and cultural coping mechanisms in response to social stressors. Coping responses are designed to ameliorate the negative impact of the stressor. For example, by becoming psychologically reserved and avoiding social encounters one can potentially minimize the impact of a crowded environment. Individual differences in the impact of crowding may provide clues regarding effective coping strategies.

Unfortunately, at present, there are no clear criteria for differentiation of coping responses from other behaviors. No clear rules are provided for discerning whether a particular behavior is a coping response, nor is it possible to easily predict which particular coping response or series of responses will be employed in a given situation. Little is known about the effectiveness of various coping strategies (see Matthews, 1979, for a detailed review of these issues).

In our studies we looked at one potential coping strategy, reduced social interaction. We obtained information from the inmates about their social behavior and involvement in prison activities. In only one prison did we find evidence for reduced social behavior (talking) in more crowded environs. Control of social contact is probably chosen infrequently in prisons because it is not a very effective technique. For example, Baum and Valins (1977) found that social withdrawal was not an effective technique in dealing with crowding in college dormitories.

One problem with social avoidance is that it does not change one's negative perception of a crowded environment. More effective strategies may include psychological strategies that change one's perception of the environment and behavioral-environmental strategies that actually change the negative nature of the environment. In a recent study by Matthews (1979), students were induced to take behavioral-avoidance or cognitive-reappraisal strategies in response to a crowded laboratory setting. He found that upon initial exposure to crowding, behavioral avoidance was more effective than reappraisal, whereas reappraisal was more effective during a second exposure. So even within a short time period, different strategies varied in efficacy at different periods of time. The Matthews study suggests the possibility that training people to reevaluate the perceived negative characteristics of their housing environment may be one effective way to reduce stress in a crowded environment. Similarly, one might deal with the social fears related to crowded conditions and reduce these fear reactions by various therapeutic techniques such as desensitization and modeling (Bandura, Blanchard, & Ritter, 1969).

An example of an effective behavioral strategy might be assertive behavior that demonstrates one's ability to control the people and events in one's environment. A dominant individual should have less to fear in a crowded environment than a submissive individual. The disadvantage of this approach is that one may become a fear stimulus for others. Other more effective behavioral strategies might involve changing the social relations and structure in the environment. For example, Baum, Harpin, and Valins (1975) and Baum and Davis (1980) suggest that dormitory suites containing four to six students foster group development that helps students reduce crowding related stress.

Another effective strategy is the modification of the physical environment to reduce crowding. Residents can achieve this by such techniques as the arrangement of their space to increase privacy, (e.g., positioning beds and use of improvised privacy screens). Modifications that require substantial architectural changes such as cubicles and the division of hallways are of course not entirely under the control of the residents but appear to be effective interventions as demonstrated by our own research (McCain et al., 1980a,b) and that of Baum and Davis (1980).

CLOSING COMMENT

The weight of the evidence cited in this chapter supports the contention that for both humans and animals crowded living conditions can be a source of stress and hence have a negative impact on health. Spatial crowding does not appear to be as influential as social crowding with regard to health. However, it would be overstating the case to suggest, as Freedman (1979) does, that spatial crowding has no negative impact on health. Effects of crowding have been found in a wide variety of settings such as individual homes, cities, dormitories, and prisons. The impact of crowding appears to be more dramatic in severely crowded conditions such as those found in prisons.

A number of psychological, behavioral, and environmental strategies may help reduce this negative impact of crowding. From a health perspective, it would be desirable to employ such strategies as well as to develop methods of identifying individuals most susceptible to crowding.

The importance of these findings are magnified by the ever-increasing populations in urban settings and the accompanying increased level of crowding. Psychology has an opportunity to make an important contribution to the solution of this problem.

ACKNOWLEDGMENTS

Our own research presented in this chapter was supported by grants from the Law Enforcement Assistance Administration, The Hogg Foundation for Mental Health, and the University of Texas at Arlington Organized Research Fund. The opinions expressed in this chapter are our own and do not necessarily reflect the views of the sponsoring agencies. We would also like to acknowledge the U. S. Department of Justice Civil

Rights—Public Accommodations Section and the U. S. Bureau of Prisons, for their assistance throughout the various phases of our research.

REFERENCES

Aiello, J. R., Epstein, Y. M., & Karlin, R. A. Effects of crowding on electrodermal activity. *Sociological Symposium,* 1975, *14,* 42–57.

Altman, I. *The environment and social behavior.* Monterey, Calif.: Brooks/Cole, 1975.

Arnow, P. M., Hierholzer, J. C., Higbee, J., & Harris, D. H. Acute hemorrhagic conjunctivitis: A mixed virus outbreak among Vietnamese refugees on Guam. *American Journal of Epidemiology,* 1977, *105,* 68–74.

Baldassare, M. *Residential crowding in urban America.* Berkeley: University of California Press, 1979.

Bandura, A., Blanchard, E. B., & Ritter, B. Relative efficacy of desensitization and modeling approaches for induction of behavioral, affective, and attitudinal changes. *Journal of Personality and Social Psychology,* 1969, *13,* 173–199.

Baron, R. M., Mandel, D. R., Adams, C. A., & Griffen, L. M. Effects of social density in university residential environments. *Journal of Personality and Social Psychology,* 1976, *34,* 434–446.

Baum, A., & Davis, G. E. Reducing the stress of high-density living: An architectural intervention. *Journal of Personality and Social Psychology,* 1980, *38,* 471–481.

Baum, A., Harpin, R. E., & Valins, S. The role of group phenomena in the experience of crowding. *Environment and Behavior,* 1975, *7,* 185–198.

Baum, A., & Koman, S. Differential response to anticipated crowding: Psychological effects of social and spatial density. *Journal of Personality and Social Psychology,* 1976, *34,* 526–536.

Baum, A., & Valins, S. *Architecture and social behavior: Psychological studies in social density.* Hillsdale, N. J.: Lawrence Erlbaum Associates, 1977.

Booth, A. *Urban crowding and its consequences.* New York: Praeger, 1976.

Booth, A., & Cowell, J. Crowding and health. *Journal of Health and Social Behavior,* 1976, *17,* 204–220.

Booth, A., & Johnson, D. R. The effect of crowding on child health and development. *American Behavioral Scientist,* 1975, *18*(6), 736–749.

Brain, P., & Benton, D. The interpretation of physiological correlates of differential housing in laboratory rats. *Life Sciences,* 1979, *24,* 99–116.

Brayton, A. R., & Brain, P. F. Studies on the effects of differential housing on some measures of disease resistance in male and female laboratory mice. *Journal of Endocrinology,* 1974, *61,* XLVIII–XLIX.

Cassel, J. The relation of the urban environment to health: Implications for prevention. *Mount Sinai Journal of Medicine,* 1973, *40,* 539–551.

Cassel, J. An epidemiological perspective of psychosocial factors in disease etiology. *American Journal of Public Health,* 1974, *64,* 1040–1043.

Christian, J. J. The potential role of the adrenal cortex as affected by social rank and population density on experimental epidemics. *American Journal of Epidemiology,* 1968, *87,* 255–264.

Cox, V. C., Paulus, P. B., McCain, G., & Schkade, J. K. Field research on the effects of crowding in prisons and on offshore drilling platforms. In J. R. Aiello & A. Baum (Eds.), *Residential crowding and design.* New York: Plenum, 1979.

D'Atri, D. A. Psychophysiological responses to crowding. *Environment and Behavior,* 1975, *7*(2), 237–252.

Dean, L. M., Pugh, W. M., & Gunderson, E. K. E. Spatial and perceptual components of crowding: Effects on health and satisfaction. *Environment and Behavior,* 1975, *7*(2), 225–236.

Dean, L. M., Pugh, W. M., & Gunderson, E. K. E. The behavioral effects of crowding: Definitions and methods. *Environment and Behavior*, 1978, *10*(3), 417–431.

Desor, J. Towards a psychological theory of crowding. *Journal of Personality and Social Psychology*, 1972, *21*, 79–83.

Dubos, R. *Man adapting*. New Haven, Conn.: Yale University Press, 1965.

Duke, M. P., & Nowicki, S. A new measure and social learning model for interpersonal distance. *Journal of Experimental Research in Personality*, 1972, *6*, 119–132.

Duvall, D., & Booth, A. The housing environment and women's health. *Journal of Health and Social Behavior*, 1978, *19*, 410–417.

Dye, T. R. Population density and social pathology. *Urban Affairs Quarterly*, 1975, *11*(2), 265–275.

Edwards, E. A., & Dean, L. M. Effects of crowding of mice on humoral antibody formation and protection to lethal antigenic challenge. *Psychosomatic Medicine*, 1977, *39*, 14–19.

Essen, J., Fogelman, K., & Head, J. Children's housing and their health and physical development. *Child: Care, health and development*, 1978, *4*, 357–369.

Factor, R. M., & Waldron, I. Contemporary population densities and human health. *Nature*, 1973, *243*, 381–384.

Fanning, D. M. Families in flats. *British Medical Journal*, 1967, *18*, 382–386.

Freedman, J. Reconciling apparent differences between the responses of humans and other animals to crowding. *Psychological Review*, 1979, *86*, 80–85.

Freedman, J. L., Heshka, S., & Levy, A. Population density and pathology: Is there a relationship? *Journal of Experimental Social Psychology*, 1975, *11*, 539–552.

Galle, O. R., Gove, W. R., & McPherson, J. M. Population density and pathology: What are the relations for man? *Science*, 1972, *176*, 23–30.

Giel, R., & Ormel, J. Crowding and subjective health in the Netherlands. *Social Psychiatry*, 1977, *12*, 37–42.

Gove, W. R., Hughes, M., & Galle, O. R. Overcrowding in the home: An empirical investigation of its possible pathological consequences. *American Sociological Review*, 1979, *44*, 59–80.

Gruchow, H. W. *A study of the relationships between catecholamine production, crowding, and morbidity in humans*. Unpublished doctoral dissertation, University of Wisconsin, 1974.

Gunderson, E. K. E., & Rahe, R. H. (Eds.). *Life stress and illness*. Springfield, Ill.: Charles C. Thomas, 1974.

Hamburgh, M., Mendoza, L. A., Rader, M., Lang, A., Silverstein, H., & Hoffman, K. Malformations induced in offspring of crowded and parabiotically stressed mice. *Teratology*, 1974, *10*, 31–38.

Henry, J. P., Meehan, J. P., Stephens, P. The use of psychosocial stimuli to induce prolonged systolic hypertension in mice. *Psychosomatic Medicine*, 1967, *29*, 408–432.

Henry, J. P., & Stephens, P. M. *Stress, health, and the social environments*. New York: Springer-Verlag, 1977.

Jacobson, J. A., Chester, T. J., & Fraser, D. W. An epidemic of disease due to serogroup B Neisseria meningitidis in Alabama: Report of an investigation and community-wide prophylaxis with a sulfonamide. *The Journal of Infectious Diseases*, 1977, *136*(1), 104–108.

Johnson, D. R., & Booth, A. Crowding and human reproduction. *Milbank Memorial Fund Quarterly*, 1976, *54*, 321–337.

Karlovac, M., Paulus, P. B., Cox, V. C., & McCain, G. *An analysis of crowding in a prison environment*. Manuscript in preparation.

Koopman, J. S. Diarrhea and school toilet hygiene in Cali, Columbia. *American Journal of Epidemiology*, 1978, *107*, 412–420.

Lazarus, R. S. *Psychological stress and the coping process*. New York: McGraw-Hill, 1966.

Lazarus, R. S., & Cohen, J. B. Environmental stress. In I. Altman & J. F. Wohlwill (Eds.), *Human behavior and environment* (Vol. 2). New York: Plenum, 1977.

Levy, L., & Herzog, A. N. Effects of population density and crowding on health and social adaptation in the Netherlands. *Journal of Health and Social Behavior,* 1974, *15,* 228-240.

Manton, K. G., & Myers, G. C. The structure of urban mortality: A methodological study of Hanover, Germany, Part II. *International Journal of Epidemiology,* 1977, *6,* 213-223.

Matthews, R. W. *Coping with crowding: Reappraisal versus avoidance.* Unpublished doctoral dissertation, University of Texas at Arlington, 1979.

McCain, G., Cox, V. C., & Paulus, P. B. The relationship between illness complaints and degree of crowding in a prison environment. *Environment and Behavior,* 1976, *8,* 283-290.

McCain, G., Cox, V. C., & Paulus, P. B. The relationship between crowding and manifestations of illness in prison settings. In D. J. Oborne, M. M. Gruneberg, & J. R. Eiser (Eds.), *Research in psychology and medicine* (Vol. II). London: Academic Press, 1980. (a)

McCain, G., Cox, V. C., & Paulus, P. B. *The effect of prison crowding on inmate behavior.* National Institute of Justice, 1980. (b)

McCarthy, D. P., & Saegert, S. Residential density, social overload, and social withdrawal. In J. R. Aiello & A. Baum (Eds.), *Residential crowding and design.* New York: Plenum, 1979.

McGlashan, N. D. Viral hepatitis in Tasmania. *Social Science and Medicine,* 1977, *11,* 731-744.

Mechanic, D. The experience and reporting of common physical complaints. *Journal of Health and Social Behavior,* 1980, *21,* 146-155.

Mechanic, D. Stress, illness, and illness behavior. *Journal of Human Stress,* 1976, *2,* 1-6.

Milgram, S. The experience of living in cities. *Science,* 1970, *167,* 1461-1468.

Monto, A. S. A community study of respiratory infections in the tropics, 3. Introduction and transmission of infections within families. *American Journal of Epidemiology,* 1968, *88,* 69-79.

Myers, K., Hale, C. S., Mykytowycz, R., & Hughes, R. L. The effects of varying density and space on sociality and health in animals. In A. H. Esser (Ed.), *Behavior and environment: The use of space by animals and men.* New York: Plenum, 1971.

Naggan, L., Morag, B., Bar-Shany, F., Egoz, N., & Brachott, D. A study of hepatitus B. antigen carriers among school children. Netanya, Israel. *American Journal of Epidemiology,* 1976, *104,* 263-271.

Paulus, P. B. Crowding. In P. B. Paulus (Ed.), *Psychology of group influence.* Hillsdale, N. J.: Lawrence Erlbaum Associates, 1980.

Paulus, P. B., Cox, V. C., McCain, G., & Chandler, J. Some effects of crowding in a prison environment. *Journal of Applied Social Psychology,* 1975, *5,* 86-91.

Paulus, P. B., McCain, G., & Cox, V. C. A note on the use of prisons as environments for investigation of crowding. *Bulletin of Psychonomic Society,* 1973, *1,* 427-428.

Paulus, P. B., McCain, G., & Cox, V. C. Death rates, psychiatric commitments, blood pressure, and perceived crowding as a function of institutional crowding. *Environmental Psychology and Nonverbal Behavior,* 1978, *3,* 107-116.

Pennebaker, J. W., Burnam, M. A., Schaeffer, M. A., & Harper, D. C. Lack of control as a determinant of perceived physical symptoms. *Journal of Personality and Social Psychology,* 1977, *35,* 167-174.

Plaut, S. M., & Grota, L. J. Effects of differential housing on adrenocortical reactivity. *Neuroendocrinology,* 1971, *7,* 348-360.

Quinn, R. W., Lowry, P. N., & Van Der Zwaag, R. Significance of hemolytic streptococci for Nashville school children: Clinical and serologic observations. *Southern Medical Journal,* 1978, 71(3), 242-246.

Rapoport, A. Toward a redefinition of density. *Environment and Behavior,* 1975, *7,* 133-158.

Rogers, M. P., Dubey, D., & Reich, P. The influence of the psyche and the brain on immunity and disease susceptibility: A critical review. *Psychosomatic Medicine,* 1979, *41,* 147-164.

Saegert, S. High density environments: Their personal and social consequences. In A. Baum & Y. Epstein (Eds.), *Human responses to crowding.* Hillsdale, N. J.: Lawrence Erlbaum Associates, 1978.

Sales, S. M., Guydosh, R. M., & Iacono, W. Relationship between "strength of the nervous system" and the need for stimulation. *Journal of Personality and Social Psychology*, 1974, *29*, 16–22.

Selye, H. *The stress of life*. New York: McGraw–Hill, 1956.

Sengel, R. A. A graph analysis of the relationship between population density and social pathology. *Behavioral Science*, 1978, *23*, 213–224.

Seta, J. J., Paulus, P. B., & Schkade, J. K. The effects of group size and proximity under competitive and cooperative conditions. *Journal of Personality and Social Psychology*, 1976, *34*, 47–53.

Sims, D. G., Downham, M. A. P. S., McQuillin, J., & Gardner, P. S. Respiratory syncytial virus infection in northeast England. *British Medical Journal*, 1976, *2*, 1095–1098.

Singer, J. E., Lundberg, U., & Frankenhaeuser, M. Stress on the train: A study of urban commuting. In A. Baum, J. E. Singer, & S. Valins (Eds.), *Advances in environmental psychology* (Vol. 1). Hillsdale, N. J.: Lawrence Erlbaum Associates, 1978.

Stewart, G. T., & Voors, A. W. Determinants of sickness in Marine recruits. *American Journal of Epidemiology*, 1968, *89*(3), 254–263.

Stokols, D. On the distinction between density and crowding: Some implications for future research. *Psychological Review*, 1972, *79*, 275–278.

Stokols, D. The experience of crowding in primary and secondary environments. *Environment and Behavior*. 1976, *6*, 49–86.

Stokols, D. S., Smith, T. E., & Proster, J. J. Partitioning and perceived crowding in a public place. *American Behavioral Scientist*, 1975, *18*, 792–814.

Sundstrom, E. Crowding as a sequential process: Review of research on the effects of population density on humans. In A. Baum & Y. Epstein (Eds.), *Human response to crowding*. Hillsdale, N. J.: Lawrence Erlbaum Associates, 1978.

Szklo, M., Tonascia, J., & Gordis, J. Psychosocial factors and the risk of myocardial infarctions in white women. *American Journal of Epidemiology*, 1976, *103*, 312–320.

Tessler, R., & Mechanic, D. Psychological distress and perceived health status. *Journal of Health and Social Behavior*, 1978, *19*, 254–262.

Weber, H. W., & Van Der Walt, J. J. Cardiomyopathy in crowded rabbits: A preliminary report. *South African Medical Journal*, 1973, *47*, 1591–1595.

Weiner, H. *Psychobiology of human disease*. New York: Elsevier, 1977.

Welch, B. L. Psychophysiological response to the mean level of environmental stimulation: A theory of environmental integration. Symposium on medical aspects of stress in the military climate. U. S. Government Printing Office Publications, 1964, 39–99.

Wicker, A. W., & Kirmeyer, S. From church to laboratory to national park: A program of research on excess and insufficient populations in behavior settings. In D. Stokols (Ed.), *Perspectives on environment and behavior*. New York: Plenum, 1977.

Wyndham, C. H., Gonin, R., & Reid, R. D. W. Seasonal variation in acute respiratory diseases and meningitis in Black miners living in hotels. *South African Medical Journal*, 1978, *54*, 353–358.

Yarnell, J. W. G. Do housing conditions influence respiratory morbidity and mortality in children? *Public Health*, 1979, *93*, 157–162.

Yodfat, Y., Fiedel, J., Cohen, D., & Eliakim, M. Chronic bronchitis and bronchial asthma in a rural community in Israel: Relation to socioenvironmental factors. *Israel Journal of Medical Sciences*, 1979, *15*(7), 573–578.

Zlutnick, S., & Altman, I. Crowding and human behavior. In J. F. Wohlwill & D. H. Carson (Eds.), *Environment and the social sciences: Perspectives and applications*. Washington D. C.: American Psychological Association, 1972.

11 Community Noise, Behavior, and Health: The Los Angeles Noise Project

Sheldon Cohen
University of Oregon

David S. Krantz
Uniformed Services University of the Health Sciences

Gary W. Evans, Daniel Stokols
University of California, Irvine

Over 70 million Americans live in neighborhoods with noise levels sufficient to interfere with communication and cause annoyance and dissatisfaction (U. S. Environmental Protection Agency, 1974). Sources of noise in these neighborhoods include aircraft overflights, traffic, construction and industrial machinery, as well as the sounds of neighbors, children, and pets. Are high levels of community noise detrimental to residents' health and well-being? This is a question we are only beginning to answer.

The potentially deleterious impact of high-intensity noise on hearing has been widely accepted by scientists and policy makers alike. Acceptable noise standards used in both national and local statutes are based on data that establishes the relationship between the intensity and duration of noise and temporary or permanent losses of hearing (Kryter, 1970). Research completed during the last 10 years also indicates that noise can affect nonauditory systems as well as auditory ones. For example, accumulating evidence suggests that prolonged exposure to high-intensity noise is associated with increased risk of cardiovascular pathology and disturbing psychological symptoms (Cohen & Weinstein, 1981). Moreover, increased levels of community noise have been repeatedly associated with greater dissatisfaction and annoyance by community residents (Borsky, 1980). Despite numerous studies of the possible deleterious effects of routine noise exposure on aspects of behavior and health other than hearing loss and annoyance, inferences concerning these other effects are generally considered tenuous.

It is difficult to reach firm conclusions based on naturalistic studies of the effects of community noise. Invariably, the possibility exists that people who choose (or are forced) to work or live in a noise-impacted area are somehow different from those who work or live elsewhere. Moreover, environments that suffer from serious levels of noise often have other characteristics (e.g., pollution, poor housing, high levels of population density) that may also affect health and behavior.

Laboratory research provides another source of data from which to speculate about the effects of routine noise exposure. This research suggests that high-intensity noise can affect at least three types of nonauditory processes. Firstly, exposure to noise can lead to a *narrowed focus of attention*. This decrease in one's breadth of attention presumably occurs either as a reaction to a noise-induced increase in arousal (Broadbent, 1971) or as a strategy to decrease the amount of information being processed when the presence of noise taxes processing capacity (Cohen, 1978). A narrowed focus of attention during noise exposure is assumed to have detrimental effects on performance of complex tasks (i.e., those requiring a wide range of attention), but not on tasks that are simple or intermediate in complexity.

A second effect of exposure to noise—at least noise that is unpredictable and uncontrollable (cannot be escaped or avoided)—is a reduction in one's perception of control over the environment (Glass & Singer, 1972; Krantz, Glass, & Snyder, 1974). This loss of control is often accompanied by a depressed mood and a decrease in one's motivation to initiate new responses (Seligman, 1975). Loss of control has also been associated with aftereffects, that is, deficits in performance that occur after the noise stimulus is terminated.

A third effect of exposure to noise suggested by experimental evidence is an alteration in physiological arousal characteristic of a generalized stress reaction (Kryter, 1970; Welch & Welch, 1970). This effect includes increased blood pressure, elevated skin conductance levels, and increased excretion of hormones indicative of sympathetic nervous system activity. There is also convincing evidence that prolonged exposure to noise can produce long-term changes in cardiovascular function in animal subjects (Peterson, 1979; Peterson, Augenstein, Tanis, & Augenstein, 1981). Most of these reactions in humans have been documented in laboratory studies involving short-term exposure to relatively high sound levels; thus, the implications of this research for those suffering prolonged exposure at home or at work are questionable.

The respective shortcomings of laboratory and field research on nonauditory effects of noise can be overcome by a strategy that combines experimental and naturalistic studies. Such a strategy examines whether effects of short-term noise exposure found in well-controlled laboratory studies generalize to settings where people are routinely exposed to high-intensity noise. Laboratory studies serve to direct our attention to categories of behavior and health that may be affected by noise, and to establish a causal link between noise and these behaviors. Naturalistic research helps to establish whether particular effects found in the laboratory also occur in real-life settings. Accordingly, this chapter reviews research on the cardiovascular and behavioral effects of community and industrial noise on humans with particular emphasis placed on health-related cardiovascular responses, noise-induced shifts in attention, and feelings of personal control. In conjunction with this review, we report results of a collaborative longitudinal study, the Los Angeles Noise Project, designed to examine the course of adaptation to noise, and the impact of a noise-abatement intervention on a variety of physiological and psychological measures (Cohen, Evans, Krantz, & Stokols, 1980; Cohen, Evans, Krantz, Stokols, & Kelly, 1981).

NOISE AND PHYSICAL HEALTH

Is noise harmful to the human body? Many would argue that outside of the effects of high-intensity sound on hearing (Kryter, 1970; Miller, 1974) there is little convincing evidence for a causal link between noise and physical disorders. As mentioned earlier, several noise-induced physiological changes have been reported in laboratory research. Such changes, if extreme, are often considered potentially hazardous to health. These studies are usually of short duration, making it tenuous to generalize these results to situations where people are routinely exposed to noise. However, epidemiological research in industrial and community settings provides some suggestive evidence of deleterious health effects.

A recent review of the foreign industrial-noise literature by Welch (1979) concludes that there is increased prevalence of a variety of specific nonauditory diseases (e.g., cardiovascular disorders, gastrointestinal complaints, infectious disease) among people who have been exposed at work to sound levels of 85 db(A) or greater for at least 3 to 5 years. Moreover, the morbidity associated with exposure to relatively high intensities of sound increases with advancing age and years of employment for both men and women. Disease prevalence tends to be greater among those exposed to sound that is unpredictable or intermittent, compared to periodic or continuous noise. Both absenteeism and accident rates are higher for those working in intense noise as compared with unexposed workers or workers wearing ear protection (A. Cohen, 1976). Many of the aforementioned studies unfortunately do not control for relevant confounding factors such as education, income, and job demands. It is also important to note that several industrial surveys failed to find a relationship between noise and ill health (Finkle & Poppen, 1948; Glorig, 1971).

The strongest case for routine industrial noise impacting health derives from research on cardiovascular problems (Cohen & Weinstein, 1981; Welch, 1979).

Impaired regulation of blood pressure (including especially hypertension) is the best documented of these effects. Other concomitants of prolonged exposure to intense industrial sound include additional clinical cardiac symptoms (e.g., arrhythmia) and vascular disorders. The impressive amount of data linking cardiovascular disorders to exposure to high noise levels at work must, nevertheless, be viewed with caution. All these studies suffer from the methodological problems associated with correlational field research, and many do not include adequate control groups. Our confidence in the relationship between prolonged exposure to high-intensity industrial noise and cardiovascular problems would be significantly increased if similar effects were obtained in well-designed prospective research.

The effects of community noise on cardiovascular problems and physiological risk factors for cardiovascular disease have also been examined. In a series of studies conducted in the neighborhoods adjacent to an airport in Amsterdam, Knipschild (1977) reports that residents in areas with high levels of aircraft noise were more likely to be under medical treatment for heart trouble and hypertension, more likely (especially among women) to be taking drugs for cardiovascular problems, and also more likely to have high blood pressure and other cardiac abnormalities than an unexposed population. Whereas these differences could not be explained by age, sex, smoking habits, or obesity, the noisy and quiet areas did differ in socioeconomic status. A final study, not subject to this alternative explanation, reports that increases in the purchase of cardiovascular drugs were positively correlated with the number of aircraft overflights at night. Similarly, a Russian study (Karagodina, Soldatkina, Vinokur, & Klimukhin, 1969) suggests that children (9–13 years old) in noise-impacted areas around nine airports show blood pressure abnormalities, higher pulse-rate lability, cardiac insufficiency, and local and general vascular changes. Unfortunately, the report does not provide any information on the nature of the quiet-control population or any details of the measurement procedures.

Studies of the effects of traffic noise on cardiovascular measures are less consistent. A German study of children in the seventh through tenth grades (Karsdorf & Klappach, 1968) reports higher systolic and diastolic pressure for children from noisy schools, whereas a Dutch study (Knipschild & Salle, 1979) found no evidence for increased risk of cardiovascular disease in middle-aged housewives living on streets with high levels of traffic noise as compared with their neighbors living on quieter streets. Overall, like the industrial studies, the studies of community noise suggest that such noise is associated with increases in the incidence of cardiovascular disease and factors related to risk of cardiovascular pathology.

One striking aspect of these data is the evidence that children as well as adults show noise-associated cardiovascular effects. In fact, based on existing theory and evidence, there is reason to expect that exposure to high-intensity noise is a greater threat to children than to adults. Physiological development may be disrupted by unusual demands of external stressors. As we describe later, children may also be psychologically less able to deal with a continuous stressor, because of a limited repertoire of coping strategies, or because they lack the opportunity to control or manipulate their own outcomes (Cohen, Glass, & Phillips, 1979). During the formative years of childhood, noise may also have a particularly detrimental effect on learning or cognitive development.

EFFECTS OF CHRONIC NOISE EXPOSURE ON ATTENTIONAL PROCESSES

A number of years ago, it was proposed that young children continuously exposed to noise adopt an attentional strategy to help them cope with their acoustic environment (Deutsch, 1964). Moreover, it was suggested that this strategy, although successful in the sense of helping the children cope with the noise, has the adverse effect of causing children reared in noisy environments to become inattentive to acoustic cues; that is, they "tune out" their acoustic environment. Children who tune out noisy environments are not likely to distinguish between speech-relevant and speech-irrelevant sounds. Thus, they will lack experience with appropriate speech cues and generally show an inability to recognize relevant sounds and their referents. The inability to discriminate sound is presumed to account, in part, for subsequent problems in learning to read.

Recent research suggests that children living and attending school in noisy neighborhoods are poorer at making auditory discriminations even when tested in quiet settings. For example, S. Cohen, Glass, & Singer (1973) studied third-through fifth-grade children living in apartment buildings built on bridges spanning a busy expressway. When tested in a *quiet* setting, children living in noisier apartments showed greater impairment of auditory discrimination and reading ability than those living in quieter apartments. The magnitude of the correlation between noise and auditory discrimination increased with the length of residence. Race, social-class variables, and hearing losses were ruled out as possible alternative explanations. Similarly, Moch–Sibony (in press) compared children from a quiet (soundproofed) elementary school in the air corridor of Orly (Paris) Airport to a nearby noisy (without soundproofing) school population matched on socioeconomic variables. Results indicated that children from the noisy school showed poorer auditory discrimination, but there were no differences between schools in reading achievement.

A third study of 4½- to 6½-year-old children from homes described by their parents as either noisy or quiet (Heft, 1979) indicates that when tested in *quiet,* children from noisy homes performed more poorly on both a matching and incidental memory task than those from quieter homes. Analyses controlled for age, preschool experience and income level of parents. It should be noted, however, that self-reports of noise level do not usually correlate highly with objective noise measures (Kryter, 1970) and thus limit the generality of these findings.

The results obtained in the aforementioned studies may be termed *aftereffects*, because task performance was measured outside the stressful environment. In contrast to the previous research, Bronzaft & McCarthy (1975) tested children *in* their respective noisy and quiet classrooms. Children in classrooms on the side of a school facing train tracks performed more poorly on a reading achievement test than children in classrooms on the quiet side of the building.

Although the evidence suggests that children living and attending school in noisy environments are poorer at making auditory discriminations and in reading performance, there is no direct evidence for the selective inattention mechanism as a mediator of these effects. Another equally plausible explanation for the auditory discrimination and school achievement results is that noise masks parent and teacher speech, similarly resulting in the child's lack of experience with appropriate speech cues and, as a consequence, reading deficits. It has also been suggested that attentional strategies employed to tune out noise stimuli may be persistently employed after termination of the stimulus (Cohen, 1980). Clearly, more research is needed to choose among these various hypotheses.

NOISE, PERSONAL CONTROL, AND HELPLESSNESS

Laboratory research on personal control over aversive stimuli (Glass & Singer, 1972) also suggests some possible long-term effects of noise exposure. The great majority of this work deals with the role of control in mediating physiological and behavioral reactivity during short-term exposure to laboratory stress (Krantz, Glass, & Snyder, 1974). Seligman (1975) suggests that motivational, cognitive, and emotional disturbances result when individuals continually encounter environmental events (especially aversive events) that they can do nothing about. This psychological state, called *learned helplessness,* results because individuals perceive themselves as incapable of exerting control over the environment.

Closely related to the work on learned helplessness is Glass and Singer's (1972) research on the effects of noise on poststimulation performance. These and other authors (Rotton, Olszewski, Charleton, & Soler, 1978; Sherrod, Hage, Halpern, & Moore, 1977) report that subjects exposed to uncontrollable noise that is unrelated to an ongoing task do more poorly on poststimulation tasks compared to subjects who perceive that they can terminate the noise at will. These effects were observed on poststimulation tasks as diverse as proofreading and measures of tolerance for frustration. Although a variety of plausible explanations for these aftereffects have been suggested (Cohen, 1980, for review), both Seligman (1975) and Glass and Singer (1972) assert that subjects unable to control or predict noise learn that there is little they can do to affect the stressor. This presumably results in lowered motivation and poorer performance on subsequent poststimulation tasks.

There is inferential data to suggest that those experiencing chronic exposure to noise in real life settings often perceive the noise as uncontrollable and show helplessness-like effects. Consider, for example, data reported by Herridge (1974) indicating that those living in "noise slums" were more likely to be admitted to a mental hospital than those living in less-noisy areas. Herridge suggests that the mental distress of those experiencing prolonged exposure to noise was largely attributable to feelings of helplessness rather than to noise per se. This assertion is supported by data indicating that residents of the noisy areas were less likely to complain about aircraft noise than residents of control areas. In other words, even though they are apparently disturbed by noise, they appear to exert minimal effort to modify or escape the unwanted stimulation. Unfortunately, the questionable demographic comparability of noisy and less-noisy areas in this study, and the low base rate of complaints from both areas restricts our confidence in this interpretation.

Although these data on the relationship between noise and helplessness are only suggestive, at least two studies supply direct evidence that, at least for children, environmental stress (noise or high levels of residential density) can result in behavioral deficits (e.g., poor performance on tasks measuring persistence). In one case these performance deficits were associated with lowered perceptions of personal control.

A study by Moch–Sibony (1979), described earlier, reported that children from a noisy school in an airport corridor also showed less tolerance for frustration than their quiet-school counterparts. Research from the crowding literature also supports the notion that chronic environmental stress can induce helplessness. A well-controlled set of studies by Rodin (1976), demonstrated that children living in presumably stressful high-density apartments were more adversely affected by a learned-helplessness pretreatment—unsolvable puzzles—than children from low-density apartments. The high-density children were also less likely to exercise their own choices when given the opportunity to do so. Thus, high chronic density can result in feelings of helplessness among children. Our understanding of the cognitive and motivational processes affected by chronic noise exposure would be advanced by a longitudinal study examining similar effects of noise stress on performance on standard helplessness measures (response to failure).

THE LOS ANGELES NOISE PROJECT

The evidence reviewed previously suggests that laboratory work on health-related cardiovascular responses, noise-induced shifts in attention, and feelings of personal control may have some generality to situations of chronic noise exposure. Whereas investigators have begun to take a closer look at the nonauditory effects of noise in naturalistic settings, methodologically tight studies are rare. This research also tends to be atheoretical and thus difficult to compare to existing laboratory work. Moreover, there are few *longitudinal* studies of people living and/or working under noise. Thus, it is unknown whether prolonged noise exposure results in increasingly deleterious effects, or whether those exposed for prolonged periods adapt to noise with effects disappearing after a while. Studies comparing measures of health and behavior of the same person before exposure, immediately after exposure begins, and at set intervals for one to several years would allow us to determine the long-term course of stress and adaptation. In addition, longitudinal studies in situations where the environmental stressor is removed or attenuated would make it possible to determine whether there are long-term aftereffects of prolonged noise exposure.

Accordingly, we conducted a controlled longitudinal study of the impact of aircraft noise on elementary school children (The Los Angeles Noise Project or LANP). The study examined the course of adaptation and the impact of a noise-abatement intervention on blood pressure, attentional processes, and feelings of personal control. (Cohen et al., 1980; 1981, for a fuller report of this study).

The subjects were children (initially third and fourth graders) living and attending schools in the air corridor of Los Angeles International Airport, and children of similar socioeconomic, age, and racial composition living and attending schools in quiet Los Angeles neighborhoods.[1] Peak sound-level readings in the noise schools were as high as 95db (A), and the schools were located in an air corridor that has approximately one flight every 2½ minutes during school hours (Lane & Meecham, 1974).

As part of a settlement of a lawsuit brought by the school systems against the airport, the interior sound levels of many of the schools in the landing corridor were lowered following the collection of data for the first testing phase of the study (T1). Thus, a large number of noise-affected children spent the following year in quieter classrooms, whereas others remained in noisy classrooms. One year after original testing, children who were still enrolled in their schools were retested (T2) on the original measures to determine whether effects of noise that occurred during the first year of the study would persist after the child was assigned to a quieter classroom. The study focused on effects occurring outside of noise exposure; thus, all measures, except school achievement tests given in classrooms, were administered in a quiet setting (a soundproof van).

Longitudinal data from subjects who were tested at both sessions (T1 and T2), and who remained in noise classrooms, were compared to children in quiet classrooms at both testing sessions. These data were used to determine if noise effects adapted—decreased or disappeared—over the 1-year interval between

---

[1]Children with hearing losses were excluded from the study. In all analyses of data, a regression analysis procedure enabled precise statistical control for number of children in the child's family, the number of years the child had lived in the neighborhood, grade in school, and race. Additional controls and multivariate analyses were used for selected dependent measures where appropriate (Cohen et al., 1980, Cohen et al., 1981).

TABLE 11.1
Overview of the Analyses in the Los Angeles Noise Project

	Title of Analysis	Sample	Classroom noise conditions during: 1977 (T1) 1978 (T2)
I.	Cross-sectional, T1	T1	noise vs. quiet
II.	Longitudinal	Subjects tested at both T1 & T2	noise[a] –– noise quiet ––vs.–– quiet
III.	Noise Abatement: Cross-sectional Analyses	T1	noise vs. abated vs. quiet
IV.	Noise Abatement: Longitudinal Analyses	Noise subjects tested at both T1 & T2	noise –– noise vs. noise –– abated

[a]The few classrooms that had had noise abatement work completed prior to T1 are included as noise classrooms in these analyses. This was done in order to make these analyses comparable to those reported in Cohen et al. (1980) and is justified by the findings reported in this paper suggesting little if any effect of abatement.

sessions. Several years before the first testing session, a number of classrooms had been treated with noise-reducing materials. Thus, because some abatement work was introduced both prior to T1 and between T1 and T2, separate analyses (both cross-sectional and longitudinal) were conducted in order to evaluate the effectiveness of the noise-abatement interventions. Four types of analyses are, therefore, discussed in this chapter: *cross-sectional* and *longitudinal* analyses to evaluate the effects of *noise* and *noise abatement*. Table 11.1 presents an overview of these analyses. In our discussion following we first consider the nature and persistence of noise effects and then discuss the effects of abatement.

AIRCRAFT NOISE AND BLOOD PRESSURE

Because chronic noise exposure might affect the cardiovascular system, a measure of cardiovascular function, resting blood pressure, was included in the LANP. The effects of noise exposure on blood pressure were decisively clear in the cross-sectional analysis of T1 data (see Fig. 11.1). Children attending noisy schools had higher systolic and diastolic pressures than their quiet-school counterparts. Moreover, the pattern of means for systolic and diastolic pressures suggest that this effect was greatest during the first 2 years of exposure, with the differences remaining consistently smaller after that point. It should be noted, however, that although these blood pressure differences were statistically reli-

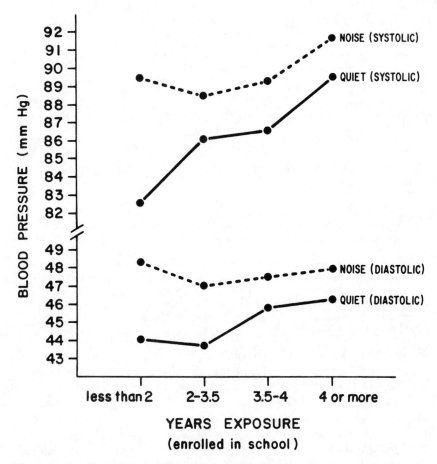

FIG. 11.1.   Systolic and diastolic blood pressure as a function of school noise level and duration of exposure for T1 sample. Each period on the years exposure coordinate represents one quarter of the sample. For example, 25% of the sample were enrolled in school less than 2 years (from Cohen, S., Evans, G. W., Krantz, D. S., & Stokols, D., 1980. Copyright 1980 by the American Psychological Association. Reprinted by permission).

able, the mean levels for children attending noisy schools do not as a group exceed normative levels for children of similar ages (Voors, Foster, Frerichs, Weber, & Berenson, 1976). The long-term health consequences, if any, of these blood pressure elevations remain unknown.

The greater difference during the first few years of school enrollment found in this cross-sectional analysis could be due to noise children habituating to the stressor as the duration of exposure increased. On the other hand, the effect could be due to some kind of subject selection bias; that is, children with noise-induced blood pressure elevations may have quickly moved out of the noise-impacted neighborhood and thus lowered the mean blood pressure for noise-school children who remained exposed for 2 or more years.

Available longitudinal data on *how long* specific noise and quiet-school children remain enrolled in their schools helped distinguish between these two explanations. Another analysis of T1 blood pressure data revealed that some form of subject selection bias was indeed operative. As depicted in Fig. 11.2, noise-school students with the highest blood pressures move out of the noise area soon (within 2 years) after the initial testing, and a reverse trend appears for the quiet children. Thus, it appears that selective attrition, *not* adaptation, is responsible for the decrease of the difference between the blood pressure of noise- and quiet-school children.

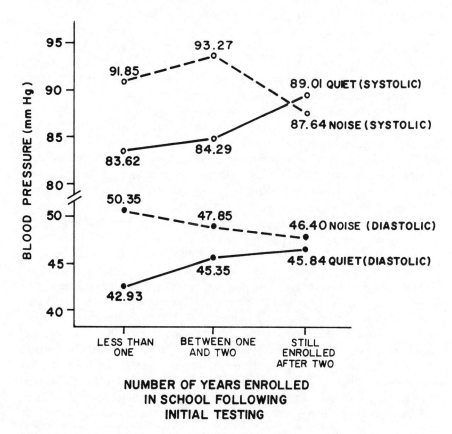

FIG. 11.2.   Systolic and diastolic blood pressure measured at T1 as a function of school noise level and the number of years enrolled in school following T1. Each period on the years exposure coordinate represents number of years students remained enrolled (from Cohen, S., Evans, G. W., Krantz, D. S., Stokols, D., & Kelly, S., 1981. Copyright 1981 by the American Psychological Association. Reprinted by permission).

It is important to emphasize that these effects occurred with race and social class partialed out of the analyses. Some possible (and admittedly speculative) explanations for the selective attrition effect among noise children are: (1) Parents of children with elevated blood pressure were sensitive to their children's experience of stress and as a consequence moved to a less-noisy neighborhood; (2) because of a familial bias (either genetic or environmentally determined), parents of children with noise-induced blood pressure elevations experienced similar stress-related reactions that motivated them to move from the neighborhood; (3) the children's elevated blood pressures were a response, not to the noise itself, but to their parents' own noise-induced stress, which motivated the parents to move from the neighborhood; and (4) some unknown third factor is related to mobility, higher blood pressure, and living in a noisy neighborhood. Although we cannot select among these possible explanations, there is recent related evidence that children of hypertensive parents show elevated cardiovascular response to stress (Baer, Collins, & Bourianoff, 1980; Obrist, Grignolo, Hastrup, Koepke, Langer, Light, McCubbin, & Pollak, in press). This reinforces the notion that parents of children with elevated blood pressure may be suffering from cardiovascular disorder. We have no ready explanation for the opposite trend for blood pressure and attrition obtained among the quiet children.

Although the analysis of the complete T1 sample indicated higher systolic and diastolic blood pressures for noise-school children, there were no effects on either systolic or diastolic blood pressure in the longitudinal analyses, which include both T1 and T2 data. Longitudinal blood pressure effects were not expected, however, because a relatively high proportion of noise-school children with higher blood pressures were lost to attrition (see earlier) and thus not included in the longitudinal analyses. Because of this attrition effect, our data do not enable us to make a definitive determination about whether the increased blood pressure levels of noise-affected children found in the initial complete cross-sectional sample habituate over time.

Figure 11.3 presents cross-sectional blood pressure data from an independent replication sample of third graders. Noise-school children had higher blood pressure levels among those exposed 2 years or less, but not among those attending noise schools for longer periods. In sum, the data from both the longitudinal study and the cross-sectional replication clearly indicate that children attending school in the air corridor have elevated blood pressures during their first few years of exposure. Although this elevation does not occur for those who have lived in the neighborhood and attended their schools for longer periods of time, data from the various longitudinal analyses argue that this is due to a bias in who moves out of the neighborhood rather than to habituation to the noise. This data is consistent with previous studies of both adults and children cited earlier, which suggest that those undergoing prolonged noise exposure show persistent elevations in cardiovascular response.

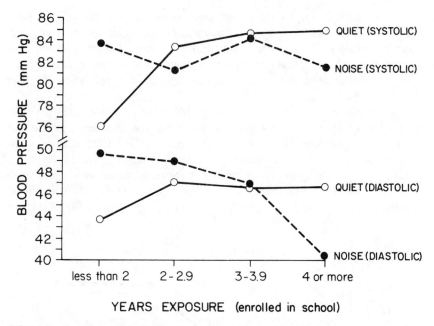

FIG. 11.3. Systolic and diastolic blood pressure as a function of school noise level and duration of exposure for cross-sectional third grade replication study. Each period on the years exposure coordinate represents one quarter of the sample (copyright in the public domain).

AIRCRAFT NOISE AND HELPLESSNESS

To determine if noise-school children behave as if they have less control over their environment, the Los Angeles Noise Project tested students on a cognitive task after a manipulated experience of success or failure. A lack of persistence after failure ("giving up" syndrome) is considered a direct manifestation of learned helplessness.

During the initial testing (T1), each child was given a treatment puzzle to assemble after the tester demonstrated the task with another puzzle. Half the children received an insoluble (failure) puzzle and half a soluable (success) puzzle. After time was up on the first puzzle, the child was given a second, moderately difficult puzzle to solve. The second (test) puzzle was the same for all (success and failure) children, and the child was allowed 4 minutes to solve it. Whether or not the puzzle was solved, time to solution, and whether the child "gave up" before the 4 minutes had elapsed were used as measures of helplessness.

Unexpectedly, during T1 a large proportion of the children receiving a soluble treatment puzzle failed to solve the treatment puzzle within the time allowed. Therefore, many children self-selected themselves into a failure condition; thus we were obliged to confine ourselves to a comparison of children from noise schools versus quiet schools, irrespective of whether they received success or failure puzzles.

Among children assigned to the success treatment condition, children from noise schools were more likely to fail to solve the first (treatment) puzzle than children from quiet schools. Secondly, there were similar effects of noise on the test (second) puzzle that occurred irrespective of whether the child received a success (solved or not) or failure treatment. Noise children were again more likely to fail the test puzzle than quiet-school children and more likely to give up than their quiet-school counterparts. Moreover, as apparent in Fig. 11.4, the

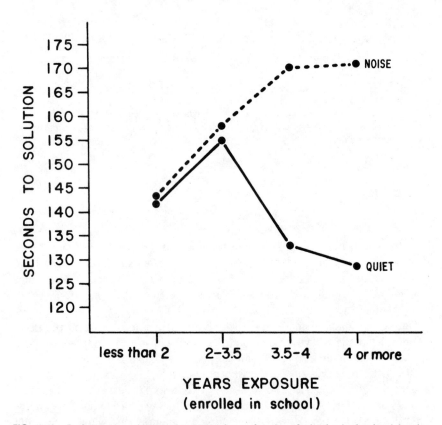

FIG. 11.4.   Performance on the second (test) puzzle as a function of school noise level and duration of exposure for T1 cross-sectional sample. Each period on the years exposure coordinate represents one quarter of the sample (from Cohen, S., Evans, G. W., Krantz, D. S., & Stokols, D., 1980. Copyright 1980 by the American Psychological Association. Reprinted by permission).

longer the child attended a noise school, the slower she/he was in solving the puzzle.

The preceding analyses indicate that children from noise schools are generally less capable of performing a cognitive puzzle task than children from quiet schools. The strongest indication that failure on these puzzles on the part of noise children is related to helplessness *per se* would be data indicating that they were more likely than quiet children to *give up* before their alloted time had elapsed. Therefore, a final analysis was conducted including only those children who failed the second puzzle. This indicated that the failures of noise children were associated with giving up more often than were the failures of quiet children. Thus, even though all these children failed to solve the puzzle, noise-school children were less likely to persist than their quiet-school counterparts.

A year later at the second session (T2) pretreatment success and failure puzzles were *not* readministered. Each child was given only the test (square) puzzle to solve. As previously, the child was allowed 4 minutes to solve the test puzzle with the same measures of helplessness assessed as in the earlier testing session. As in the analysis of the entire T1 sample, there were effects of noise on test puzzle performance that occurred irrespective of whether the child received a success (solved or not) or failure treatment. Noise children were reliably more likely to fail the test puzzle than quiet-school children, and more likely to take longer solving the puzzle.

Although these analyses suggested that noise-school children were again poorer than quiet-school children at solving the test puzzle at both testing sessions, the increased "giving up" of noise, compared to quiet-school children, did not appear in the repeated measures analysis. The disappearance of this effect in the longitudinal analysis may have occurred because of a subject attrition bias, because the children had had a previous experience with the same puzzle, or because the effect disappears (i.e., adapts out over time). It should be noted that the cross-sectional analysis of the entire T1 sample did not indicate a lessening of giving up with increased years of school enrollment; thus suggesting that the giving-up effect does not adapt out over time. In sum, the data indicate that performance deficits among noise-school children persist over a 1-year period. However, it is unclear whether the poorer performance of noise children can be interpreted as learned helplessness.

AIRCRAFT NOISE, DISTRACTABILITY, AND SCHOOL ACHIEVEMENT

Earlier it was proposed that selective inattention may result from chronic noise exposure. Because children who are relatively inattentive to acoustic cues should be less affected by an auditory distractor, distractability was used as a measure of selective inattention in the LANP. Subjects performed a crossing-out E's task under both ambient and distracting conditions. The subject's task was to cross out the E's in a two-page passage from a sixth grade reader. In a distraction condition, the child worked on one of the versions of the task while a tape recording of a male voice read a story at a moderate volume. In the no-distraction condition, the alternative form of the task was completed under ambient sound conditions. The criterion measure was performance (percent E's found) on the distraction task after these scores were adjusted for no-distraction performance. It was expected that children from noise schools would be less affected by distraction. Because selective inattention is a strategy that develops over time, it was also predicted that this "tuning out" strategy would increase with exposure (Cohen, Glass, & Singer, 1973).

It can be seen in the cross-sectional (T1) data presented in Fig. 11.5 that children in noise schools did better than the quiet group on the distraction task

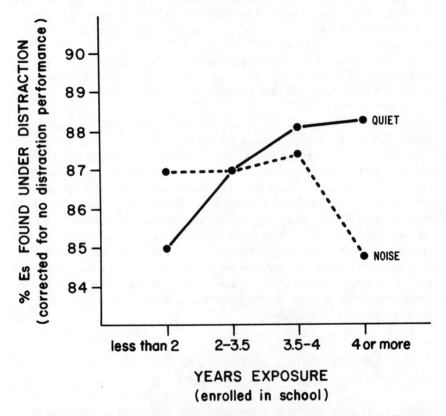

FIG. 11.5.   Distraction as a function of school noise level and duration of exposure for T1 cross-sectional sample. Each period on the years exposure coordinate represents one quarter of the sample (from Cohen, S. Evans, G. W., Krantz, D. S., & Stokols, D., 1980. Copyright 1980 by the American Psychological Association. Reprinted by permission).

during the first 2 years of exposure and unexpectedly worse after 4 years. Contrary to earlier evidence, this finding suggests that as the length of noise exposure increases, children are *more,* rather than less, disturbed by auditory distractors. One possible explanation for this effect is that at first, the children attempt (somewhat successfully) to cope with the noise by tuning it out. Later, however, as they find that the strategy is not adequate, they give it up. This interpretation is consistent with the helplessness data. Alternatively, it is possible that as the duration of exposure increases, the children become more discriminating in terms of the kinds of sounds that they tune out; that is, initially they tune out a wide range of acoustic stimuli (including the distractor used in the present study) but later tune out only aircraft sounds.

Figure 11.6 presents longitudinal data based only on those subjects who returned for testing at both T1 and T2. It can be seen that there was a pattern similar to the T1 data reported previously, except that noise children enrolled for 2-4 years also appear to be less distractable than their quiet counterparts. Furthermore, the T2 noise sample continues to show the pattern of better performance which becomes equivalent to the quiet group after 4 years of enrollment.

Auditory discrimination and reading achievement were assessed in an attempt to replicate previous work and to establish if there is an association between these measures and the children's attentional strategies. Standardized reading and math tests (administered during the second and third grades by the school system) were gathered from school files, and an auditory discrimination test (Wepman, 1958) was administered individually to children in the soundproof van. Results indicated that math, reading, and auditory discrimination were all unrelated to noise or duration of noise exposure.

Further correlational analyses, however, did suggest that those children who were better at auditory discriminations were also better on both the reading ($r = .19$) and math ($r = .18$) tests. However, there were no significant relationships between these variables and the selective inattention measure. In sum, there was no evidence in the initial analysis of the T1 data that aircraft noise affected reading and math skills, nor that these skills are related to a selective inattention strategy.

It should be noted that the failure of this study to replicate the previously reported relationship between community noise and reading ability (Bronzaft & McCarthy, 1975; Cohen, Glass, & Singer, 1973) may be attributable to an experimental design insensitive to noise-induced differences in school achievement. In both the earlier studies, all students attended the same school. Moreover, in the Cohen et al. (1973) study, students from both noisy and quiet apartments were taught in the same classrooms by the same teachers. In the present study, noise and quiet children attended different schools, were in different classrooms, and had different teachers. It is likely that these factors add substantial error variance to the equation making the detection of a small effect of noise quite difficult.

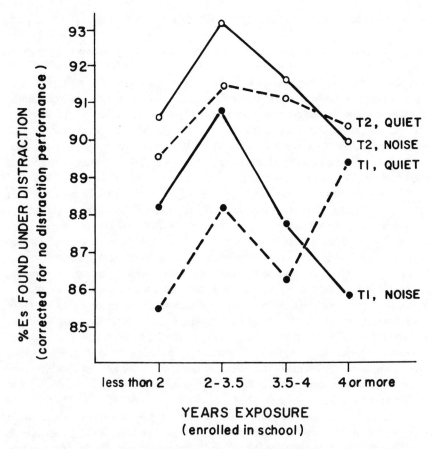

FIG. 11.6.   Distractibility at T1 and T2 as a function of school noise level and duration of exposure for the longitudinal study. Sample includes only those subjects present for both sessions (from Cohen, S., Evans, G. W., Krantz, D. S., Stokols, D., & Kelly, S., 1981. Copyright 1981 by the American Psychological Association. Reprinted by permission).

NOISE ABATEMENT AND NOISE-STRESS REDUCTION

Do noise abatement interventions (and the resulting reduction in classroom noise levels) decrease or ameliorate the effects of noise in impacted classrooms? Both cross-sectional data collected during the first testing session and longitudinal data looking at changes in response of children moved from noisy to quiet classrooms are relevant to this question. T1 cross-sectional abatement analyses, based on the entire sample, were collected during the first testing session and compare children who were in noise-abated classrooms to those in noisy (nonabated) rooms and those from quiet schools. (Recall that prior to T1, a number of noise-impacted schools had been treated with sound-reducing materials). Longitudinal abatement analyses look at the changes in response of children who moved from a noise to noise-abated classroom in contrast to those children who spent both years in noise-impacted rooms. As outlined in Table 11.1, longitudinal data are based only on those subjects available for retesting at T2.

To examine effects of abatement, data from T1 were reanalyzed with classrooms categorized as noisy, abated, and quiet. The mean peak noise level for noise classrooms was 79 dB(A); for abated, 63 dB(A); and for quiet classrooms, 57 dB(A). Analyses suggested only a minimal impact of the abatement intervention. Childrens' perceptions of noise and noise interference, blood pressure, and the auditory distraction measure were apparently *unaffected* by abatement.

On the other hand, abatement seemed to provide at least slight improvement on two factors. Firstly, abatement had a marginal effect of increasing the number of children who were able to solve the moderately difficult test puzzle in the helplessness task irrespective of whether they received a soluble or insoluble first puzzle. It is noteworthy, however, that giving up, the measure designed to provide a direct assessment of feelings of helplessness, was affected only by the noise-school versus quiet-school distinction. Secondly, although reading achievement and auditory discrimination ability were unaffected by abatement, there was evidence that math achievement was higher for children in abated than for those in noise classrooms. It is important to consider, however, that unlike all other measures that were administered in a relatively quiet setting, the achievement tests were actually taken in the classroom. Thus, the relative deficit in math performance of the children from the noise as opposed to noise-abated classrooms may be attributable to noise interfering with test performance, rather than to an aftereffect of noise that we would expect to occur even outside of the noise-impacted environment.

The longitudinal data similarly provides little evidence that children who had been enrolled in a noise impacted school show improvement in their performance and/or health following a 1 (school)-year experience in a noise-abated classroom (even though sound attenuation had a substantial effect on interior sound levels). In contrast to the cross-sectional analysis, the longitudinal data did not even indicate improvement in ability to solve the moderately difficult puzzle on the part of children in noise-abated rooms. This failure to mimic the cross-sectional findings may be due to an attrition bias or to the marginality of the effect itself. Unfortunately, school achievement data were not available during the second testing session, and thus there was no opportunity to reevaluate the ameliorative effects of noise abatement on school achievement found in the cross-sectional analyses.

In sum, the evidence for ameliorative effects of classroom-noise abatement were neither substantial nor did they cover a wide range of measures. Behavior in the classroom, however, was affected by the sound attenuation as was school achievement test performance. Both of these measures likely reflect a remediation of the effects that occur during noise, rather than after exposure.

IMPLICATIONS AND FUTURE DIRECTIONS

The data from our study of aircraft noise indicated that the noise resulting from chronic exposure to aircraft overflights affects a variety of cognitive, motivational, and physiological processes in a manner generally consistent with previous laboratory findings on the nonauditory effects of noise and other stressors. Blood pressure was relatively higher in noise-impacted children, there was evidence for poorer cognitive functioning in the form of lowered puzzle-solving performance and math achievement, and noise children were less distractable during the early, but not later, years of exposure. With the exception of math achievement scores, all these effects occurred outside of noise exposure and may therefore be termed aftereffects. Moreover, these effects cannot be attributed to confounding economic or social variables or to hearing loss. Because the effects were also stable over a 1-year period, there was very little evidence that children habituated or adapted to the noise stressor over time.

Although this chapter has concerned the physical intensity of sound as it might affect health and behavior, it is also important to note that noise is a psychological concept. The meaning of noise to the individual (termed *cognitive appraisal*) and the context in which noise occurs play important roles in determining effects on annoyance, performance, and health (Cohen & Weinstein, 1981; Lazarus, 1966). In accord with these principles, recently completed analyses of LANP data have revealed that after controlling for the physical intensity of noise, the *child's ratings* of noise annoyance predict a variety of dependent measures. For example, diastolic blood pressure is relatively higher among children who rate classroom noise as more bothersome. In addition, noise levels at home and school have an interactive effect, with school noise abatement making less of a difference on blood pressures of children from noisier than quieter homes.

Pending further replications of these results in other settings, it is difficult to draw definitive conclusions about the clinical or policy significance of these data, and we favor a cautious approach toward interpreting our findings. To this end, our own research program is longitudinal in design and includes an ongoing replication of this study with a population exposed to traffic noise. However, from a policy point of view these data do support the need for noise-abatement work in noise-impacted settings, but they also suggest that short-term protection by sound insulation in the classroom may not be enough. Although there was evidence that abatement affects behavior in the classroom, the ameliorative effects of noise insulation were neither substantial nor did they cover a wide range of measures. This relative ineffectiveness may have occurred because the effects of previous noise exposure are relatively long lasting; that is, it takes more than a 1-year reprieve from the noise for a return to more normal levels of behavior and health. Secondly, because the children are all exposed to the noise outside the school—in their homes, on the playground, etc.—a quieter classroom may not have been a sufficient intervention. Finally, in evaluating the abatement results, it is also important to remember that most of the children attending noise schools spent previous years in nonabated classrooms. Thus, although abatement interventions were not entirely effective for this population, it is possible that children who start to attend school after the entire school has undergone noise abatement (and are thus always in relatively quiet classrooms) would benefit from the interventions. Therefore, it is likely that a more effective noise abatement in schools (bringing overall levels closer to those in quiet schools) and decreased noise exposure *outside of school* would have an increased ameliorative impact. Decreasing overall community noise levels by creating buffer zones between airports and other sources of high-intensity noise and the surrounding communities would be one way of providing more adequate protection for community residents.

A research strategy of studying effects that are closely linked to laboratory findings, together with the use of both cross-sectional and longitudinal approaches in the field, has important benefits. In particular, it helps establish the scientific validity and practical value of work with potential implications for social issues. The research reviewed in this chapter clearly suggests lending additional weight to the possible impact of aircraft noise on psychological adjustment and on nonauditory aspects (particularly cardiovascular) of health. As converging laboratory and naturalistic approaches eliminate alternative explanations for noise-associated effects, the potential for increasing scientific knowledge and for affecting the formation of public policy increases.

ACKNOWLEDGMENTS

Portions of this paper were adapted from an article by the authors in *American Scientist,* September, 1981. Their collaborative research reported in this chapter was supported by grants from the National Science Foundation (BNS 77-08576 and BNS 79-23453), the National Institute of Environmental Health Sciences (ES0176401), the Society for the Psychological Study of Social Issues, the University of Oregon Biomedical Fund and the Uniformed Services School of Medicine (C07214). The authors are indebted to Sheryl Kelly and the staff, children and parents of participating schools.

REFERENCES

Baer, P. C., Collins, T., & Bourianoff, G. G. The heart rate orienting response in children of hypertensive fathers. *Psychosomatic Medicine, 1980, 42,* 74 (Abstract).

Borsky, P. N. Research on community response to noise since 1973. In J. V. Tobias (Ed.), *The proceedings of the third international congress on noise as a public health problem.* Washington, D. C.: American Speech and Hearing Association, 1980.

Broadbent, D. E. *Decision and stress.* New York: Academic Press, 1971.

Bronzaft, A. L., & McCarthy, D. P. The effects of elevated train noise on reading ability. *Environment & Behavior,* 1975, *7,* 517-527.

Cohen, A. The influence of a company hearing conservation program on extra-auditory problems in workers. *Journal of Safety Research,* 1976, *8,* 146-162.

Cohen, S. Environmental load and the allocation of attention. In A. Baum, J. E. Singer, & S. Valins (Eds.), *Advances in Environmental Psychology,* (Vol. 1). Hillsdale, N. J.: Lawrence Erlbaum Associates, 1978.

Cohen, S. The aftereffects of stress on human performance and social behavior: A review of research and theory. *Psychological Bulletin,* 1980, *88,* 82-108.

Cohen, S., Evans, G. W., Krantz, D. S., & Stokols, D. Physiological, motivational, and cognitive effects of aircraft noise on children: Moving from the laboratory to the field. *American Psychologist,* 1980, *35,* 231-243.

Cohen, S., Evans, G. W., Krantz, D. S., Stokols, D., & Kelly, S. Aircraft noise and children: Longitudinal and cross-sectional evidence on adaptation to noise and the effectiveness of noise abatement. *Journal of Personality and Social Psychology,* 1981, *40,* 330-345.

Cohen, S., Glass, D. C., & Phillips, S. Environment and health. In H. Freeman, S. Levine, & L. G. Reeder (Eds.), *Handbook of medical sociology.* Englewood Cliffs, N. J.: Prentice-Hall, 1979.

Cohen, S., Glass, D. C., & Singer, J. E. Apartment noise, auditory discrimination, and reading ability in children. *Journal of Experimental Social Psychology,* 1973, *9,* 407-422.

Cohen, S., & Weinstein, N. Nonauditory effects of noise on behavior and health. *Journal of Social Issues,* 1981.

Deutsch, C. P. Auditory discrimination and learning: Social factors. *The Merrill-Palmer Quarterly of Behavior and Development,* 1964, *10.*

Finkle, A. L., & Poppen, J. R. Clinical effects of noise and mechanical vibrations of a turbo-jet engine on man. *Journal of Applied Physiology,* 1948, *1,* 183-204.

Glass, D. C., & Singer, J. E. *Urban stress: Experiments on noise and social stressors.* New York: Academic Press, 1972.

Glorig, A. Nonauditory effects of noise exposure. *Sound and Vibration,* 1971, *5,* 28-29.

Heft, H. Background and focal environmental conditions of the home and attention in young children. *Journal of Applied Social Psychology,* 1979, *9,* 47-69.

Herridge, C. F. Aircraft noise and mental health. *Journal of Psychosomatic Research,* 1974, *18,* 239-243.

Karagodina, I. L., Soldatkina, S. A., Vinokur, I. L., & Klimukhin, A. A. Effect of aircraft noise on the population near airports. *Hygiene and Sanitation,* 1969, *34,* 182-187.

Karsdorf, G., & Klappach, H. Einfluesse des Verkehrrlarms auf Gesundheit und Leistung bei Oberschulern einer Grofzstadt. *Zeitschrift fur die Gefamte Hygiene,* 1968, *14,* 52-54.

Knipschild, P. Medical effects of aircraft noise. *International Archives of Occupational and Environmental Health,* 1977, *40,* 185-204.

Knipschild, P., & Salle, H. Road traffic noise and cardiovascular disease: A population study in the Netherlands. *International Archives of Occupational and Environmental Health,* 1979, *44,* 55-99.

Krantz, D. S., Glass, D. C., & Snyder, M. L. Helplessness, stress level and the coronary-prone behavior pattern. *Journal of Experimental Social Psychology,* 1974, *10,* 284-300.

Kryter, K. D. *The effects of noise on man.* New York: Academic Press, 1970.

Lane, S. R., & Meecham, W. C. Jet noise at schools near Los Angeles International Airport. *Journal of the Acoustical Society of America,* 1974, *56,* 127, 131.

Lazarus, R. S. *Psychological stress and the coping process.* New York: McGraw-Hill, 1966.

Miller, J. D. Effects of noise on people. *Journal of the Acoustical Society of America,* 1974, *56,* 729-764.

Moch-Sibony, A. Study of the effects of noise on the personality and certain psychomotor and intellectual aspects of children, after a prolonged exposure (French). *Travail Humane,* in press.

Obrist, P. A., Grignolo, A., Hastrup, J. L., Koepke, J. P., Langer, A. W., Light, K. D., McCubbin, J. A., & Pollak, M. H. Behavioral-cardiac interactions in hypertension. In D. S. Krantz, A. Baum, & J. E. Singer (Eds.), *Handbook of psychology and health: Cardiovascular disorders.* Hillsdale, N. J.: Lawrence Erlbaum Associates, 1982, in press.

Peterson, E. A. Some issues and investigations concerning extraauditory effects of noise. Paper presented at Annual Meeting of American Psychological Association, 1979.

Peterson, E. A., Augenstein, J. S., Tanis, D. C., & Augenstein, D. G. Noise raises blood pressure without impairing auditory sensitivity. *Science,* 1981, *211,* 1450-1452.

Rodin, J. Crowding, perceived choice, and reactions to controllable and uncontrollable outcomes. *Journal of Experimental Social Psychology,* 1976, *12,* 564-578.

Rotton, J., Olszewski, D., Charleton, M., & Soler, E. Loud speech, conglomerate noise, and behavioral aftereffects. *Journal of Applied Psychology,* 1978, *63,* 360-365.

Sherrod, D. R., Hage, J. N., Halpern, P. L., & Moore, B. S. Effects of personal causation and perceived control responses to an aversive environment: The more control, the better. *Journal of Experimental Social Psychology,* 1977, *13,* 14-27.

Seligman, M. P. Helplessness: *On depression, development, and death.* San Francisco: W. H. Freeman, 1975.

U. S. Environmental Protection Agency. *Information on levels of environmental noise requisite to protect public health and welfare with an adequate margin for safety* (EPA 550/9-74004). Washington, D. C.: U. S. Government Printing Office, 1974.

Voors, A. W., Foster, T. A., Frerichs, R. R., Weber, L. S., & Berenson, L. S. Studies of blood pressure in children, ages 5-14 years, in a total biracial community. *Circulation,* 1976, *54,* 319-327.

Welch, B. L. Extra-auditory health effects of industrial noise: Survey of foreign literature. Aerospace Medical Research Laboratory, Aerospace Medical Division, Air Force Systems Command, Wright-Patterson, June, 1979.

Welch, B. L., & Welch, A. S. *Physiological effects of noise.* New York and London: Plenum, 1970.

Wepman, J. *Manual of directions: Auditory discrimination test.* Chicago: Author, 1958.

Author Index

Numbers in *italics* denote pages with complete bibliographic information.

Subject Index

329